PRAISE FOR *LEARNING WHILE CARING*

"*Learning While Caring* reflects knowledge, wisdom, and insight from fifty-plus years of teaching and practicing medicine. A dedicated physician, researcher, and academic leader, Dr. Hellman illuminates the highlights as well as the frustrations and ethical dilemmas of caring for patients and conducting research. His essays on medical ethics and the rights of the individual patient contain indispensable information for clinical investigators, physicians, and the general public. His discussion of the policy implications of current biomedical discoveries and the delivery of health care in a cost-conscious environment will be of interest to policy makers and health care consumers alike.

Dr. Hellman deals with difficult issues in academic medicine with wisdom, wit, compassion, and common sense. *Learning While Caring* is a wonderful, insightful, and wide-ranging look at medicine, disease, and public policy; I recommend it highly."
—Robert J. Zimmer
President, University of Chicago

"In *Learning While Caring*, we are introduced to the ethical basis of the role of the physician in the era of great change arising from medical and scientific discoveries, and more recently, the nascent revolution in 'affordable care.' Hellman provides sound philosophical arguments to judge the ethics of current trends in medicine—for example, why prospective, randomized controlled clinical trials place the physician in an ethical dilemma. By analogy, practicing in a managed care environment creates perverse incentives for doctors to prescribe what may be best for society to control health care costs, yet may be at odds with what the doctor believes is best for his particular patient. Hellman articulates the ethical basis for which the physician should resist these trends in order to serve the patient well.

Through 40 years of learning and practicing medicine in roles from student, resident, director of the Joint Center for Radiation Therapy at Harvard, to physician-in-chief at Memorial Sloan Kettering Hospital, to Dean of the Pritzker School of Medicine at Chicago, Dr. Hellman has a unique platform from which to view the evolution of medicine, through his lens as a physician caring for an individual patient. Such a view frequently places him in the role of an unappreciated contrarian or curmudgeon. But his arguments are clear and his voice needs to be heard, now more than ever."
—William R. Brody, MD, PhD
President and Professor Emeritus, Salk Institute for Biological Studies

"To read this book is to take a journey through 50 years of progress in cancer science, with observations on how we know what we know, how new knowledge in medicine should be generated, and the important relationship medicine has to other areas of general knowledge and vice versa. The reader is guided by Dr. Sam Hellman, one of the most distinguished leaders in oncology and medicine, having established the department of Radiation Oncology at Harvard, led New York's Memorial Sloan-Kettering Cancer center, and served as Dean of Biological Sciences and the School of Medicine at the University of Chicago.

Dr. Hellman has challenged the ethics associated with randomized clinical trials, arguing that the treating physician cannot simultaneously be the clinical scientist enrolling that patient in a clinical study. His observations and analyses of breast cancer outcomes redefined how we view and treat breast cancer. In doing so, he postulated the concept of oligo (limited) metastatic disease, a concept that has profoundly changed the way we manage many cancers today.
There is depth and wisdom in this outstanding work which can be enjoyed by both medical professionals and the general public alike."
—Allen S. Lichter, MD, FASCO
Chief Executive Officer, American Society of Clinical Oncology

"Sam Hellman is unquestionably one of the most distinguished cancer physician-scientists of our era. This book meticulously collects his career-long unique experiences and thoughts across a range of key areas, from ethics to academics to clinical care. It provides a privileged historical perspective to the still young field of oncology, in both the understanding of the challenges of taking care of patients and cancer research in general. It is, above all, a wonderful testament to his profound love and commitment to helping patients with cancer, and reminds us why we chose to devote our lives to this fight. I am hopeful that the passion and wisdom present in this collection of writings and essays will be highly contagious and drive our best students and physicians-in-training to join our cause. Dr. Hellman and his generation have made it possible for them to finish the job."
—José Basegla, MD, PhD
Physician in Chief and Chief Medical Officer, Memorial Sloan Kettering Cancer Center

Learning While Caring

*Reflections on a Half-Century
of Cancer Practice, Research,
Education, and Ethics*

SAMUEL HELLMAN, MD

PRITZKER DISTINGUISHED SERVICE PROFESSOR EMERITUS

THE UNIVERSITY OF CHICAGO

OXFORD
UNIVERSITY PRESS

OXFORD
UNIVERSITY PRESS

Oxford University Press is a department of the University of Oxford. It furthers the University's objective of excellence in research, scholarship, and education by publishing worldwide. Oxford is a registered trade mark of Oxford University Press in the UK and certain other countries.

Published in the United States of America by Oxford University Press 198 Madison Avenue, New York, NY 10016, United States of America.

© Oxford University Press 2017

All rights reserved. No part of this publication may be reproduced, stored in a retrieval system, or transmitted, in any form or by any means, without the prior permission in writing of Oxford University Press, or as expressly permitted by law, by license, or under terms agreed with the appropriate reproduction rights organization. Inquiries concerning reproduction outside the scope of the above should be sent to the Rights Department, Oxford University Press, at the address above.

You must not circulate this work in any other form and you must impose this same condition on any acquirer.

Library of Congress Cataloging-in-Publication Data
Names: Hellman, Samuel, author.
Title: Learning while caring : reflections on a half-century of cancer practice, research, education, and ethics / Samuel Hellman.
Description: Oxford ; New York : Oxford University Press, [2017] | Includes bibliographical references.
Identifiers: LCCN 2016029436 | ISBN 9780190650551 (hardcover)
Subjects: | MESH: Hellman, Samuel. | Medical Oncology | Physicians | Neoplasms—therapy | Professional Practice | Physician-Patient Relations | Biomedical Research | Collected Works | Personal Narratives
Classification: LCC RC262 | NLM QZ 7 | DDC 362.196/994—dc23
LC record available at https://lccn.loc.gov/2016029436

This material is not intended to be, and should not be considered, a substitute for medical or other professional advice. Treatment for the conditions described in this material is highly dependent on the individual circumstances. And, while this material is designed to offer accurate information with respect to the subject matter covered and to be current as of the time it was written, research and knowledge about medical and health issues are constantly evolving and dose schedules for medications are being revised continually, with new side effects recognized and accounted for regularly. Readers must therefore always check the product information and clinical procedures with the most up-to-date published product information and data sheets provided by the manufacturers and the most recent codes of conduct and safety regulation. The publisher and the authors make no representations or warranties to readers, express or implied, as to the accuracy or completeness of this material. Without limiting the foregoing, the publisher and the authors make no representations or warranties as to the accuracy or efficacy of the drug dosages mentioned in the material. The authors and the publisher do not accept, and expressly disclaim, any responsibility for any liability, loss or risk that may be claimed or incurred as a consequence of the use and/or application of any of the contents of this material.

To Allison, Julianna, Justine, and Michael

Another side of Poppa Sam

CONTENTS

Preface	*xi*
Acknowledgments	*xli*
Introduction	1
Commentary	1
The Aims of Education; an annual address to The University of Chicago freshman class; published in *Perspectives in Biology and Medicine*, 1990	6
A Doctor's Dilemmas; Commencement Address, Allegheny College, 1984	20
The End of Inevitability, or Frankenstein and the Biological Revolution; published in *Pharos*, 1994	25
1. Medical Ethics and Learning	33
Commentary	33
Randomized Clinical Trials and the Doctor–Patient Relationship: An Ethical Dilemma; published in *Cancer Clinical Trials*, 1979	38
Of Mice but Not Men: Problems of the Randomized Clinical Trial; published in *New England Journal of Medicine*, 1991	44
Ethics of Randomized Clinical Trials; from a series of Ethics Grand Rounds, Dana Farber Cancer Institute, edited by E. J. Emanuel and W. Bradford Patterson; published in *Journal of Clinical Oncology*, 1998	54
The Patient and the Public Good; published in *Nature Medicine*, 1995	70
On First Looking into Kutcher's *Contested Medicine*: Ethical Tensions in Clinical Research; published in *Perspectives in Biology and Medicine*, 2010	79

Managed Care and the Doctor–Patient Relationship: A Ménage
  à Trois; unpublished essay, 1997   *93*
Fin de Siècle Medicine: Avoiding the Unintended Consequences
  of Health Care Reform; published in *Brookings Review*, 1994   *100*
Premise, Promise, Paradigm, and Prophesy; published in *Nature
  Clinical Practice Oncology*, 2005   *107*
Learning While Caring: Medicine's Epistemology; published
  in *Journal of Clinical Oncology*, 2014   *109*

2. Academic Medicine   *123*
Commentary   *123*
Medicine: A University; Pritzker School of Medicine,
  The University of Chicago, 1999   *128*
Comments on the Presentation by President Don Randel,
  The University of Chicago Symposium, "University of the
  Future," 2001   *132*
The Intellectual Quarantine of American Medicine; published
  in *Academic Medicine*, 1991   *135*
Tales of the Unnatural: Return From the Dean(d); published
  in *Journal of the American Medical Association*, 1998   *144*
A Lamentation on the Death of Collaboration; unpublished essay,
  2002   *150*
Irwin Freedberg and the Changing Times of Academic
  Medicine: from "Remembering Irwin Freedberg,"
  published in *Journal of Investigative Dermatology*, 2006   *154*
Ivar, Michael, and Zvi: Celebrating the Diversity of Our
  Friends and Colleagues; published in *Nature Clinical
  Practice Oncology*, 2005   *158*

3. Research   *161*
Commentary   *161*
Reflections of a Radiation Oncologist as President of the American
  Society of Clinical Oncology; published in *Journal of Clinical
  Oncology*, 1987   *170*

Technology, Biology, and Traffic; published in
    Acta Oncologica, 2001   *177*
Karnofsky Memorial Lecture. Natural History of Small
    Breast Cancers; published in *Journal of*
    Clinical Oncology, 1994   *185*
Dogma and Inquisition in Medicine: Breast Cancer as
    a Case Study; published in *Cancer*, 1993   *199*
Darwin's Clinical Relevance; published in *Cancer*, 1997   *208*
Oligometastases; published in *Journal of Clinical Oncology*, 1995   *224*
Oligometastases Revisited; published in *Nature Reviews Clinical*
    Oncology, 2011   *231*

4. Perceptions of Cancer   *245*
   Commentary   *245*
   Evolving Paradigms and Perceptions of Cancer; published
      in *Nature Clinical Practice Oncology*, 2005   *248*
   Oncologists and Their Patients; unpublished essay, 2016   *262*

5. Heroes   *269*
   Commentary   *269*
   Thomas Hodgkin and Hodgkin's Disease. Two Paradigms
      Appropriate to Medicine Today; published in *Journal of the*
      American Medical Society, 1991   *272*
   Curies, Cure, and Culture; published in *Perspectives in Biology*
      and Medicine, 1992   *284*
   The First Century of Cancer Chemotherapy; published in
      Journal of Clinical Oncology, 1998   *292*

Summing Up   *297*
Index   *309*

PREFACE

This book is about three major themes of my career in academic medicine and oncology: the ethics of clinical experiments and how we learn in medicine; how medicine fits in academia; and my particular research interests. As you will see, these seemingly different motifs are all part of a continuum rather than being separate and discrete. They occurred during an exceedingly dynamic and changeful period in biological and medical research and clinical practice. To appreciate my experiences and the bases of my interpretations of them requires that you are familiar with my background and education; therefore, I begin with a brief biographical sketch so that you, the reader, can understand the basis of my worldview.

Western health care delivery separated into two forms, with Western Europe and Canada embracing universal access guaranteed by governmental programs, while in the United States private health care persists, though with increasing government involvement and oversight. All of these changes occurred during my career and inform the essays collected here. They are by no means comprehensive of those times, but rather they are reflective of my interests and are the product of my upbringing, education, and experience.

I was born in 1934 in the nadir of the Great Depression to a Polish Jewish immigrant mother who came to the United States in 1920 at the age of 11, and a first-generation Jewish severely hearing-compromised father. While I heard discussions of my father's difficulties in making a living during those times, my memories are rather of a rich and pleasant childhood, living in a nice residential apartment building located on a small block between Van Cortlandt and Mosholu parks. Most residents neither had, nor did they require, an automobile. I was educated at PS 94 (K–6), PS 79 (7–9), and DeWitt Clinton High School (10–11). These were very pleasant years, with friends having very similar backgrounds and family values. I remember World War II, but as a young child I was more concerned with the maps published in the newspapers showing the progress of our forces. It was viewed as a game. However, I remember my parents and grandmother worrying about my two uncles, one in the Navy and the other in the Air Force, the latter receiving the Purple Heart on three occasions. I also remember the crying at the table as the horrors of the Holocaust were revealed.

This all changed when in 1948 my father won a car in a raffle. Neither he nor my mother knew how to drive, and so one of my mother's brothers took on the teaching responsibilities, but with only the mixed success characteristic of people learning to drive later in life. Both got driver's licenses but neither was very proficient. With this new capacity and the increased postwar prosperity, their horizons enlarged with individual home ownership becoming a realistic goal achieved in time for my senior year of high school (1950–1951). I went from a New York City school with about 5,000 boys to a much smaller coeducational high school in an affluent Long Island suburb. It was not possible to walk to stores or even to visit what friends I made in this neighborhood of single-family dwellings. My schoolmates had cars, friendships developed since grade school, and most important, they were used to a more affluent lifestyle—one that I resented. My self-identification never changed, despite the move from the middle-class Bronx to postwar suburban Long Island.

Because I wanted to attend a small coeducational liberal arts college, my mother found Allegheny College in western Pennsylvania and a few other Pennsylvania schools for us to visit. Allegheny was my choice, and so I left Long Island to take the train from New Jersey to the town of Meadville in the northwest corner of Pennsylvania in September 1951. It was an inspired choice, exposing me to the WASP values and culture reflecting those of mainstream America of the 1950s. There was an expectation of success, security, and easy acceptance into society consistent with the majority culture. Like most male students, I joined one of the seven fraternities. Two of the fraternities did not admit Jews, this becoming my first exposure to the overt institutional anti-Semitism prevalent at that time. Since the most attractive fraternities were open to all religious denominations, this restriction was educational but not inconvenient. As an aside, much later in life I met another Jewish fraternity brother who could not understand my continuing involvement with the college since he remembers it as a quite prejudiced institution. Rather, I remember it as a reflection of America of that time, a place where Jews were a minority, and anti-Semitism existed but the majority culture was open to us. This was quite different from my predominantly Jewish Bronx neighborhood, but resulted in a re-evaluation of my worldview; I was not part of the majority, and my minority status required notice but need not hinder me. My fellow students were open, welcoming, and nice, resulting in extremely pleasant daily living as well as a number of important lifelong friendships. My exposure to higher education was exhilarating due to the broadly based required curriculum, small classes, and the quality and interest of the faculty. I had been interested in being a physician for as long as I can remember, I was a good student, and so consistent with the stereotype, my middle-class Jewish parents encouraged this career path. I majored in chemistry, but the required humanities courses piqued my interest in philosophy, causing me to avail myself of more philosophy offerings. There were many opportunities for personal interaction with faculty within these areas as well as many others. Among the most important was Lewis Pino, a young chemist who became a friend and mentor, as well as my providing "Lew" and his wife, Carol, with a babysitter for their young family. Alfred Kern, an English professor, was a budding novelist and with Pino taught a senior seminar exploring the connections between science and the humanities. Al and I connected again later in life when I joined the Allegheny Board of Trustees. Horace Lavely, a religion professor, was also responsible for teaching philosophy. He offered me a private reading course concerned with reconciling philosophy and religion with science. While I never became convinced of this latter reconciliation, there was much in the study of philosophy that prepared me for my career as a physician and scholar. Perhaps the most meaningful course was "Philosophy in Literature" taught by the Dean, Julian Ross. Dr. Ross was the most respected member of the faculty by his students as well as his peers. His book on this subject still adorns my bookcase; while only occasionally browsed, it still serves as a reminder of this treasured learning experience. Philip Benjamin was the school librarian and an unlikely pre-med advisor who worked diligently in helping me gain admission to a New York State medical school so that I could use a Regents Scholarship that I had just won, which was restricted to schools within New York State. Raymond Shafer, then the Crawford County district attorney and who, later in life, became the governor of Pennsylvania, was the alumni advisor to our fraternity chapter. As president of the fraternity chapter, I had some positive dealings with him, and my appreciation of him was enhanced later in life when we served together on the Allegheny College Board of Trustees. The only negative impression I have of my Allegheny experience was of the dean of students who, I have been told, wrote a negative reference for me to medical school, apparently because of a party at my off-campus apartment during my sophomore year at which alcoholic beverages were served. It was Philip Benjamin, the librarian/pre-med advisor, who intervened on my behalf to ameliorate the damage.

Some 25 years after graduating I returned to Allegheny as a trustee. It was recommended that new trustees tour the college. While doing so, I was passed in the hall by a professor whose required course "Ideas and Institutions of Western Society" I took in my freshman or sophomore year. He stopped me, remembered me, and also remembered that I went to medical school in upstate New York. He thought it was at the University of Rochester rather than State University of New York Upstate Medical School at Syracuse. This episode epitomized for me the interest and involvement of faculty with students, even those to whom they had only limited exposure.

The Allegheny board experience introduced me to the nature of nonprofit institutional governance and the important responsibilities of trustees. Before joining the board I asked a colleague who was serving on another college board what the duties of board membership were. He replied with an old saw of the three Gs—"Give, Get, or Get off"—but the experience turned out to be much more than that. Most pleasurable was meeting many of my former college friends and acquaintances as well as others committed to the college. Friendships were refreshed or new ones made, providing a view of successful mature products of the college as well as others involved with the institution. I served as chairman of the Board from 1987 to 1993 and was involved in selecting a new president and presiding over major discussions among faculty, students, and trustees concerning divestment of college endowment investments in companies having significant business investment in South Africa due to the policies of apartheid. Eventually we did divest, but the process and discussion were almost more important than the outcome for all involved. Divestment was being considered on many campuses at that time. The Board of Trustees at Allegheny, as well as many others, prioritized their fiscal responsibilities in the selection of investments, while the faculty and students were more concerned with expressing the moral unacceptability of apartheid. I believe all parties profited from these discussions. While the Bronx and my parents provided the base for my worldview and ethics, Allegheny provided the liberal education so important to my values, responsibilities, and appreciation of our culture.

I chose SUNY Upstate rather than a New York City medical school because of the similarity to western Pennsylvania. This was a particularly fateful and fortuitous decision since it enabled me to meet my future wife and lifetime companion Marcia (Rusty) Sherman. We met in December 1955 as a result of a "blind date" organized by a close childhood friend, Rhea Topal, to whom I am forever grateful. I would not have applied to this medical school were it not for the Regents scholarship. The conditions of the scholarship required accepting admission to a New York State medical school within 30 days of receiving notification of the award, which came on Christmas Eve 1954. My pre-med advisor, Philip Benjamin, contacted Dr. William Faloon, a young faculty member at Upstate, who facilitated my application processing and became my medical faculty advisor, and later my laboratory research mentor. Research under his guidance enabled me to win the research award at graduation. Fate, kismet, whatever! Rusty and I were wed at the end of my second year of medical school, at the time of Rusty's graduation from Syracuse University. She supported us teaching high school history during my last two years of medical school, my internship, and the first year of my residency. An older classmate, Jerry Scanlon, who became a lifelong friend was my guide to entering marriage. We followed—with only occasional cheating—his suggestion of dividing each paycheck into separate envelopes devoted to food, rent, and other necessary expenditures, leaving the remainder for entertainment. This frugality served us well but was hard for Rusty to revise when times were better. I did not find that a problem. Another older medical school classmate, Jack Garnish, and I shared an apartment with four other classmates. Jack was just back from four years of active duty in the US Air Force and served to help temper my freshman-year nerdiness with his maturity gained from that experience. Jack and Jerry, both native upstate New York residents, introduced us to skiing and we shared many vacations with one or both of them with their spouses, Jackie and Barbara. However, my medical school years also began with a great tragedy; my closest friend Martin Topal (brother of Rhea, who arranged my date with Rusty) developed severe polio, which invalided him for the rest of his life. He probably was exposed to the virus when Rhea, Martin, and I went for a summer weekend to the Tanglewood Music Festival. This was at the end of the summer epidemics of this terrible disease before the wide acceptance of the Salk vaccine. This is but one of the examples of my good fortune; all three of us were there together, but both Rhea and I were spared.

These medical school years were full with study, companionship with my colleagues, and of course with the carefree beginning of our marriage and a lifetime love affair that continues to grow. I well remember warning Rusty that "medicine is my life"—how naïve—but Rusty embraced it. Of course, family became, as it should be and still is, my first priority and I am devoted to it. I was a good student and Bill Faloon encouraged me to apply for an internship at one of the Harvard teaching hospitals, resulting in my being accepted as a medical intern at Beth Israel Hospital. Again a fortuitous choice: this one-year experience resulted in five lifetime friendships, two with fellow interns, one nurse (also wife of one these fellow interns), and two neighbors during that seminal year. These two intern colleagues had very distinguished careers: Allan Rosenfield as an outstanding dean of the Mailman School of Public Health at Columbia University for 20 years; H. Richard Nesson, president of the Brigham and Women's Hospital and then president of Partners Healthcare. His wife, Lois Nesson, was the "charge nurse" on my first internship rotation and nurtured me through those early internship challenges. She remains a dear friend of the family who continues to be in regular contact with Rusty these 58 years. Fred and Ruth Stavis, upstairs neighbors during that eventful year, also remain dear friends in regular contact with us. We bought a vacation home in New Hampshire in 1982, shortly followed by the Nessons and Stavises as neighbors. This continued until Dick Nesson's death and later our sale of our New Hampshire home in 2012.

The Beth Israel internship began my education in the art of medicine: from how to communicate with the patient and his or her family, to how to present oneself, to how to unravel multiple complaints and triage them in order of importance and urgency, to when to call a consultant, to consulting with diagnostic imaging and pathology colleagues. The opportunity to witness real masters of the art on both the full-time and private staff was a real glimpse of academic leaders and masterful practitioners, often in the same person. Some doctors who made lasting impressions were the chief of medicine, Hermann Blumgart, a distinguished cardiologist; Louis Wolff, another distinguished cardiologist who is recognized eponymously in the "Wolff-Parkinson-White Syndrome"; Milton Hamolsky, an endocrinologist who later became chairman of medicine at Brown University. A. Stone Freedberg, another cardiologist, early in his career recognized the bacteria causally associated with gastric diseases but was discouraged from diverting from heart disease to follow this up: I learned later that Freedberg was likely to have had a bacteria related to gastric illnesses named after him if he had pursued this association, but he didn't because his chairman advised him to focus on cardiology, rather than follow up his novel identification of a then unknown bacteria in the stomachs of patients with gastric disease. In 2005 Barry Marshall won the

Nobel Prize for fulfilling Koch's postulates, confirming the association of that bacterium with diseases of the stomach. He later commented that Freedberg would have won the prize had he continued his studies.

At that time I also met Howard Hiatt, a young faculty member just back from the Pasteur Institute, then the center of understanding how genes are organized and function. This was my first exposure to molecular biology related to health and disease, a harbinger of things to come. The World War II Viennese refugee chief of radiology, Felix Fleischner, was a master clinician and wonderful showman, making radiology rounds a focus of our days. This was my first personal exposure to individuals whose names are associated eponymously in medicine: Wolff of the Wolff-Parkinson-White Syndrome and Fleischner of Fleischner's Sign and the Fleischner Society. Later in my career I studied and cared for patients with Hodgkin Lymphoma and wrote about the history of this disease; I found that Malpighi was really the first to describe the disease and Hodgkin's contemporary, Wilks, attributed the discovery of the disease to Hodgkin for reasons discussed in my selected essays to follow.

Equally important in my admiration for Beth Israel Hospital was the attention and concern not only with the patient but her family, social structure, and emotional wellness. This was an integrated effort of nursing, social work, physicians, and hospital administration. It was and remains the best example of integrated patient care in my American experience, equaled in my experience only at the Royal Marsden Hospital in the United Kingdom, and the Antoni Van Leeuwenhoek Hospital in the Netherlands, both cancer hospitals within a national health service. During this intern year I became disenchanted with internal medicine and unsure as to what direction my career should take. I decided to try a radiology residency, perhaps stimulated by Fleischner, and in any case radiology experience would be useful in most clinical career paths.

I was accepted to a radiology residency at Yale New Haven Hospital. In those days, the residency comprised two years of diagnostic imaging and one year of radiation oncology. My first nine months of diagnostic imaging, while interesting and useful, kept me too far from the patient and medical decision-making. I was a consultant but was not directly caring for the patient. I knew then that this would not be my career choice, but I was in the midst of my residency and so rotated to radiation oncology, a field to which I had very limited exposure in medical school. I found it very exciting! It had hands-on patient care, opportunities for cure, required making important therapeutic decisions, used my interest in the physical sciences, and used my newfound diagnostic imaging training. It also exposed me to molecular biology during the early years of the biological revolution, revitalizing my nascent laboratory research interests. I completely immersed myself in the field of oncology and have never looked back, nor did I return to complete my general radiology training. I found that it was possible to be certified in Radiation Oncology by completing a more extensive training program. Oncology in 1960 was practiced primarily by general surgeons, general radiologists, and hematologists. Radiation oncology in the United States was just beginning to be a separate specialty, and similarly so were surgical oncology and medical oncology. By chance, I was able to be involved in these exciting and important developments and they became essential to my career within oncology, medicine, and academic leadership.

At that time, the chairman of radiology, Morton M. Kligerman (known to all as "Klig"), was a dynamic leader and a radiation oncologist. He had just received one of the first NIH training grants and I was to be his first trainee. I completed the fellowship, including a year in the laboratory, first studying DNA repair and then I started my own lab studying hematopoietic stem cells. I was offered a faculty position at Yale but I thought I should widen my experiences, and so Klig arranged and, through the NIH grant, supported an additional year seeing and to some extent participating in radiation oncology at the Royal Marsden Hospital in London, led by Sir David Smithers, that included some of the leaders of our field, notably Julian Bloom and Emmanuel Lederman. This allowed me to observe and often participate in the care of patients in this most distinguished internationally recognized cancer hospital. The staff were all extremely good physicians because they understood the natural history of the specific cancers they treated. The emphasis on the nature and predilections of the disease was characteristic of the doctors I encountered there. The specialty was and still is called "clinical oncology" rather than, as in the United States at that time, "radiation therapy" and now radiation oncology. Their knowledge and behavior were epitomized in the British title. Much more than competent practitioners of a medical craft, they were primarily oncologists with a deep understanding of the specific cancers they cared for and an understanding of all treatment-related modalities relevant to them. At that time, we Americans were to a much greater extent the recipients of the newest advances in diagnostic imaging and the equipment required. It was remarkable how the British used the history and physical exam without these technological tools to properly diagnose and fashion appropriate treatments. It was this view of the specialty that I tried to emulate in my clinical practice and what I tried to teach to my students. Included in my fellowship was participation in the laboratory of the biophysicist, Professor Leonard Lamerton, who led a laboratory of scientists utilizing the rigorous methods of physics to study biological problems. Nicholas Blackett was also interested in hematopoietic stem cells, so Lamerton suggested that we collaborate. We did quite successfully, culminating with Nick joining me many years later at Harvard.

This became my "Wanderjahr," a year in which an apprentice traveled and improved his skills before settling down to the practice of his profession, such as enjoyed by some medical practitioners in Britain in the nineteenth century. I was not alone, as many of my American medical colleagues in other fields interested in academic careers did such a year, as did some from other English-speaking countries. This experience was a revelation for me, allowing me to see the cultural differences between the United States and Britain, both in general and in medicine specifically. I saw and participated in the National Health Service, believed it to be a better system than ours, and thus expected it to be adopted soon in the United States. So much for my predictions, but I still favor that system and so lament our failure to adopt such a national health care program. Perhaps the Affordable Care Act will bring us closer to this, but it seems only a small step, very late in coming. We came to London with our two very young children and it was a challenge that fell especially on Rusty to make a home in the UK still recovering from World War II. But all considered, it was a Wanderjahr from which I profited greatly.

During that year I visited a number of centers in the UK and on the continent, allowing me to separate those accepted parts of medical dogma and procedure that were universal rather than those that were just local custom. These differences were primarily in the details of treatment, but occasionally there were important differences in medical care. These observations produced a healthy skepticism of dogma, and the resulting certainty served me well in my subsequent professional life, some of which will be the subject of a number of my academic contributions to be considered later in this volume.

Returning to New Haven at the beginning of 1966, I began my faculty career as an assistant professor. I received some NIH research support for my stem cell research, as well as developing an active practice of radiation oncology and resident teaching. Yale at that time had an outstanding department of medicine, chaired by one of the giants of American medicine of the time, Paul Beeson. I tried to faithfully attend medical grand rounds to see him in action, as well as to keep up on medical advances with such erudite and convivial medical colleagues. At one of these rounds there was a discussion of a breast cancer patient whose major symptom was bone pain caused by extensive metastatic cancer. The ensuing discussion focused on the excess of calcium in her blood, the result of her bony metastases. When the discussion concluded, I pointed out that the reason the patient was admitted was bone pain, but there was no mention of how that was being addressed. Dr. Beeson was taken aback by this omission and used this to emphasize that our primary responsibility is to the patient and her particular symptoms. That I still remember and have tried to teach this patient-centered orientation to my students is a tribute to my Yale experience.

I enjoyed being a young faculty member very much and was productive in both clinical and laboratory research and looked forward to staying at Yale for an extensive period of time, but was surprised to hear, about a year and a half later, that Harvard Medical School wanted to consider me for a new position. They were in the process of developing a combined center of radiation oncology to provide service for the six patient care facilities in close proximity to the medical school. Concomitant with this venture, a new chairman of radiology for Harvard and the then Peter Bent Brigham Hospital, Herbert L. Abrams, was recruited. Radiation oncology was a part of that department and Herb was leading the search. Abrams came from the radiology department at Stanford University, led by the premier academic radiation oncologist in the United States, Henry S. Kaplan, so he recognized the value of a strong program in that field. This new endeavor was intended to be a collaborative venture of the member hospitals as well as an academic home for Harvard's radiation oncology efforts. Much to both my surprise and pleasure, I was selected to lead this effort, and so with Rusty and our six- and four-year-old children we moved to Newton, a Boston suburb, at the beginning of March 1968. While six institutions were involved in discussions of participating in such a center, we began with four members: Peter Bent Brigham Hospital, Beth Israel Hospital, Boston Hospital for Women, and New England Deaconess Hospital. After about two years the other two institutions involved in the initial planning, Boston Children's Hospital and what has now become the Dana Farber Cancer Institute, joined the Joint Center for Radiation Therapy (JCRT) at Harvard Medical School (HMS).

While it was an exciting time starting a new collaborative enterprise, the very nature of the center not being a single physical facility, but depending on the willingness of the members to cooperate, made the arrangement fragile. Unfortunately, this arrangement came apart after a successful collaboration for more than a quarter of a century, and more than 10 years after I had left Harvard. The JCRT was very much an HMS project brokered by the dean's office, but as I was to learn later, the dean had only limited leverage over its member hospitals. Coming to HMS at 33 years of age and having been an assistant professor at Yale for only two years was a somewhat intimidating but exalting experience, and, as Klig described to me, it could lead to "Harvarditis." As I understood, this disease was characterized by the "symptoms" of fully requited self-love and difficulty separating delusions of grandeur from reality. It may also be associated with smugness and arrogance. During my time on the Harvard faculty, I felt that, to my peers, all educational experiences not at Harvard were equally discounted, with the exception of that at Boston University and Tufts, those neighboring institutions being even further denigrated. A Harvard colleague referred to me as being "anointed" because I was given a tenured position even though all my previous experience (except that at Beth Israel Hospital) was not at HMS-affiliated institutions. While this may be a playful exaggeration, such were the prejudices of many of my colleagues.

Unexpectedly, to be the leader of a new Harvard enterprise was an exciting challenge and turned out to be great fun. Since there were no such multi-institutional collaborative programs under the school's aegis that were housed and supported by the member hospitals, we could be as creative as possible without having any concern for past precedence. Having so many masters, effectively I had none. What counted to all was performance: providing modern radiation therapy and an academic research and teaching program without being a financial drain on any of the member institutions. Governance consisted of monthly meetings of the hospital directors with our administrator and me. They were an amicable group as long as the plaudits significantly outnumbered complaints and the finances were in order. This was a time of cost-based reimbursement, plentiful research funding, and only modest and decorous conduct of the hospital executives with each other—quite far removed from the aggressive competition among hospitals and health plans now so prevalent.

Most urgent was the need for personnel both professional and technical, as well as modern equipment, then sorely lacking. Martin Levene, an experienced radiation oncologist who worked in both the Brigham and Beth Israel hospitals, was well thought of by the Beth Israel Hospital leaders as well as referring physicians. He agreed to join us and turned out to be a great addition. I was 33 years old and not far from completing my training, while Martin was in his mid-forties. He quickly became my deputy and a great complement to me. Two young physicians came from the Yale training program with me, as well as a recent graduate of the Princess Margaret Hospital in Toronto. Jim Belli, a radiation biologist from Dallas, physicist Bengt Bjarngard from Lund, Sweden, and chief technologist Leon Graff from Halifax, Nova Scotia, completed the initial professional component of the JCRT. I came to Boston in March 1968 and the others in time for our starting the clinical program in July. Some of these new colleagues came with their families and lived with us temporarily until they got settled. Rusty was completely engaged with this latter effort while busy with our new digs and two young children.

We wanted the radiation treatment facility to be within the individual hospitals as much as possible, while not unnecessarily duplicating equipment and profiting from the economies of scale offered by multiple hospitals in close proximity. This was a novel concept so that we centralized administration, research facilities, and some treatment-planning activities, with the actual treatment being delivered as much as possible in the member institutions from which the patient originated. This was necessary for inpatients and desired for outpatients so that they would be close to our doctors and the local referring or collaborating physicians. This was largely adhered to, except for some specialized equipment or expertise located only in one institution being sufficient and avoiding unnecessary duplication. We recruited junior staff, developed training programs for resident physicians, medical physicists, and radiation technologists (now referred to as radiation therapists, a title formerly used for the caring physician, who now is called a radiation oncologist).

Gustavo Montana and John Chaffey, immediately after finishing their Yale fellowships, became the leaders of the JCRT efforts at New England Deaconess Hospital and Peter Bent Brigham Hospitals, respectively. Martin Levene continued at Beth Israel and also covered the Boston Hospital for Women. Jim Belli served as first substitute when needed, as well as starting his laboratory, which with mine, formed the nidus of basic research in the nascent academic enterprise. After the first year, Gus Montana was recruited to chair the program at the University of North Carolina and was replaced by Stanley Order, who had just finished his fellowship at Yale. By 1970, the Children's Hospital and the Jimmy Fund, the forerunner of the Dana Farber Cancer Institute, joined, and J. Robert Cassady was recruited to lead pediatric radiation oncology after finishing the radiation oncology fellowship at Stanford Medical School.

These were heady times for this young group. Eventually the changes in health care delivery in the US ended the collegiality of the member institutions necessary for the JCRT to continue, but for more than 25 years the collaborative venture prospered, the first 15 years under my leadership. My angst with the dissolution of the JCRT is described in one of the essays to follow.

My research interests begun at Yale reached their full flowering during these years in Boston. I continued my clinical studies of Hodgkin Lymphoma—the current preferred usage for Hodgkin's disease—and became very interested in Thomas Hodgkin. He was remarkable for both his personal and professional activities, many in my judgment more important than the eponymous disease that brings him to our attention. I discuss these facets of his life more fully in the section devoted to my heroes. My interest in breast cancer was primarily concerned with studying methods of treatment that allowed the patient to retain her breast without compromising the outcome. This brought me into conflict with many surgeons who advocated the then prevailing treatment, radical mastectomy, an operation that leaves the patient without the breast and underlying muscles and often results in debilitating and disfiguring swelling of the arm on the side of the breast removal. These were vigorous discussions and debates that I discuss more extensively later, and they led to me being a co-editor of five multidisciplinary texts on this disease. The commitment to a multidisciplinary rather than a competitive approach to cancer care has been a major feature of my career, started in my early studies of combined surgery, radiation, and chemotherapy for tumors of the head and neck. My stem cell research continued as I, with Leslie Botnick and Peter Mauch, who both began when they were fellows and continued when they joined the faculty, tried to learn how stem cells gave rise to mature blood cells, how they circulated in the blood, determined what type of blood cell to produce, and how they responded to aging, radiation, and certain drugs.

It was also during these years that Vincent DeVita, Steven Rosenberg, and I created the first truly multidisciplinary cancer textbook. We designed the book and chose experts to write individual chapters, although we wrote some as well. We then edited all these contributions so as to result in a comprehensive and consistent manuscript appropriate for all doctors involved in cancer treatment. The first of the seven editions in which I participated appeared in 1982, and the eighth, done by Vince, Steve, and Ted Lawrence replacing me, was published in 2008; thus for more than a quarter of a century, I spent a significant part of my life working on this textbook with my co-editors. Although others attempted to replicate our text, throughout that time ours was the most popular by far. A friend with extensive academic textbook experience gave me the excellent advice that we should stipulate that the publisher support two meetings for each edition: the first to decide on content, organization, and possible authors of the chapters; the second to review, modify, and edit as needed all the chapters. He said that this was best done away from home at a nice location pleasing to our spouses. These arrangements were accepted by Lippincott, our publisher, and served us well. Alice and Steve, and Mary Kay and Vince bonded with Rusty and me at the meetings, and we have continued our friendships.

Vince, at that time the director of the National Cancer Institute, made an unusual request of me, then the chairman of the Board of Scientific Counselors of the Division of Cancer Treatment (DCT) in the early 1980s, to bring James Curran of the Centers for Disease Control and Prevention (CDC) to our meeting. Jim described a new disease in horrific terms. Vince explained the need for funding an effort to understand and control this disease. He asked permission to divert DCT funds for this urgent effort, despite it not being directly related to cancer. Of course we did. This was my first knowledge of what is now called AIDS. Later it was appreciated that AIDS was cancer-related since it was associated with an increased incidence of some cancers. This and my subsequent experience as physician-in-chief at Memorial Sloan-Kettering Cancer Center, to be described later, involved me in the responses of the medical community to this disease. Despite Memorial being a cancer hospital, we had a large number of AIDS patients, both because of the particular tumors associated with AIDS and our staff's extensive experience and knowledge of immunosupression produced by anti-cancer drugs. While there was some apprehension of possible contagion by some staff, we accepted the obligation of all the medical community to caring for patients with this new disease. I was particularly gratified but not surprised with the positive response of the hospital's Board of Directors to this responsibility.

A particularly meaningful, somewhat related experience was a visit to Tanzania in 1981 to help in setting up a cancer center in Dar es Salaam. Claudia Henschke, a friend and radiologist, asked me to join her in visiting Dar to help in this effort, especially to visit with US diplomatic officials there to help to ensure continued American funding support for this effort. Ronald Reagan had just become president, and Claudia and others were concerned that the change in administration might deleteriously affect the cancer center's development. Claudia's interest in this was a part of her determined effort to do what she could to secure her recently deceased father's work in setting up cancer centers in the developing world. Ulrich Henschke was chairman of radiation oncology at Howard University in Washington, DC. He had previously asked me to accept a resident from his training program from Tanzania, Jeff Luande, for training in pediatric oncology since Henschke felt this was not varied enough at Howard. Dr. Luande stayed far longer than was originally intended and participated in far more than just pediatric cases. He completed his training and returned home to develop a cancer center affiliated but separate from the Muhimbili Medical Center (MMC). This center was conceived by Dr. Henschke, but unfortunately shortly thereafter Henschke was killed in a private plane crash. Dr. Luande originally was to be guided by him, so my additional charge was to provide some advice and guidance. My visit provided me an opportunity to see medicine practiced by qualified physicians but with limited resources involving extensive triage by the patients, their family, and the doctor before even coming to MMC. For example, while liver cancer is quite common in Tanzania as well as much of Africa, it was hardly seen at MMC because, I was told, it was well known in the predominantly rural country that the disease was incurable and not worth the trip to Dar es Salaam. I also saw patients with what was called "Slim Disease," thought to be due to some invading unknown gastrointestinal organism. Later it was recognized as AIDS. While I was never directly involved in its treatment, these early encounters with information about

AIDS stimulated Vince, Steve, and me to edit the first AIDS textbook, which subsequently went through four editions.

Jeff was seeing a very different patient population than that he was exposed to at the JCRT. Rather than a concern for breast preservation in women with early stage breast cancer, his patients presented with much more advanced cancers of many types. The principles of treatment remained the same, but the application needed to be consonant with the extent of the disease and the social arrangements allowing rural patients to be cared for in his urban facility. A side benefit of the visit was a trip with Claudia and Jeff to Moshi at the base of Kilimanjaro, to Arusha, and then to a number of game reserves, highlighted with a visit to the extensive game preserve in the Ngorongoro Crater.

At home, our social life to some extent resumed, despite being away from Boston for eight years. The Stavises and Nessons were true Bostonians: Fred Stavis with his brother were running the family seafood business and Dick Nesson was a trusted associate of Howard Hiatt, then the chair of medicine at Beth Israel Hospital. Dick continued to have increasing responsibilities in the Harvard medical organizations, including being a founding co-medical director of the Harvard Community Health Plan; then he became the director of ambulatory care at the Peter Bent Brigham Hospital, then president of a merger of the Peter and Robert Bent Brigham Hospitals with the Boston Hospital for Women into what is now known as The Brigham and Women's Hospital. His last presidency was of Partners Health Care, initially including the Brigham and Women's Hospital and the Massachusetts General Hospital, and more recently including other affiliated facilities.

An extremely close new family friendship developed during these years with Jan and Frank Morgan and their children. Frank was the Boston bureau chief for Newsweek and a marvelous companion, involving me in many activities of the nonmedical community. Through Frank, I joined the St. Botolph Club and enjoyed regular poker games, dinners, and pleasant companionship. The two families celebrated the Spring holidays together at their house for Easter and at ours for Passover. This friendship was interrupted by both families moving away, the Morgans to Hawaii and us to New York City. Sadly, both have died, Frank just this year.

PREFACE

By the time our daughter was in high school, Rusty was ready to return to full-time employment. This occurred at the full flowering of the feminist movement and Rusty was invigorated by this and wished to enter graduate school to prepare for a new career. She received her master's degree in counseling and consulting psychology from Harvard at the same time as our daughter Debbie's graduation from high school. Rusty then began working at Northeastern University and continued full-time employment and a gratifying career in consulting, counseling, and training, in New York City at the Association of Junior Leagues, then in Chicago at Michael Reese Hospital and then, for the majority of her career, at The University of Chicago, until we both went part-time and later retired.

An unexpected invitation to be considered for appointment as the physician-in-chief at Memorial Sloan-Kettering Cancer Center came from Paul Marks, then its newly appointed president. Most remarkable to me was being interviewed by the three leaders of MSKCC Boards of Directors: Honorable Chairman Laurance Rockefeller, Chairman Benno C. Schmidt, and Chairman of Memorial Hospital, James Robinson III. These were captains of finance and industry of the highest order, but all completely devoted to MSKCC and to eradicating cancer. Association with these three gentlemen and the other board members during my tenure at MSKCC was a treasured singular experience in my career, marked by their stature in their fields while being completely immersed in what was to be my home institution for the next 5 years.

Before leaving my descriptions of Harvard, I must note the amazement of many of my colleagues that someone would leave a Harvard professorship for almost any position elsewhere. This was highlighted by the recommendation of a surgeon colleague and friend that before doing anything irrevocable I should seek psychiatric consultation. This may well be an extreme example of the previously mentioned "Harvarditis."

Paul Marks was determined to lead MSKCC in a major saltation of its academic faculty and physical facilities. My responsibilities were to develop these efforts with regard to patient care and clinical research. Of course I knew a great deal of the general reputation of the doctors already at the institution, but actually seeing them practicing their respective specialties was revelatory. The level of expertise demonstrated was of the highest quality with only the rarest of exceptions. I saw great medicine during my Harvard and Yale experiences, but these were not all concentrated on a single disease. Early in my stay at Memorial, we were invited to a Hellman family wedding where I visited with our family's longtime physician who was a role model to me. He assured me that he knew why I had come to the institution. He said it was because I had had a lymphoma as a teenager. I was shocked to learn that two operations—described to me as an appendectomy and a few months later lysis of adhesions—were really for diagnosis and removal of the tumor. In fact, I had seen an eminent Memorial surgeon in his private office outside the institution sometime after these procedures for advice as to whether further treatment was required. He did not recommend it. My family physician was astounded that I knew nothing about the diagnosis of lymphoma. My parents were not pleased that this was revealed to me since they had not planned to ever inform me of it. I also think that my doctor believed that I must have known at some level but if I did, it was completely sublimated. Many years later I returned to Memorial for treatment of another cancer. This experience as a patient and cancer survivor, while not recommended, offered me the opportunity to see the disease from different perspectives. It highlighted the different ways cancer was perceived not only for patients and the general public, but also for different medical specialties and in the arts and the media. This is discussed in the collected essays that follow.

What was needed at MSKCC was not improved clinical care since the staff was of the highest quality, but rather enhanced academic activities in clinical and translational research. It was my job to make a plan to achieve these goals, recruit academic leaders, and develop the facilities needed for these programs. During those years, I was fortunate to attract from elsewhere, promote from current staff, as well as retain some departmental leaders, many of whom became internationally recognized as leaders of their respective disciplines. All seemed to flourish and many became great friends. There is always a risk in mentioning some that one might inadvertently omit others, but I must do it because it was such an illustrious group: radiation oncologist Zvi Fuks; medical oncologist John

Mendelsohn; pediatric oncologist Richard O'Reilly; surgical oncologist Murray Brennan; neuro-oncologist Jerome Posner; and medical physicist Clifford Ling. They in turn recruited an extraordinary staff. This excellence helped further recruitment in other fields of importance in a cancer center such as diagnostic radiology and pathology. There were outstanding leaders in special fields of expertise, especially valuable in a cancer hospital, who were already present, such as Kathleen Foley in pain management and Marguerite Lederberg in psychiatry. It was at MSKCC that I appreciated what are today the early fruits of precision, personalized medicine, and immune methods of treating cancer. John Mendelsohn was among the first to develop and use therapeutic agents based on the newfound genetic alterations seen in cancer. Lloyd Old, a scientist at the center, was a pioneer in cancer immunology and quickly convinced me of its promise in cancer treatment.

Being at Memorial and in New York City is different from other places. New York is the center of media, finance, and the cultural life of America, and MSKCC is considered the apogee of such institutions in the world. Some of the patients were very famous, or at least, very well known and/or very wealthy. The board members of the center and hospital were, as is to be expected, selected from the most respected, influential, and wealthy, as is also true of most eleemosynary institutions, but here in the great commercial mecca that is New York City, they were the *ne plus ultra*. For me (with no experience except for participating on the Allegheny College Board of Trustees), involvement with this board was a rare and never to be repeated experience. The least pleasant aspect of my position was being expected to attend social events of the institution, or of the board members themselves. The novelty wore off quickly. I would not like to leave this discussion of the board without recognizing those three leaders who first interviewed me for the position of physician-in-chief as special trustees whose dedication to the institution was remarkable. Laurance Rockefeller was the *eminence grise* while being quite polite and self-effacing. Memorial Hospital was supported by his family, and he was the Rockefeller brother most involved with MSKCC. Benno Schmidt was the long-time managing partner of the venture capital firm, J. H. Whitney & Co. He was the most knowledgeable layman about cancer whom I have ever met and one of the prime movers in the creation of the National Cancer Act in 1971. Benno had an interesting anecdote about how this legislation came to be. Mary Lasker, a devoted philanthropist with great influence with congress, and Benno led the lay contribution to the effort while Edward (Ted) Kennedy, senator from Massachussets, was the prime mover in Congress in getting the bill passed. Benno relates that when he discussed the proposed act with President Nixon, the president agreed to support the bill, but only if Senator Kennedy's name be removed. Benno had to go to the senator and tell him of this. Kennedy took this disrespectful snub with such good grace that Benno related that, despite their considerable political differences, he remained a friend and admirer of the senator.

Jim Robinson, then the CEO of American Express, was chair of Memorial Hospital, a couple of years younger than me, and very helpful and supportive. Rusty and I were friendly with Jim and his wife Linda Robinson during that time and later, but as often the case when moving away, this has reduced largely to holiday greetings. I was privileged to have these board leaders at that time. Working for and with Paul Marks was complicated. Paul was an extremely effective visionary, a recruiter par excellence, an excellent fundraiser, but he could occasionally be difficult dealing with staff or consultants. He was fine with me, but it sometimes required me to provide some remedial care to others.

The social highlight of our time in New York City was to awaken a previous friendship with Irene and Irwin Freedberg that began when Irwin and I were training at Beth Israel Hospital in Boston. Irwin became a leading academic dermatologist, founding a combined dermatology department serving several of the Harvard teaching hospitals near the medical school. Seem familiar? It was modeled after the JCRT. Irwin left Boston to found a new Department of Dermatology at Johns Hopkins. Seem familiar? We both left tenured positions at Harvard Medical School to accept leadership positions at other leading American medical schools. Irwin was then recruited to New York University, which at that time had the largest and best-supported dermatology department. When first considering going to MSKCC, I called Irwin to discuss living and working as

PREFACE   xxxiii

academic physicians in New York City. He described an essential difference with this observation: in Boston or in Baltimore, when going to the symphony or opera you always saw people that you knew, but in New York City that was rarely the case. That turned out to be true for us as well. We did meet old acquaintances, Joan and Gus Montana, but they were visiting from Chapel Hill, North Carolina. The message was that New York City was very big and impersonal. Once coming to the city, we and the Freedbergs renewed and reinvigorated our friendship. We all loved opera and the symphony, loved to ski, and had houses in New Hampshire as a result of living in Boston. Common interests, similar family closeness, and mutual affection reinforced each other. Linda Robinson, Jim's spouse and a public relations guru, was an active supporter and fundraiser for the NYU dermatology department that Irwin chaired. This dual connection came together when both couples were guests together at our New Hampshire home and then when we attended the wedding of Jim's son. The Freedbergs remained among our closest friends until their premature deaths. My memorial remembrance of Irwin is presented in the essays to follow because we both lived in a golden age of academic medicine, as described in Chapter 2 on this subject.

After 5 years at MSKCC, much of my recruitment and facility renewal program was well underway, and life in New York City was not as enjoyable as we had hoped. I missed being an integral part of a medical school and a university. I was not actively looking to change my position when what seemed to be an excellent opportunity was presented to me by a superb recruiter, then President Hanna Gray of The University of Chicago. The position she wanted to discuss was vice president of The University of Chicago and dean of the Biological Sciences Division (BSD), which included the deanship of the Pritzker School of Medicine. This seemed manna from heaven: return to academia at a distinguished university with BSD and the medical school being physically contiguous with the rest of the university. There was one problem: the hospital and its leader responded to a separate board. This included some members of the university's Board of Trustees, the president, the provost, and me, as well as an equal number of independent trustees. This duality of governance and perceived mission troubled me. I feared that the hospital board would be guided more by financial risks and opportunities, rather than the missions of an academic medical center adjoining an impoverished minority neighborhood. After considering the opportunities and the assurance of the support of President Gray as well as my high, but as it turned out, overestimation of my abilities in dealing with boards, I accepted. The university has lived up to my high expectations. It is a wonderful institution, and extremely collaborative both within and outside traditional boundaries. When I left the deanship 5 years later and when Rusty and I both retired, we much preferred staying in Chicago and at The University of Chicago rather than returning to New York City or Boston. It was not until after my eightieth birthday that we moved to be closer to our daughter, Deborah, now a professor of law at the University of Virginia, and her young family.

During my career I have had the opportunity to either join or participate with boards of directors of both philanthropic organizations and those of commercial companies, some as startups, and one large medical equipment manufacturer. I have discussed Allegheny, MSKCC, and The University of Chicago boards elsewhere in this volume, but not my for-profit boards both big and small. Varian Associates was the leading medical linear accelerator manufacturer in the world but this was only one of its products. The others included devices for making electronic chips, large chemical analysis instruments, and an X-ray tube manufacturing facility. I joined the Board of Directors after a new CEO was appointed and was in the process of making significant changes to the company, including adding some board members familiar with the particular products. For me it was a window into a completely new world. The bulk of the BOD were senior business executives familiar with not only the roles and responsibilities of board membership but more importantly how boards actually worked. As an aside, this activity was somewhat incongruous with my working-class Bronx background. Even so, I was impressed with the quality of my colleagues and how they went about affecting the company. With the medical business there seemed to be two goals: maximizing profits and improving medical care. Often they appeared to be in parallel, but occasionally these goals could diverge. Maximizing profits was much more focused on the quarterly financial performance, but this could slow research and development aimed at better methods of treatment. Walking this line was a measure of leadership by the executives as well as the board. It was quite different from academic medical research or even medical center management. The splitting of Varian into three new corporations because the businesses were quite different and not synergistic was thought to be advantageous for all the resulting entities. But most important, it was felt that the stock price did not reflect the company's true value because the metrics for evaluating the different businesses were different, and stock analysts could become confused. Varian Associates split into three separate companies. Board members were allocated to the different businesses, and so I now joined the board of Varian Medical Systems, the new corporation manufacturing radiation therapy and diagnostic X-ray equipment. The split turned out to be an excellent decision, for we could now focus on our individual businesses and the sum of the stock prices after the split grew markedly. This experience opened my eyes to how large corporations are run, as well as to the vagaries of the stock market.

I also became a member of the boards of two startups: InSightec, an MRI-guided focused ultrasound company, and Vantage Oncology, a community-based supplier of radiation therapy services. Both companies had enthusiastic and highly competent leadership. The focused ultrasound device is disruptive technology. The experience on this board taught me how resistant the status quo is to radical change. The invention is outstanding, its value clear with many possible future uses in cancer, neurological diseases, and targeted drug delivery; despite this, getting it accepted as a part of medical practice can be quite frustrating. This is in stark contrast to Varian making important improvements on accepted devices that are already utilized in medical practice. Vantage was in a middle position; its goal of bringing major cancer center–level care to the community as a for-profit enterprise is unusual but not really disruptive. Its development seems very promising except that, like the oft-cited Chinese admonition, it is very difficult to navigate and prosper in "interesting times."

Much to my surprise, I was asked to be on the Board of Trustees of The Brookings Institution when I was the Dean of Medicine at The University of Chicago. This was at a time when then First Lady Hillary Clinton was actively involved in health care reform. My friend and MSKCC leader Jim Robinson was a Brookings trustee, and he was the likely reason that I was chosen in order to add medical leadership experience to the board. I had known of Brookings as the prototype "think tank" providing studious analysis to government. I knew of it mainly for its economic studies. Seeing it in its fullness was somewhat surprising: economics was important, but so were foreign affairs and governance studies, which were followed during my tenure by a new program in metropolitan policy. Meeting and hearing from these various areas expanded my horizons from primarily health issues. Brookings had a very different kind of mission with different kinds of scholars and trustees. I found it very broadening and, despite my limited background, I felt I could contribute to some discussions other than those germaine to health primarily as they related to organizations and logic and, of course, my left of center political leanings. I believe that I was useful in elevating health care delivery as an important area for Brookings, but I gained much more than I gave. I enjoyed it greatly.

Before leaving describing my board service I must mention my deep and enthusiastic commitment to the Ludwig Institute for Cancer Research (LICR) and subsequently Ludwig Cancer Research, a fusion of all of Daniel K. Ludwig's cancer philanthropic efforts. Lloyd Old, my MSKCC colleague and noted cancer immunologist, invited me to be on the Scientific Advisory Committee (SAC) of the institute. LICR is different from more traditional philanthropically-based medical research organizations. It is international, and does not give out competitively sought individual grants but rather supports whole units residing in health care enterprises devoted to cancer-related research. Our SAC not only advised but also reviewed our far-flung units from Melbourne, Australia, to Sao Paulo, Brazil, including Western European and American centers. The committee was composed of internationally distinguished scientists and physicians, including two Nobel Laureates during my time on the committee. While the funds were considerable, they were small compared to those awarded by the National Cancer Institute, so not only did we seek excellence, but we also had to search for promising research areas not otherwise well funded. Two areas stood out as attractive targets for our efforts: an area of molecular biology called signal transduction, and tumor immunology. It is a great satisfaction to see how both of these fields are now well recognized for their importance and exciting new possibilities for improved cancer treatment. We played a significant role in making this possible. Later in my involvement with LICR, I was asked to relinquish my committee membership to join the Board of Directors of the Institute and eventually be a trustee of the institute and of Mr. Ludwig's Testamentary Trust. Daniel K. Ludwig was a shipping magnate who used about half of his then assets to form LICR and later left the remainder in trust for six US institutions for cancer research. These two different funding sources form the basis of a coordinated and synergistic organization, Ludwig Cancer Research, now in the full flower of its research for possible clinical benefits. Being involved with Ludwig efforts was and still continues to be a special delight of my medical career.

I enjoyed leading a program of renewal and elevating our academic enterprise but did not relish participating in some of the necessary parts of being a dean. Meetings, committees, personnel issues, and fundraising were more burdensome than I expected. Five years after completing my deanship I wrote a facetious piece about this experience that is presented in Chapter 2, "Academic Medicine." I planned to continue my deanship beyond my 5-year appointment if some changes could be made to the organizational relationship of the Division of Biological Sciences to the leadership of the hospital and its board. The restructuring of the dean/vice president position was not to occur for many years, and only after two other deans served. I am pleased to note that the current dean's relationship to the hospital and a change in the board's responsibilities seem much more satisfactory, but perhaps that is just how it appears to me now as an outside observer. As I was completing my term, President Gray was replaced as The University of Chicago president by Hugo Sonnenschein, who did not share my views concerning the structure, and so I stepped down as dean but did not leave the university. I returned to what I loved most in my career: teaching, research, and patient care. I then had the best university position possible, a tenured faculty member whose department chairman was a former student of mine, Ralph Weichselbaum, whom I greatly admire and am fond of, in a great university in my favorite city. After 5 years as an academic administrator and before returning to the clinic, I spent 6 months refreshing and retooling at centers of excellence that I admired and where I was welcomed: most notably at the Antoni von Leeuwenhoek Hospital and Netherlands Cancer Center. During this time I decided to limit all my clinical and research efforts primarily to breast cancer, its natural history, and by extension to that of other cancers. Rusty continued her job at the university and then we both gradually and progressively diminished our responsibilities until moving to Charlottesville 22 years later. Although I am more retired than not, I still contribute some advice and discussion at periodic retreats of Ralph's lab. Because I am an occasional (4+ times a year) visitor and not in any position of authority, the participants feel free to accept or reject my advice. I enjoy doing this, and Ralph and his colleagues tell me that I am helpful. Whether or not this is true or just good manners, I am pleased to continue this involvement. I am also still quite involved as a board member of the Ludwig Institute for Cancer Research, which keeps me abreast of exciting new research developments.

After returning to The University of Chicago from the Netherlands, I resumed my breast cancer research with a young faculty member, Coral Quiet, who helped me resume work begun at MSKCC on breast cancer natural history using the long-term databases in both institutions. Later, Ruth Heimann shared this effort with me. Ralph Weichselbaum, my nominal boss and former student, made every effort to make this time productive and pleasant. Further, he and I embarked on collaborative research in metastatic spread, especially postulating a state of limited metastatic spread that might be amenable to regional treatment. We called this "oligometastases," with the prefix *oligo* meaning few. This research has been very fruitful, with many others now recognizing the entity and Ralph's lab finding molecular markers of this state of limited metastatic spread. He also invited me to participate in a minor way in his other laboratory efforts. I think I help some, but I know I enjoy it and continue today to visit Chicago at regular intervals to meet with the lab and Ralph to review and discuss some projects of mutual interest, especially those related to metastatic spread.

Now to the collected essays and talks. These are organized into five chapters: Medical Ethics and Learning; Academic Medicine; Research (both clinical and laboratory); Perceptions of Cancer; and finally, Heroes, on two historically important and especially admirable people whose careers I have learned to admire during my professional life, Thomas Hodgkin and Marie Curie. The ethical essays were stimulated by my involvement in clinical research during a time of societal reconsideration of research on humans. Medicine has long been a part of higher learning and the university. My experience as a faculty member, department chair, physician-in-chief, and dean all stimulated my writings on this subject. My research efforts occurred at times of great changes in both fundamental knowledge and clinical care. Breast cancer treatment was being changed dramatically and I was involved in the changes in limiting the extent of surgery and preservation of the breast while maintaining and in some cases improving cancer curability. My laboratory research on bone marrow stem cells preceded the current explosion of study of these seminal cells of both cell renewal systems and cancer. Cancer is a weighty metaphor in our society. This affects its care and treatment in profound ways. My essay on this subject illustrates these effects. I end the collections with my heroes because of their contributions and examples, not primarily scientifically, but as members of society.

ACKNOWLEDGMENTS

This work has had important contributions from Amy Huser at The University of Chicago and from Andrea Knobloch and Allison Pratt at Oxford University Press. But none of this would have happened without my lover, life partner, friend, advisor, and counselor, my wife Rusty (Marcia) Hellman.

Learning While Caring

Introduction

COMMENTARY

I cannot remember a time when I did not want to become a doctor. Our family physician was an early role model, but I believe this predilection was a naïve romantic one that viewed physicians in heroic terms, as in the prevailing media and books read in my youth. Of course the view evolved as medicine changed, so that by the conclusion of my professional career, medicine was much more scientifically based and more institutionally located, and was consuming almost one-fifth of the US economy. Despite these huge changes, certain things remain the same, especially the primary obligation of the doctor to the patient. This requires loyalty and honesty to the patient. We are currently at the end of the beginning of the revolution in biology and medicine that has resulted from the understanding of how genetic information is passed generationally. Our capacities are far greater now, but the essence of medical practice remains the same, even though there are many more restrictions on how we practice and document our patient encounters.

I began my postgraduate training in 1959 and formally became an emeritus professor in 2006, but I still continue, 10 years later, to perform some research advisory and teaching activities (thus the half-century referred to in the title of this book). I was born and grew up in the Bronx, one of the "outer boroughs" of New York City, where my worldview was largely formed. "You can take the boy out of the Bronx but you can't take the Bronx out of the boy" is an expression I have also heard about another outer borough, Brooklyn. It may be true for both places, as it implies the importance of the early formative years. While I believe that I have modified my manner and general decorum, many of my current values were formed at that time. So these are the reflections of a middle-class, first-generation college graduate from the Bronx who went on to a medical career in cancer research, patient care, and teaching.

Following my postgraduate training and education, I began a career taking care of cancer patients and simultaneously doing research concerned with improving cancer treatment. These endeavors started at Yale University School of Medicine, where I did my postgraduate medical training, followed by 15 years at Harvard Medical School as professor and chairman of the Department of Radiation Oncology and director of the Joint Center for Radiation Therapy. Subsequently, I was the physician-in-chief at Memorial Sloan-Kettering Cancer Center and then dean of Biology and Medicine at The University of Chicago. Surprising to many, after completing the deanship I returned to taking care of cancer patients, teaching, and cancer research.

These were particularly exciting times for medicine, starting with the revolution in biology begun in 1953 by the discovery and publication that year by Watson and Crick of how genetic information was passed on. More than 60 years later, we are still in the thrall of this discovery and its ethical, social, and political consequences, as well as its medical implications. During this half-century there was a less heralded but equally important change in medicine resulting from technical innovations in the methods of diagnosis and the availability of new treatment techniques and pharmaceuticals. Some of the fruits of the biologic revolution may be here today, but these are the "low-hanging fruits," with many more forthcoming. We will continue into the full flower of constantly improving medical technology and new genetic and epigenetic information, resulting in insights into diagnosis, prognosis, disease prevention, and molecularly-targeted drug development.

Following the exposure of the medical abuses by the doctors of the Third Reich and then the 1972 revelation of the Tuskegee syphilis experiments, the new field of medical ethics emerged. As I engaged in clinical research, I became acutely aware of the dual and potentially conflicting roles of personal physician simultaneously being a clinical investigator. My uneasiness with current practices is presented in Chapter 1 of this book, "Medical Ethics and Learning."

My career included a small but active medical practice, laboratory and clinical research, teaching and academic leadership. This collection of my writings considers both the science that I performed and the ethics of doing research on human beings. There have been great changes in how clinical research is performed, as well as in the methods used. My experiences in leading academic medicine in various capacities provide the basis for my essays concerning the place of medicine in the university, as well as the place of biology in a general education. Cancer has been the subject of my patient care efforts, clinical research, and basic science laboratory work, but this book also considers the academic setting in which these endeavors occurred.

Cancer can lurk undetected in the body and in the genome. It can metastasize silently until it grows large enough to produce deleterious symptoms. But these characteristics have been so metaphorically used and emphasized that all too often one cannot consider the disease for what it is: a variety of illnesses varying from highly curable to incurable and fatal. Taken in aggregate, cancer is the most curable of the serious chronic diseases. Currently, diabetes, multiple sclerosis, Lou Gehrig's disease, coronary artery disease, Lupus, and many others are not curable, but many cancers are. This is also discussed in some of the essays included in this collection.

These essays provide a perspective of the various aspects of my professional life. I have tried to organize them into coherent themes. This collection of essays and the accompanying commentaries were written for a number of reasons. First, to respond to Socrates' admonition that an unexamined life is not worth living, I reflect upon the major aspects of my professional career and the times in which they occurred. Obviously, existing concomitantly with my professional activities, there has been the more important personal and family life. As much as possible, my home life shall remain private since it is personal and well known to those who are concerned, but I mention it here to recognize its priority. Second, these activities in my academic life, while well known to my son and daughter, are not to my grandchildren—thus the dedication to them. Perhaps most important, my professional activities in the last half-century occurred in the midst of great changes both in medical science and the practice of medicine and so may be of significance and interest to a larger audience. While medical science may be exciting and important, it is not all of medicine, but rather it is a necessary precondition for some of medicine. Science is emphasized in medical education, but the practice of medicine requires much more. A former medical student of mine was one of three daughters of a distinguished biological scientist (not a doctor), all of whom received medical educations. I asked Jennifer why this was so, and her response was that their father, whose opinion they greatly respected, felt that the best general education was that of a physician. It is that education leavening my worldview that provides the basis for the practice of medicine, medical research, and academic leadership that this book is about. This is best expressed in a series of topics to which I have devoted my intellectual efforts and writings. I have organized them into chapters, each with a Commentary, followed by some essays that I have published, written, or expressed in talks related to these subjects. These comprise those clinical medical and laboratory research writings, history, and philosophy that I believe are appropriate for a generally educated audience. There may be some specific medical or scientific material in a few, but I believe the general sense of the essays will be well understood by a general audience. Only in Chapter 3, "Research," will some essays contain unfamiliar jargon or concepts. I will try to prepare the reader in the commentary and will discuss separately some research not included in the essays.

The book's title and subtitle describe the subject, both attending to the ill patient—in this case with cancer—and the context in which these reflections were made. The five chapters may seem quite separate and unrelated, but they are not; they are closely interrelated in an academic physician's career. As a physician, the relationship with the patient is paramount, while as an investigator learning how to improve such treatment for future patients is the goal. Both occur in institutional settings, primarily the university, the hospital, and the outpatient clinics. Thus ethics and learning are first discussed since these different goals—treating individual patients, the essence of medical practice—in different settings may have different and sometimes conflicting aim and methods. The Research chapter tries to give a flavor of that research. My two heroes were chosen as they reflect the best of efforts in science and medicine at much earlier times as a way of illuminating our current times and responsibilities.

The initial essays attempt to demonstrate the importance and interrelationship of ethics and epistemology to healthcare. I believe I was prepared to be aware of these issues by my undergraduate philosophy teachings. That is the purpose of undergraduate teaching: to create what Pasteur in a different context called "a prepared mind." Education should provide factual and intellectual context but, most important, methods of critical thinking. This is true in undergraduate education but equally so in teaching residents. One of the nicest comments about my teaching was when I overheard one resident tell a younger trainee that not only did I teach them about the disease, but most important, how to think about an individual case as well as a report in a medical journal. My medical experience then becomes the subject for these philosophic inquiries.

The essays I have chosen to be a part of the Introduction come from talks I have given. The first was one of a series of annual lectures given to all incoming first-year college students at The University of Chicago. The series is called "The Aims of Education," and this title comes from a well-known talk by Alfred North Whitehead almost a century ago. My purpose in this lecture was not only to address the title, but also to place the importance of biology to students not majoring in that subject, as well as to emphasize the importance of the humanities to the biology students. The second is a commencement address to my Alma Mater, Allegheny College, and the third talk was given to graduating medical students emphasizing the societal and ethical issues raised by medical and biological advances. I hope that they provide my view of academic preparation of both future doctors and members of society in general. The remainder of this volume reflects on these interactions of the humanities, social sciences, and biology that I encountered in my career as an academic oncologist.

THE AIMS OF EDUCATION

Copyright © 1990 The University of Chicago. This article was first published in *Perspectives in Biology and Medicine* 1990;33(4):469–479. Reprinted with permission by Johns Hopkins University Press.

This lecture is historically given to the matriculating freshman class. "The Aims of Education" derives its title from an address by Alfred North Whitehead in 1917. To follow such a famous philosopher and such an ambitious title just begins to suggest the pretentiousness possible in this lecture. The possibility that the three P's—pretention, pomposity, and platitudes—may form the substance of this presentation causes me to approach the subject with trepidation. I do not wish to be guilty of any of the P's, but, in attempting to avoid them, I do not want to be guilty of the three T's—triviality, triteness, and timidity. I shall try to walk a road between these consonants, expecting to step occasionally to either side, while I verbalize what I believe to be the aims of this portion of your educational experience. We Americans have a curious view of the beginnings and ends of portions of the educational experience. Graduation is often called "commencement" to signify that it is the beginning of the next phase of life. Speeches given on that occasion usually do not reflect on previous education but, rather, emphasize the future and the graduates' place within it, although occasionally describing how the educational experience has prepared the student. It is this forward, optimistic view that so characterizes the American system with its special emphasis on progress, change, and the future. It is of interest that graduation usually occurs in the spring, a time of new growth and renewal in nature.

What, then, are we to do with this event? Matriculation or enrollment is clearly a time of beginning; however, it occurs in the autumn of the year. Shall we contrast it with graduation being commencement by suggesting that matriculation into college is the end of something? It, like graduation, is both an end and a beginning. It marks the end of that part of education concerned with providing the rudiments necessary to be adequately prepared to function in society. What is beginning is higher education, to be experienced in a different way. You will be expected to accept much greater responsibility for yourself and your education. This greater freedom, accompanied by responsibility, is characteristic of adulthood. If you are to enter this period of your life it is appropriate for you to ask the purpose of college; thus, a talk entitled "The Aims of Education."

Of course, you realize that the undergraduate years are only a small part of the educational experience; but these are special years. Before going any further, you should understand that it is my belief that all views of education are largely autobiographical. This one will be no different. I believe that this personal view of what is best in education prevails because education in itself, especially undergraduate education, is so exhilarating, pleasant, and exciting. We remember it with such affection that we want others to share such an experience. We believe our educational experience to be the paradigm for undergraduate education in general. Second, since all of our educational experiences are limited, we know best that which we have observed and in which we have participated. Within the multitude of institutions of higher education, the undergraduate curriculum is organized in many different ways. The stuff of undergraduate education is so intrinsically compelling that it is, in my experience, very difficult to offer an unsatisfactory collegiate experience.

This brings great solace to educators, especially when engaging in curricular reform. It should, one hopes, give you some sense of security. It will be difficult for us to make these college years unattractive. There is even the reasonable possibility that the mix of substance and pedagogy will be synergistic and enhance the experience.

Now, a word or two about The University of Chicago as the site of your undergraduate education. My vantage point is that of a relative newcomer, as this begins my second academic year at this institution. Since I have chosen to come to this university, I am prejudiced in my view, which is that you have made an extremely wise choice. Why do I feel this to be the case? First, while this is a great institution whose mission is the discovery and transmission of knowledge, its center is the undergraduate college. The college is not separate from the rest of the university, nor is it the college alone that defines the institution. Rather, the college is an integral part of all the divisions of the university and they of it. Each of the four divisions has major responsibility for and involvement in the college. The organization of this university is consistent with a continuum of education, especially emphasizing the connections of undergraduate, graduate, and professional education. As a physician, I am particularly pleased to find that the medical school is incorporated into the university in a way not often found. Rather than being a separate facility on a separate campus, the Pritzker School of Medicine is embedded within the Division of the Biological Sciences. This division is responsible for education in undergraduate and graduate study in biology and in the study of medicine. This organization of medical education emphasizes the academic, the intellectual, and the scholarly rather than the trade or craft nature of professional preparation. It is also beneficial to collegiate education. It allows the participation of many in the life of the college who otherwise might be considered only medical faculty. It provides a larger, more diverse faculty for undergraduate education than otherwise would be possible. It assures the heterogeneity of views and vantage points so invigorating to the educational experience.

What of this new environment—its people and its culture? This beautiful campus provides, with its peaceful collection of collegiate gothic buildings amid open green spaces, an atmosphere for study, reflection, and a sense of defined community. The architecture reminds us of the tradition and roots of the university, of the importance of the continuum of learning. The solidity is reassuring. Even the new buildings, while reflecting modern ideas and thought, pay homage, by materials or design elements, to the past. New and old together in this special place are all closely applied to the hub of the quintessential American city, Chicago, full of life, excitement, culture, and beauty. The city reflects American optimism, productivity, and even brashness, but without being arrogant or smug; in fact, if anything it is a little overly humble.

William James wrote after visiting our city in 1896, "I wish you were here with me to see Chicago and its institutions. It is a stupendous affair—'storm centre' of our Continent, already outstripping New York in civilization, size and importance.... It is a place of vast ideas and titanic energy, and the largeness and ambitiousness of its beginnings must determine its character for all time." The essential natures of the city and this institution persist.

Our university community has dominant features that describe its mission: the libraries, laboratories, and classrooms of all sizes and shapes; places for culture, communion, and entertainment, as well as study, new friends, fellow students with similar goals but often quite different backgrounds, and faculty of great talent and diversity; all of this with a meter of its own, a calendar of quarters with punctuation—academic, cultural, and social. This is a new universe in which to enjoy learning.

I should like now to make a brief comment about some of the subjects to be included in the substance of undergraduate education. I will begin with a parochial view of why I believe that a knowledge in biology is so essential to a liberal arts education. We are living during a revolution in biological knowledge that has been compared to that seen in nuclear physics in the 1930s. This comparison may prove to be conservative. A more apt one may be with the Industrial Revolution. Biology has been transmogrified from a descriptive science to one able to probe the basic mechanisms of genetics and development. Further technical advances are coming so rapidly that new possibilities for learning and creating are occurring faster than they can be incorporated into the discipline or to useful application. Truly, we live in interesting times. The tremendous increase in biological understanding makes many formerly abstract or theoretic questions quite susceptible to scientific analysis with quite urgent practical consequences. Without spending much time on this, I suggest you think about: in vitro fertilization, test-tube babies, determination of many genetic details of the unborn—not only those concerning significant illnesses but also, for example, those of gender, intelligence, or appearance. What qualities of the embryo or fetus do we want to know about, and what shall we do with the information? Scientific progression in these areas has been considerable and will continue. How these developments are to be incorporated into our lives is a question for us all. To fully consider these, one must understand the underlying biology.

Thought has a history, makes progress, and is informed by discovery; thus, philosophic thought is enriched by discoveries in science. We need this information to deal with complicated social, moral, and political issues. Many of the great concerns of humans are involved with biological phenomena: living, dying, parturition, thought, perception, love, emotions in general, and social behavior, to name but a few. I am not suggesting that biology alone is a liberal arts education. I am suggesting, however, that without the knowledge of biology it seems to me extraordinarily difficult to be liberally educated today.

Let us begin to consider what the title of this talk, "The Aims of Education," has to do with the undergraduate experience. First, you must recognize that, while education neither begins nor ends during these four years, they are especially important and worthy of separate consideration. This period begins what is called "higher education" to separate it from the basic rudiments supposedly taught in primary and secondary schools. Much has been said about the purpose of undergraduate education. Surely it is to develop and nurture habits that will allow us to continue to learn throughout our lives. It must expose us to a broad spectrum of disciplines, present some of the exciting universe of ideas, and whet our appetites for further discovery. Perhaps this is the most exciting part of our education—to encounter more different fields and new ideas than we had thought possible.

I believe that a glossary of terms is necessary when we consider education. We might begin with "memory"—the ability to remember or to recall past experience. Learning means to gain knowledge, to fix in memory, to acquire through experience, or to become informed. In biology, one describes learning as the modification of behavior by experience. Memory has a short-term and a long-term component, both of which may be used for learning. "Knowledge" is the state of knowing, of understanding through experience or study, and "education" is concerned with imparting and acquiring knowledge. This latter is a rather limited definition. The subject of this lecture (and those that preceded it) is to elaborate on this limited view. What about these terms? You will need memory. You will be expected to learn using this mechanism. Some of what you learn will, it is hoped, use long-term memory; thus, you will retain the information you acquire longer than is required for a particular examination. We recognize that much of this learning will use only short-term memory that, if not reinforced, will not remain. What we hope will persist will come from the process. Learning in the biological sense requires behavior modification as a result of experience. We expect that your behavior will be changed by the college experience. Knowledge, the state of knowing or understanding, is a goal of education. What has not been mentioned, but is perhaps the main goal of education, is wisdom. This is described variously as understanding what is true, right, or lasting; it is common sense and sagacity, and it is erudition. While we are ambitious for you, we do not expect wise, sagacious, erudite individuals at the end of this experience. That is a lifetime's work, to be achieved only in degrees but to be in quest of always. We hope that by the time of your commencement you will feel committed to this quest and, to some extent, prepared for it.

Our education must provide the necessary rudiments and tools required to partake of certain disciplines. For example, we must understand the French language if we are to fully understand the French culture and literature. Similarly, mathematics is a language of physics, and it seems ludicrous to discuss genetic engineering if we do not understand what a gene is.

Education must provide insight into the relationships of what appear to be separate subjects. In many ways the separation of disciplines is misleading; they are, in fact, interactive. Some of the better courses you will take will consider the relationships of different fields or will be concerned with ideas that are between traditional disciplines. For example, we should consider the relationship of philosophy to literature, to law, to religion, to science, to medicine, and to politics. Fields developed at interfaces include biophysics and psychobiology. Ideas in one field have influence on others. For example, as we look at the current federal bureaucracy, one might suggest that "chaos theory" in physics has wider applications.

Information and knowledge are necessary. Ideas alone are insufficient. We must also accumulate some necessary information and techniques, but these latter, without the study of ideas, miss the point of education. It is the mix of ideas with information, each informing and modifying the other, that leads to understanding. Preparation for a lifetime of continuing education and learning is an extensive undertaking. We cannot learn sufficiently for all of life during these four years. Little may remain but attitudes and habits. Education in different fields exposes us to various ways of thinking. We learn to be discerning, to separate the important from the trivial, to be critical, to not accept concepts without subjecting them to analysis, to perceive relationships, and to recognize the importance of new knowledge or concepts in one field for other areas of endeavor. There are many aims of education. This is not a complete list but rather some of the aims. The list must include the development of greater self-awareness with continued questioning and the opportunity for growth. Education must result in a feeling of pleasure and excitement with learning. Others at this institution and elsewhere have been concerned with the materials included in a liberal education. I take a somewhat different view. While there are texts not appropriate for study, the number of those suitable far exceeds our capacities to read and to learn. Our education should prepare us for a lifelong quest for knowledge, the critical consideration of which leads to wisdom. I worry little about whether the books considered are the best; instead, I am concerned that thoughtful, critical analysis is being emphasized.

Now, I would like to share some personal reflections regarding my own education and how it prepared me for my life as a physician and scientist. I gave you fair warning that this talk would be somewhat autobiographical. Before coming to Chicago, I was the physician-in-chief at Memorial Sloan-Kettering Cancer Center in New York City. In that role, I was responsible for all the patient care and clinical research activities at that institution. Let me present to you a few of the more vexing recent problems that I faced in that position. Acquired immunodeficiency syndrome, or AIDS, was recognized to have major consequences which affect healthcare, societal mores, and resource allocation. We had to consider how we would cope with this epidemic, what it would do to our ability to perform our primary mission of cancer research and patient care. There were questions about whether it was proper to identify patients with the disease or to label samples of blood or urine taken from them. Should such patients be isolated from other patients? Should these other patients know the diagnosis of patients with AIDS? These are questions that deal with the rights of the individual as compared to those of the group. These may be conflicting or coincident. How to consider them has been the stuff of philosophic consideration usually a part of undergraduate education. Consideration in the abstract prepares one for the practical circumstance. What of the staff? Should staff with AIDS be restricted in their activity? Should all staff or patients be tested to see if they have the virus? AIDS has brought to public awareness two sociological phenomena that society had been reticent to consider openly: homosexuality and intravenous drug use. To deal successfully with AIDS, this plague of our time, we must understand the sociology of the groups that constitute these phenomena. To address questions related to how the disease is caused, transmitted, and may best be treated or prevented, one needs scientific and medical knowledge, but this is hardly sufficient. Sociological, ethical, and political considerations are also necessary.

Our hospital tried to offer all that we could to seriously ill cancer patients. Such very aggressive therapy is not always successful. Unfortunately, this is not known until well into the therapy, at which time the patient is receiving expensive treatment, being cared for by large numbers of highly trained healthcare workers, and often is relying on sophisticated instruments for continued survival. This required us to consider when treatment should be withheld or terminated. To answer such questions, we had to consider the rights and wishes of patients, their families, and the staff. We also had to consider the implications of the decision on our ability to care for other patients. Resources are always finite. Their utilization in one circumstance may prevent their availability for another, so, again, we needed to consider the conflicting rights of the individual and those of the group. In this instance, the equitable distribution of societal resources is not an abstract but a practical consideration to be dealt with in an atmosphere charged with emotion. These problems are difficult at best, but without having considered the general principles previously, they would seem overwhelming. Robert Maynard Hutchins instructs us, "Education is not a substitute for experience. It is preparation for it."

What about research on humans? This is an area of conflicting responsibilities. One does such research to help future patients without detrimentally affecting today's patients. What are the responsibilities to today's patient compared to the experiment with its resulting benefit to the patient of tomorrow? The currently accepted procedure is to conduct a randomized prospective clinical trial. This is an experiment in which eligible patients who consent to be in the trial are randomly allocated to either of the two treatment groups. One group receives the best available treatment for the disease studied, while the second group receives the experimental treatment. The trial is continued until there is statistical evidence that a predetermined difference between the two groups is, or is not, established. Statistical analysis will reveal the number of patients required in each group to determine whether there is a meaningful difference at some level of statistical likelihood. Most studies require that the likelihood of the difference being due to chance is less than 5 percent. Consider what should be done when one is comparing a treatment administered to one group of patients with that given to a second group of patients, and one begins to see a difference. When should the study be stopped? When one has a hunch that one treatment is better than another, a "gut feeling," or statistical proof? The problem here is that of providing each individual patient with what one believes to be the best treatment. Such beliefs change with experience in the experiment.

If one modifies treatment to individual patients before the study is concluded, then the experiment may be rendered useless, thus sacrificing future patients in the interest of the current patient. If one waits to conclude the study, one may deny current patients what one believes to be the best treatment. To consider these conflicting obligations, one should consider the license and responsibilities of the physician. Are his or her obligations solely to the individual patient? While there appears to be an implicit covenant between doctor and patient suggesting that the physician will always act in that patient's interest, there are exceptions. The law requires that certain communicable diseases and certain types of wounds must be reported. In such cases, reporting the illness or injury may not be in the patient's best interest. The confidentiality of the doctor–patient relationship is abrogated in such circumstances. This is done because we believe that the societal gain is more important than the patient's right to privacy. How are such questions of individual versus common good, of the implicit understanding of the social contract, to be resolved?

These and other important questions require far more than purely scientific considerations. While the latter are necessary, they are insufficient. To approach these issues intelligently, my colleagues and I required much more of our education than scientific knowledge; but, without the scientific knowledge, the problems could not be addressed at all. Similar questions are present in other professions, businesses, and many aspects of life. One need not go further than current newspapers to consider under what conditions, if any, we condone abortion. What are the rights of the ovum or sperm donor to a frozen embryo? Does the latter have rights? Such questions, while the result of biological and medical discovery, require much broader considerations. A general education is the best preparation for understanding the implications of scientific advance, but you must understand the advance as well.

Part of education is learning about one's predecessors, their concerns, and how they chose to live their lives. During my professional career, I studied and treated patients with Hodgkin's disease, a malignancy of the lymph nodes. In the course of these studies, I became interested in Thomas Hodgkin. In preparing this talk, I found myself reflecting on Hodgkin, a man to be much admired but largely unknown except for the eponymous reference in medicine.

Thomas Hodgkin was born in 1798 to a devout Quaker family. He became and remained strongly committed to the Quaker beliefs throughout his life. He was unable to study medicine in England because membership in the Church of England was required. Following his medical education in Edinburgh, he continued his studies in Paris, where great advances in medicine were being made. Not only did he study with the great French physician Laennec, but he also sought out Baron Alexander von Humboldt, the scientist, explorer, and sociologist about whom Hodgkin quoted the Roman slave Terence. "He always thought that among all things, nothing belonging to man was foreign to him."

This emphasis on the breadth of one's interests formed a credo for Hodgkin's life and is inscribed on his grave. Von Humboldt explored

South America, making contributions in botany, astronomy, volcanology, and archaeology, as well as those in geography and meteorology for which he is most well known. Hodgkin was most interested in von Humboldt's concern for the treatment of the natives in the New World. This coincided with Hodgkin's great life's interest—his overriding concern for those people not benefited by Western civilization but rather threatened by it.

After his time in Paris, Hodgkin returned to London, where he made his major contributions to science and medicine, including the description of the disease that bears his name. Were he aware of it, I am sure he would minimize his role in this accomplishment and would not agree with the appropriateness of this achievement to memorialize his life. His medical career was effectively ended in 1837 as a consequence of his strongly held social concerns. His career depended on his receiving a permanent appointment as physician at Guy's Hospital. This was controlled by the powerful secretary of the hospital, Benjamin Harrison, who was also a member of the board of directors of the Hudson Bay Company. Hodgkin was agitated by the mistreatment of natives by the company. He implored Harrison to use his position to change company policy. Rather than do this, Harrison successfully blocked Hodgkin's appointment at the hospital and his future medical career. While Hodgkin continued some of his medical interests, increasingly he devoted himself to the underprivileged. He was a cofounder of the Aborigines Protection Society and the Syrian Medical Aid Association, both concerned with the welfare of peoples native to areas colonized by Western Europe. He was active in the movement promoting the abolition of slavery in the New World and providing Liberia as a home for former slaves. He made extensive tours of the Middle East with his friend, the great philanthropist Moses Montefiore, concerned with the health and social welfare of the peoples of this area. He died in 1866, a probable victim of a cholera epidemic, and is buried in Jaffa.

Hodgkin was a medical scholar who used observation and careful organization to discern relationships. He was vigorous in his attempts to learn from both the leading scholars and his own observation. He was an effective teacher and writer. As a physician, he accepted the responsibility of providing medical care for the poor. He wrote on health promotion and disease prevention. Health, rather than illness, was the emphasis here, presaging today's renewed interest in health promotion. But I find him most exemplary, and recommend him to you, for his general concerns and actions as a human being. He considered issues both within and outside of his profession to be his concern. He pursued his views with passion and commitment, even when the possible consequences for himself were uncertain. These personal and professional actions formed a continuum of behavior that described him as a person. He was not always successful in pursuing his beliefs, but, even when he was not successful, I believe that his life must have been personally fulfilling because of these efforts. I do not mean to suggest that the grand gesture or the noble pursuit of futility is the desired goal, but rather that active participation in life in service of one's commitment is rewarding in itself, almost regardless of outcome. Browning tells us:

> For thence—a paradox
> Which comforts while it mocks—
> Shall life succeed in that it seems to fail:
> What I aspire to be
> And was not, comforts me.

What has this to do with "The Aims of Education?" I would argue, a great deal. In Thomas Hodgkin we find great breadth of interest, vigorous championing of one's views, great moral strength, and a willingness to participate in the events of his time. Our education should prepare us for all of these. It should stimulate new interests, foment commitment, encourage social responsibility, and invite active participation in life.

Let us now return to the undergraduate experience. What are the aims of this education? I believe that there are four classes of educational aims. The first we might title self-realization or self-fulfillment. This is one of the most frequently mentioned aims when higher education is the subject. It is important for our inner life, to make us reflective, aware of our place in the world and our relations to others. Questions concerning existence, purpose, and the meaning of events need to be contemplated if we are to be fully realized as individuals. A second aim is career preparation. While careerism is often condemned when it is the only goal, the fact is that much of our time and energy is spent in our work. This can be a source of tremendous fulfillment or a significant burden. Career choice and preparation are important, but they should not dominate the college experience. Third, education prepares us to act as intelligent members of the larger community. We must consider our place and responsibility to our community and society. This preparation is necessary for our life in a civilized society. Finally, there is preparation for those parts of our vocation that do not depend on special knowledge but rather on general knowledge, attitudes, wisdom, and understanding, so that we may recognize the important questions that appear in the course of our work that have much broader implications. I have tried to present you with some examples of this from my experience. AIDS, prolongation of life, clinical experiments, and resource allocation are examples from my profession. Other careers may present different questions. They are present as a part of living. The values systems, knowledge, and ideas necessary for making wise choices require a general rather than a limited education. Thus, the aims of education are to develop habits of learning, to provide personal fulfillment, to make life meaningful, and to be important for one's career. Such education is required for being an informed citizen and for acting as a wise and just individual.

I began this discussion by commenting on commencement and matriculation. This is the beginning of your collegiate education. There is a crispness in the air presaging an invigorating climate not only meteorologically but intellectually. New ideas, new experiences, and new responsibilities await you. I am reminded of a former professor of mine who, when informed by a student that the test being administered was identical with that given last year, responded that, while the important questions do not change, the answers do. We look forward to your providing even more stimulating answers to important questions.

READINGS

Ashmore, H. S. *Unseasonable Truths*. Boston: Little, Brown, 1989.
Beadle, M. *Where Has All the Ivy Gone*. Garden City, NY: Doubleday, 1972.
Browning, R. "Rabbi ben Ezra."
Kass, A. M., and Kass, E. H. *Perfecting the World*. Boston: Harcourt Brace Jovanovich, 1988.
Rose, M. *Curator of the Dead*. London: Peter Owens, 1981.

A DOCTOR'S DILEMMAS

Commencement Address, Allegheny College, 1984

I have entitled this address "A Doctor's Dilemmas" because I would like to present to you some of the problems which recently faced me and for which I believe the traditional liberal arts education prepares one well.

As you go out from this place, it is appropriate to reflect on what this education was all about and how you are likely to use it. I am a physician, researcher, and educator concerned with the improvement of medical treatment and the reduction of mortality and morbidity due to cancer. This scientific and medical problem may seem removed from much of that which is studied in a liberal arts education.

One might expect that my Allegheny scientific background was appropriate for medical training—and so it was. I felt well prepared for the rigors of medical school and surely those graduates of the large universities who were offered more specialized courses seemed to have no significant advantage over me. Some of them took courses very similar to those which later were a part of our medical school curriculum. While this made the latter course easier initially for them, the emphasis on specialized courses limited student breadth, resulting in a much narrower view of science. But, Allegheny is known as an excellent pre-professional school with outstanding scientific credentials—so excellence of scientific preparation is surely no surprise.

Former Dean at Allegheny, Julian Ross, in his book *Philosophy in Literature*, commented on some differences between science and what he broadly called "philosophy." He emphasized that a good scientist must specialize. He said it is misleading to say that the aim of any scientist is the discovery of truth. His or her aim is rather the discovery of some particular fact or law relating to some particular subject matter. A philosopher may also specialize, but when she does so, it is done at the expense of understanding the whole and therefore, Dr. Ross tells us, she is likely to be less effective as a philosopher. You might consider the philosopher to be a wise person and the scientist as described by Dr. Ross to be a technical expert. This is a time of increasing reliance on technology and general understanding becomes all the more important.

Secondly, Dr. Ross tells us that the "technical expert" prefers to work with precise measurement and feels uneasy without it, while the philosopher cannot possibly do so. These dealings with uncertainty are important in dealing with life in general.

Thirdly, and most importantly, he suggests that science is not primarily interested in the value or worth of what it discovers. That is not to say that science has little value—its benefits of course are incalculable—but rather, that those benefits may be a byproduct rather than the direct concern of the scientific discovery. The one value in which science is interested is truth. Whether the discovery has the potential for harm or great good for mankind is not a person's concern as a scientist, it is very much his or her concern as a human being. This last point is easily illustrated with the important advances in physics resulting in atomic energy and, of course, in the new biologic revolution.

How then did this liberal arts education prepare me for my scientific career? Let me illustrate this with a few recent dilemmas that medical research and medicine face.

First, there are those concerned with living and dying. What is the definition of life? When does it begin? When is the fetus viable? When does life end? These questions can be answered in scientific, ethical, social, and religious terms and one cannot act on any one of these exclusively. As our skills increase, the circumstances and age at which viable human life begins may be considered to become earlier and earlier. With the life-sustaining instruments available in modern hospitals, prolongation of bodily functions may persist far in excess of meaningful consciousness. These problems must be dealt with. So, we in medicine are concerned with the problems in birth control and abortion. My most recent personal involvement has been to develop guidelines to determine under what circumstances it is appropriate not to offer mechanical life-sustaining assistance to terminally ill patients. Such seeming medical decisions have significant ethical, social, and religious implications. One is best prepared to consider them by a broadly based liberal education.

Medical care is becoming increasingly expensive. It is very difficult to read the newspaper without seeing an article concerned with this increasing use of our financial resources. In learning to restrict expansion of medical expenses, of course we must be first concerned with reducing unnecessary expenses. However, when these are done, we find many valuable procedures and techniques which are quite expensive. An example of this might be heart transplantation. This extraordinarily expensive procedure obviously has value. Under what circumstances should it be done? These are not purely medical questions, but require a diversity of knowledge and understanding. Great Britain does not offer "artificial kidney" treatment for patients who have chronic renal failure. They feel it is just too expensive. I would suggest to you that that is a societal, rather than a medical decision, but it has clear medical consequences and thus must be a concern for doctors.

The traditional relationship of patient to physician might be considered a covenant in which the physician is expected to do or advise the patient as to all that he or she thinks might be of benefit. The physician should have no other motives or goals. This may be difficult to reconcile with medical research in which it is sometimes important to offer patients alternative treatments. If one does not know or have an informed opinion as to which treatment is better these patients may be randomly allocated to the alternative treatments. Such random allocation studies are powerful techniques for learning which treatment may be better. But rarely does the physician not have an opinion as to which treatment is better. Further, as the study proceeds, the physician may develop some opinion as to which alternative serves the patient better. What should the doctor do? If the study is not done or is stopped before completion then the knowledge and potential benefits to future patients are lost, but continuing the study may be in conflict with the traditional doctor-patient relationship. Lastly, the preconceived opinion may be incorrect. Without an appropriate study this misconception may continue.

There are no simple answers to questions like this and there are many others like it in medical research. How medical research or patient care is interpreted depends on the circumstances of the research and patient care. The community hospital is different than the research institute. The nature of the doctor–patient relationship requires consideration of these differences.

Social mores and changes in them may have profound medical effects. Dealing with these in order to influence disease requires skills, knowledge, and judgment far removed from purely "technical" medical competence. To offer an example, if I told you that cancer-related deaths could be reduced by 30% today, many of you might be surprised. The mechanism is simple—stop all smoking of tobacco. While we know this to be true, we in medicine have failed in achieving this objective. The successful achievement of this goal requires understanding of sociological, ethical, legal, psychological, and public relations considerations that are not part of a narrowly defined technical education.

So Dr. Ross has described the technical specialist far too narrowly for this person to function effectively in this society. We physicians and scientists need a heavy dose of what he calls the philosopher. Since most of these questions are societal, we all as citizens need the philosopher's skill to make wise decisions.

A liberal arts education prepares us for uncertainty. It prepares us for both new questions and perhaps even more importantly, for changing answers to old questions. I am reminded of a former Allegheny professor who was in the habit of repeating examination questions from year to year. When asked about this, he suggested that the questions in life rarely change; it is the answers that do.

Sometimes I am sure you may have felt during your education that it was not practical enough. Recently I chaired the Academic Policy committee of the Board of Trustees and a student member concerned with job interviews wondered whether there should be a course specifically concerned with preparing students for job interviews. While some advice and help in interviewing skills surely would be helpful, we must be concerned about being too practical or narrowly focused in our career preparation.

It is of course a great honor to receive an honorary degree from Allegheny College and an especial pleasure is that I am to be sponsored for this from the faculty by Prof. Alfred Kern and from the trustees by Gov. Raymond Shafer. Prof. Kern is an Allegheny graduate who exemplifies the true liberal arts tradition. He is a teacher, a writer, and an intellectual. Gov. Shafer, also an Allegheny graduate, is perhaps the paradigm of what we hope for from such a graduate. His contributions to our community, society, and college offer very high standards for our graduates. Both were at Allegheny when I was a student—Al as a young faculty member and aspiring writer with whom, during a seminar course, I had fascinating discussions—Ray, as the Crawford County District Attorney and head of the corporation which was responsible for the fraternity house in which I lived and of which I was president. In this latter capacity I met Ray and learned to respect and admire him. In my judgment they represent the best of the liberal arts tradition.

What is my advice to you today? I suggest you realize that the future is change and uncertainty. Machiavelli, who is sometimes maligned but as a guide often gave his Prince quite good advice, said,

> There is nothing more difficult to take in hand, more perilous to conduct, or more uncertain in its success, than to take the lead in the introduction of a new order of things.

I suggest that the future which will be in your hands will be "a new order of things" as that which was in our hands was "a new order of things," quite different from that which our parents faced.

Remember the values taught in a liberal education. Your responsibilities are both to act on them and to preserve them.

Use the reasoning and analytic skills honed in this rigorous education. Much of the liberal education is in knowing how to think.

Continue the concern for others and the bonds that bind, so natural and fostered during these college years and in this place.

Preserve, expand, and replenish our important institutions. Shortly they will be in your charge.

THE END OF INEVITABILITY, OR FRANKENSTEIN AND THE BIOLOGICAL REVOLUTION

Samuel Hellman, "The End of Inevitability, or Frankenstein and the Biological Revolution," *Pharos Alpha Omega Alpha Honor Med Soc* 1994;57(2):41–43.

The author (AΩA, State University of New York at Syracuse, 1958) is A. N. Pritzker Distinguished Service Professor, Department of Radiation and Cellular Oncology, The University of Chicago. This paper is based on Dr. Hellman's commencement address at the SUNY Health Sciences Center in Syracuse in May 1993.

Human life consists of dynamic tensions between increasing and decreasing capacities and between health and disease. Our bodies grow and develop, increasing our capacities, and then the process is reversed: first, with regard to physical prowess; then with diminishing mental faculties. All through this growth and diminution we are at risk for disease and untimely death. Even if we escape such, we accept senescence and, ultimately, "natural" death as the normal order. Many feel that it is dangerous and even evil to attempt to alter certain basic processes of nature. It is what the townspeople rose against in the book *Frankenstein*. Written in 1818 by Mary Shelley, with the express purpose of frightening the reader, this novel evokes a basic reverence for the current condition of human frailty and a fear of the consequences of change. This apprehension is the heart of the objections to genetic engineering and biotechnology today, which in Cambridge, Massachusetts, resulted in the city council considering limiting such activities at Harvard University and the Massachusetts Institute of Technology.

The title of my paper, "The End of Inevitability," refers to those assumptions we make about the relationships of human beings to health, disease, and the biological conditions of life. While many hold these conditions of life to be fixed and unchanging, I believe that a great revolution in biology and medicine is occurring that requires fundamental reconsideration of what has been accepted as inevitable. What concepts were thought to be fixed may be on the brink of being altered in fundamental ways.

There have been other times in history when such important changes in our knowledge have occurred that the very paradigm for societal arrangement and human understanding has changed. The Ptolemaic view of the centrality of Earth and of humans was transformed into the Copernican view of the solar system, in which our world is but one of nine planets and not an especially distinguished one at that. This concept was not merely new knowledge but a historical discontinuity that changed the ways in which we consider ourselves, the world, and our relation to the universe. Similar changes should be expected consequent to discoveries and inventions in biology and medicine.

The Current Consensus

What is the biomedical model generally accepted today? Our concepts of disease and health accept progress within limits. The discovery of antibiotics for bacterial disease has pointed to our eventual dominance of these known pathogens. We expect there to be similar therapeutic agents for viruses, protozoa, and other perhaps even as yet undiscovered classes of agents. Even more success may result from preventive measures such as vaccination. Despite this optimism, we believe that some forms of infectious diseases will be with us always. We expect that new diseases will continue to plague us, as AIDS, genital herpes, and Legionnaires' disease do today. These disorders are the result of changes in lifestyle or, more importantly, are due to a continued dynamic tension between host and pathogen, both adapting, with neither capable of eventual dominance. The details of the relationship may change as the host or any specific pathogen gains a temporary advantage, but the very relationship is considered to be permanent. We accept the notion that nature's fundamental variety and adaptability will produce new conditions and disease even as progress is being made with the older ones.

In viewing chronic disease we hope that such conditions can be significantly modified so that life will be more pleasant. We expect that heart disease, cancer, diabetes, arthritis, multiple sclerosis, and other chronic diseases will gradually be controlled by a mixture of modern medicine, surgery, and changes in lifestyle, but we anticipate that some chronic diseases will always be with us as a consequence of societal living. We understand that these diseases may result from our own activities. Our requirements for food, energy, and other conditions of comfortable living cause environmental changes that result in undesirable medical consequences. In a certain sense, civilization can be considered detrimental to health.

Perhaps the most firmly embedded of the current assumptions is the one that there are a series of age-related changes that result in the gradual diminution of our faculties. We believe these changes to be inevitable. We hope at the most to live well, possessed of as many of our faculties as possible, until it is time for us to die. What is certain is mortality, even if disease and some diminution of our abilities and powers are forestalled. The most optimistic goal of today's expectations is for one to live well until succumbing to a quick and painless death before one's faculties become too limited.

Preparation for the Future

With some temerity, but with the certainty of the necessity of such considerations, I say we must question these assumptions. Not confronting them will affect scientific progress little. Changes will certainly occur. How prepared we are for new scientific developments will, in large measure, determine their effect on us as individuals and as a society. We will have two roles, both exciting, challenging, and traditional. While we all accept our primary responsibility as healers, we sometimes forget our responsibility as teachers. If we are to gain from the new biology while eliminating many of its pitfalls, we must educate the public to the implications and power of these scientific discoveries.

Fundamental changes in a medical paradigm occur abruptly, concomitant with a new discovery or innovation. For example, surgery has been changed completely by the effective development of anesthetic agents and the understanding of the importance of aseptic technique. Before these discoveries, major surgery was reserved as a desperate measure, accompanied often by grave consequences. A great premium was placed on procedures that took little time, and great value was placed on the speed of the operator. Infection was considered to be an inevitable accompaniment of a surgical procedure. Surgery precluded the use of prosthetics, grafts, and transplantation. It was only with asepsis and anesthesia that the potentials of surgery could be explored. A similar shift in the medical paradigm is occurring today.

What are our expectations for future medical advances, and do they require a major alteration in our model of health and disease? Difficult to contemplate is the notion that we shall be able to modify inherited or congenital diseases and characteristics. Genetic engineering, *in vitro* conception and growth, and prenatal diagnosis and description all exist today, making it clear that we must, at the very least, consider the consequences of eliminating inherited diseases. This concept is not at all straightforward, for the social, ethical, and economic considerations of genetic manipulation are quite different from those of prenatal screening. While society is having difficulty developing guidelines for the termination of pregnancy, it is completely unprepared to deal with altering or modifying the concept us to ensure certain desired genetic presentations. Considerations for genetic diseases that manifest themselves early may be different from those whose consequences are not present until late in life. Examples of the tremendous opportunities and excitement associated with such genetic discoveries may be seen in a recent issue of the *Journal of the American Medical Association,* which contains two articles on family pedigrees of carriers of the *BRCA1* gene associated with familial breast cancer and responsible for about 5% of all breast cancer.[1,2] I mention that the articles were in *JAMA,* not *Nature* or *Science,* because they have practical and immediate significance. In one instance, a 33-year-old woman scheduled for prophylactic bilateral mastectomy because her mother and two sisters had developed breast cancer at an early age was found unlikely to have the mutated gene. For a 40-year-old cousin, who had delayed having mammograms, finding the mutation led to careful mammographic examination and the discovery of a 0.5 cm otherwise occult breast cancer. Think of the issues society must face for widespread testing. What stigma is associated with finding the mutation? What happens to insurance, employment, social relations? Alternatively, how exciting it is to be a health professional during these times of great increases in our knowledge.

Eugenics, or selective breeding of humans, has been rejected by society. Predictive genetics appears to be acceptable, but what of preventive genetics or actual genetic manipulation, and, if this is to be considered, what inherited characteristics should be modified, if any? What about physical or mental abilities, appearance, emotional response, or gender, to name a few? If these attributes should be manipulated, who should decide? There are at least three different groups, each with an interest, but not always the same interest, in this question: society, the family, and those performing the procedure. These groups may be in conflict as they have different considerations or weigh the same considerations differently. Society may want fitness if it is primarily motivated by utilitarian concerns. But there will be considerations of diversity and spontaneity. Philosophical and religious views will conflict with such utilitarian concepts. Questions of enormous magnitude require serious discussion in our society. While physicians must make the public aware of these new capacities, how they are integrated into society must come from an informed public. We must accept an educational charge. Our message must also emphasize the enormity of the possibilities as well as their immediacy.

Equally difficult is the consideration of how we would deal with little or no diminution in our faculties as we aged. It is unthinkable that useful, active, life span could be significantly prolonged. We are all concerned with ways in which we can live well until our time has come to die. The most unthinkable thought is that we could modify our time to die and, perhaps, even the inevitability of dying itself. It is not my purpose to engage in a long discussion of this latter point but, rather, to emphasize that it is important that we consider the consequences of what at first might seem to be an outrageous notion, that is, the disappearance of the inevitability of the current limits on longevity, so that we can deal with such a possible development as the significant extension of life. If we accept the end of inevitability, we must help to formulate guidelines for how we should address these matters and, equally important, provide the catalyst to assure public debate and eventual development of policy. We must have greater dialogue than that between Frankenstein and the townspeople. Society must become educated in science. While physicians and scientists must consider the social, moral, and economic consequences of their discoveries, our society is not content, nor should it be, with allowing health professionals to make these decisions alone. Clearly, it is our responsibility to educate the decision-makers and inform the discussion.

For society to begin to deal with these concepts, it must be educated to the possibility of their existence. It must also recognize that not wanting such scientific "advances" does not prevent their discovery. Science moves forward, increasing knowledge. We have never been successful, nor do I believe we should be, in limiting its discoveries or in determining what they should be. The earth is not the center of the universe, regardless of how Copernicus and Galileo were treated by their peers. The Frankenstein story has persisted because it speaks to vital social concerns. We are fearful of tampering with the essence of nature and the creation of life. Frankenstein's well-meaning desires had untoward evil effects. Good intentions do not necessarily result in a good outcome. Perhaps most importantly, the story avers that there are certain things with which science should not tamper, and a scientifically ignorant society, endowed with common sense, knows best. The popular 1931 film version of Shelley's novel shows the townspeople as correct when, as a mob, they seek to limit Frankenstein's studies. The view is that there are certain subjects not appropriate to scientific inquiry. There is no doubt that those espousing this view would include many of the subjects of this discussion as taboo. While the Frankenstein parable is enduring, it is basically flawed. Technology and science are neither evil nor good, nor are their discoveries. Studying the nature of the atom did not cause radioactivity or nuclear explosion. The possibilities for constructive use of the energy resulting from implementation of discoveries in nuclear physics are great; their failure represents society's inability effectively to integrate these astounding new discoveries. Powerful forces will become available to us in biology and medicine. We cannot, and we should not, prevent their occurrence. We can, however, begin to understand them and try to use them. An optimistic view is that, while Frankenstein's monster is always a possibility, it is also possible that a great many positive things can still come from discovery. Like Adam and Eve, we have tasted from the tree. Our innocence is gone and cannot be recovered. Health professionals have a special responsibility to educate the public and stimulate public discussion. Society must come to realize that inevitability is not a useful concept with regard to the considerations of health, disease, and even longevity. We must begin to think the unthinkable if we are to harvest the possibilities of scientific discovery, rather than be victims of its undesired consequences.

REFERENCES

1. Biesecker, BB, Boehnke, M, Calzone, K, et al.: Genetic counseling for families with inherited susceptibility to breast and ovarian cancer. *JAMA* 269: 1970–1974, 1993.
2. King, MC, Rowell, S, and Love, SM: Inherited breast and ovarian cancer: What are the risks? What are the choices? *JAMA* 269: 1975–1980, 1993.

1
Medical Ethics and Learning

COMMENTARY

The first series of essays centers on my uneasiness with the randomized clinical trials that have become the *sine qua non* of clinical research. The randomized clinical trial is thought to be highest in the hierarchy of medical evidence. In this chapter I describe my ethical concerns with this method as I became increasingly concerned with this type of trial design, beginning with the essay "Randomized Clinical Trials and the Doctor–Patient Relationship," published in 1979 as randomized trials were to become the standard method. My daughter Deborah was still in high school at that time, but by 1991 she had graduated college, majoring in philosophy. She then had two postgraduate study years, first at the Sorbonne and then at Columbia University, followed by law school at Harvard. During her senior year in law school, I discussed my concerns with trials with her, and this discussion resulted in "Of Mice but Not Men," published jointly by us in *The New England Journal of Medicine*. We both continue to be vexed by these issues and to continue to write about differing aspects of research ethics. I include two further publications of mine on clinical trials; the first, "Ethics of Randomized Clinical Trials," is an Ethics Rounds held at the Dana Farber Cancer Institute in which I was the discussant. It highlights some of the ethical problems for the physician caring for a patient, as contrasted with the clinical investigator, especially when the same individual acts as both the investigator and the physician to a patient. The second essay "The Patient and the Public Good" discusses other conflicts with the doctor's primary role as caregiver to the individual patient. Today, as we learn more about the genetic profile of individual cancer, there is great interest in what is called precision medicine, matching the drug to the genetics of the cancer. In order to test such a treatment philosophy, new statistical tests are being considered, rather than those that include large numbers of clinically comparable and similarly staged patients. The new tests result in many smaller groups of genetically similar patients, making trials much more difficult because with such small numbers of patients, the differences must be very large in order to statistically determine that the difference is unlikely to be a matter of chance. The ultimate of such individualized trials is called "N of one" where N is the number of patients being tested and compares the patient against herself. This will only determine differences in initial response, but not duration of impact or overall survival. In any case, my concerns with randomized trials or any proposed trial are based on my belief that the individual patient's rights must be primary in all medical practice and must preempt utilitarian gains unless society specifically proscribes a treatment or procedure. New trial design must not prevent the physician from offering the patient the treatment that she believes to be correct for that individual patient, with appropriate caveats as to the nature and surety of the knowledge on which that recommendation is based.

The next offering concerning the ethics of clinical research is an essay review, "On First Looking into Kutcher's *Contested Medicine*," of a book concerned with medical experiments done at the height of the Cold War. This allowed me to broaden my considerations of ethics in clinical research. It is especially relevant to the conflict between the patient's rights and the common good during a national crisis. War is deemed a time in which the common good trumps individual rights—when we purposely put certain citizens in harm's way in order to achieve a greater good for our country. Was the Cold War of the 1960s such a time? The 1960s were a time of great expansion of basic human rights, including advances in civil rights and the creation of Medicare as a health right for the elderly. The Declaration of Helsinki was agreed to in 1964. The

Declaration of Geneva of the World Medical Association binds the physician with the words, "The health of my patient will be my first consideration," and further expounds that even in clinical research it is the duty of the physician to promote and safeguard the health, well-being, and rights of patients, including those who are involved in medical research. The physician's knowledge and conscience are dedicated to the fulfillment of this duty.

Despite the Nuremberg Code of 1947 (which requires the patient's voluntary compliance with any experiment, and includes other requirements protecting the patient's interests) and the Declaration of Helsinki almost two decades later, the explication and expansion of patient rights followed a more deliberate pace, with doctors slowly relinquishing the paternalistic model for one of informing and involving the patient in medical decisions. Ideally, this should involve the doctor providing information and some evaluation of its quality and then helping the patient make the appropriate choice for his or her care, based not only on the provided information, but also on the patient's particular values and social circumstances. A cautionary note here is my occasional witnessing of young doctors and medical students providing the treatment alternatives without indicating the doctor's choice and the reasons for it. This is not fair to the patient, and almost always results in some variation of "What would you do if you (your mother, child, etc.) were the patient?" Proper handling of this essential component of patient care is a critical part of the "art of medicine" and must not be lost while empowering the patient. It is important to separate these rights of patients *in* health care from those rights *to* health care; the latter, the subject of health care reform, is discussed in the sixth and seventh essays ("Managed Care and the Doctor-Patient Relationship" and "Fin de Siècle Medicine," which focus on managed care).

My consideration of patient rights and the social contract inherent in the doctor–patient relationship was greatly stimulated by the Clinical Ethics Series presented at The University of Chicago by Mark Siegler and his clinical ethics colleagues. This series was well attended not only by physicians, but also by faculty and students from many other parts of the university. I well remember commenting at one of these sessions, using the terms "rights" and the implicit "contract" between doctor and patient, when an eminent law professor followed my comment by noting that such words had especial resonance in the law and fruitfully expanded the discussion—thus another example of The University of Chicago's interactive faculties. Most recently, my wife and I have moved to Charlottesville, home of the University of Virginia, where it is almost impossible to not "hold these truths to be self-evident, that all men are created equal, that they are endowed by their Creator with certain unalienable Rights, that among these are Life, Liberty and the pursuit of Happiness.—That to secure these rights, Governments are instituted among Men," as written by Thomas Jefferson, that early inhabitant of this city who seemingly still animates the town and his university. Both life and the pursuit of happiness surely require health. Bottom line—rights are important and are becoming even more so in health care.

The last decade of the twentieth century was consumed with health care reform discussions, begun by William Jefferson Clinton during his successful election campaign for president of the United States. Shortly after his election, a task force led by First Lady Hillary Clinton made recommendations that led to the Health Security Act of 1993. This was never enacted into law but led to continuing discussion as well as the flowering of "managed care" and "managed competition." (These issues have returned to the forefront with the successful passage of the Affordable Care Act in 2010.) This first attempt, in 1993, at trying to expand medical care while controlling costs led to the essays, Managed Care and the Doctor-Patient Relationship and Fin de Siècle Medicine which are for a lay audience and should be read in the context of the ethical requirements of the doctor–patient relationship as discussed in the previous papers. The discussions of 1993 resulted in changes, which have persisted, with intrinsic conflict involving three important values: equity in medical care, quality, and cost. Managed competition was promised to be a good solution to cost concerns. Not only did this result in increasing concentration of medical care facilities and practices, but such competition decreased cooperation and collaboration in medicine—an example of which was the demise of the Joint Center for Radiation Therapy (JCRT), lamented in the next chapter. A purely capitalist model does not appear to me to be appropriate to equitable high-quality healthcare for all. A better model for medicine is that basic health care, like basic education, is a right that should be regulated and managed by government, as it is in most of the countries in Western Europe. Australia, Canada, the United Kingdom, France, Japan, and South Korea have single-payer systems. The Affordable Care Act, like the Health Security Act of the Clintons, tries to provide affordable medical care for all, but within a competitive model, with limited government involvement as either a payer or provider. However, we do have a true single-payer system for the elderly, Medicare, in which the government provides most of the funding for basic care but the care is given in many different competing private and public settings. Additional private insurance can be purchased to augment this basic coverage. It is claimed that expanding this to all people, regardless of age, would be too expensive, but I don't believe this to be true. Such hybrid systems seem to work well in the aforementioned countries, which all devote less of their gross domestic product (GDP) to health care than does the United States. Perhaps Medicare for all, or something similar, is best to achieve the right to health care in the United States. This will require releasing the current bargaining constraints placed on this program.

The final two essays in this chapter ("Premise, Promise, Paradigm, and Prophesy" and "Learning While Caring") are about inductive learning used in medicine and science and its limitations. I believe that the reliance of the scientific method on theories and testable hypotheses, as well as their conditional nature, is often not clearly understood or articulated by physicians, scientists, and the general public. The methods of science result in conditional knowledge, not certainty, and are always subject to modification or rejection. This should result in humility when espousing opinions—not necessarily a characteristic of either scientists or physicians.

RANDOMIZED CLINICAL TRIALS AND THE DOCTOR–PATIENT RELATIONSHIP: AN ETHICAL DILEMMA

Hellman S. Randomized clinical trials and the doctor-patient relationship: an ethical dilemma. *Cancer Clinical Trials* 1979;2:189–193 (*now American Journal of Clinical Oncology*).

As we have developed the scientific basis of modern medicine, tremendous advances have been made. The randomized controlled clinical trial has become the favored technique of therapeutic research. This procedure, while at times quite informative, is associated with both practical and ethical concerns. This paper deals with some of the ethical difficulties for the investigator.

The nature of the doctor–patient relationship is central to the conflicting pressures on the physician-investigator. It is my strong contention that there is an unwritten understanding in the doctor–patient relationship stating that the physician will give his or her best advice, indicating not only that which he or she is sure of (a dangerous word in medicine in any circumstance), but those things that he or she thinks probable, likely, or reasonable. From this distillation of facts and opinion, the physician advises the patient as to the most reasonable course of action. The second and equally important part of this "covenant" is that the physician will act in regard to the patient only as he or she perceives that patient's best interests with no conflicting responsibilities. There may be other parts of the doctor–patient relationship to be discussed; but at least these two make randomized prospective clinical trials extraordinarily difficult, if not impossible, at least as they are currently formulated.

It is currently dogma that prospective randomized trials are necessary in order for a new therapy to be accepted or an old therapy discarded. Other methods are considered suspect; thus, in order to advance medical knowledge, the investigator is required to consider the prospective randomized trial. Such trials have a number of difficult ethical problems, not only in the initial formulation, but in patient accrual, follow-up, and confirmation. In order to begin initial randomization, the physician must have no reasoned view as to which treatment is better. For if he or she believes that one treatment is better, surely this must be described and recommended to the patient, although one might well point out the level of certainty with which the opinion is held. The physician usually favors one form of treatment, either because it holds promise for increasing cure or because it is less toxic. Clearly, both of these are strong and compelling reasons to recommend a specific treatment for the patient. If the physician has no opinion as to which is better, this may well mean that the difference is small, perhaps trivial, and not worth studying. Sometimes in his or her exuberance to accrue patients into a study, the physician-investigator encourages the patient to accept the treatment alternative to which he has been randomized by suggesting that this may be of benefit. While this may later on be proven to be the case, if it is done to further the study rather than the patient's interests, it violates the traditional doctor–patient relationship.

Even after the trial has begun, major ethical problems persist. The participating physician will develop opinions as to which treatment is better. Can he or she continue to randomize since no longer is one as uncertain as to the preferable alternative? The usual solution to this ethical problem is to keep the results hidden from the investigators. This does not lessen the ethical problem; it just makes its solution more difficult. Even if it were an ethically acceptable solution, it is frequently impractical. While restricting outcome data is sometimes possible, often it is not since the investigators continue to observe the treated patients and form clinical impressions. Thus, the ability of the physician to randomize future patients should decrease as he or she observes previously treated patients. Since these judgments may be distorted or erroneous due to observation of only a small number of the trial patients, it is obligatory to know the results of the whole study as it proceeds, in order to better inform the next patient. Failure to do so in order to preserve the validity of the study appears to be a direct conflict of interest.

An even more obvious problem is raised by the conventional technique of analyzing the arms of the study and showing that one group is different from the other although the P value has not reached 0.05 (the conventionally accepted level of significance) while keeping the two treatment alternatives coded. One treatment is likely to be better than the other, but the investigator does not know which. The physician must learn which treatment is likely to be better before the next patient is entered into the trial in order to prevent that patient from being randomized to a probably inferior treatment. Thus, the physician should not participate in any trial that does not promulgate such data availability. When one treatment seems likely to be better than the others, not only must the physician consider it for the next patient, but he or she must also consider going back and treating all those previously randomized "control" patients so that they receive optimum treatment. Such a technique may invalidate the use of this control group for the study. Consider what would happen in the current adjuvant breast cancer programs if once the data looked suggestive, all the control groups received chemotherapy as well. The outcome of such a treatment policy would be to greatly limit or to abrogate completely the usefulness of these studies. However, this may be required in order to maintain the physician's responsibility to these patients.

It is the general view of the scientific community that independent confirmation of experimental results is required before general acceptance. This view has been extended to clinical investigation and randomized prospective trials. On the face of it, I would suggest that such confirmatory trials are ethically impossible unless the physician has sufficient reason to doubt the first trial. Even if one doubts the previous trial, the information that one treatment was shown to be better than the other in a previous trial must be told to the patient before the patient enters the trial.

The physician must choose to act in the patient's interests regardless of the informational benefit for the community. "The greatest good for the greatest number" cannot be the proper philosophy for a physician entering into the conventional doctor–patient relationship. The physician must vigorously pursue information necessary to act in the patient's best interest. That investigators have opinions as to preferable treatment alternatives seems clear. In every trial, a significant number of patients are treated off protocol. Sometimes the reason for this is that the patient is unusual by virtue of being associated with the investigators, either personally or professionally, or by being an important community leader. In my experience, rarely are such patients distributed randomly to the treatment alternatives; rather, they usually receive the one treatment which the investigators feel is to be favored. Should not all patients be treated this way?

If randomized trials are to be done, then the physician must explain to the patient that the traditional doctor–patient relationship will not obtain and, further, that while the physician is interested in this patient, the medical care he or she receives will be guided not exclusively by what is in the patient's best interest but will be balanced against the interests of the community at large and the purposes of the trial. For example, should one group of patients appear to do better than another without the difference reaching statistical significance, patients would continue to be randomized and those already randomized would not have their treatment altered. This must be understood by the participating patient, referring physician, and physician-investigator. It may be difficult for the patient to enter into such a new arrangement with a physician during catastrophic illness. Consider the patient who is referred to or seeks the "Cancer Center" with advanced disease for which all conventional therapy has been exhausted. This patient is willing to participate in "experiments" in order to be availed of new therapy; but if the therapy is to be tested using a prospective randomized trial, there is a good chance that the patient will not receive the therapy and continue to be denied it until the study is concluded. Is the patient in the "control group" happy with this treatment? Is he or she frankly informed that this treatment is no different from that available through conventional means perhaps closer to home and with much greater flexibility? Even if all this could be explained to the patient, as a society in general, we might question whether this license to abrogate the traditional doctor–patient relationship should be given to the medical community.

Because of these problems, it is worth considering what the advantages of the randomized prospective clinical trial are. Obviously, the purpose is to compare and, if present, uncover differences between alternatives. This technique of prospective randomized trial is used primarily to avoid misleading information due to either observer bias or misinformation if the alternative study groups are not comparable. Observer bias is usually avoided by having strict rules for patient entry into the study for randomization—usually that evaluation is to be done by an impartial party, the medical statistician. Group equality is usually assured by stratifying patients for as many prognostic variables as possible and randomly allocating within these subgroups. The stratification allows uniformity with regard to known prognostically important variables while randomization assumes that unknown prognostically important variables will be distributed equally between the two groups. Additional advantages often quoted for the randomized prospective clinical trial are that patients are more carefully evaluated, staged, and followed.

There are disadvantages in the current prospective clinical trials. It is clear they require large numbers of patients in order to show moderate differences. The larger the likely difference, the smaller the number of patients necessary. However, the larger the likely difference, the more ethically difficult it is for the physician to randomize patients. When the differences are considered likely to be small and large numbers of patients are required to randomize, then one must question how important the results of the study are likely to be. If in fact one is dealing with two treatments of known difference in toxicity and one is interested in finding out whether they have equal effectiveness, then one is trying to prove that there is no difference. This is impossible to prove using the prospective clinical trial; and what one operationally tries to prove is that the difference between the groups is likely to be less than some previously agreed upon amount. If that difference is relatively small, then very large numbers of patients must be placed into the study.

From this brief consideration, there appear to be overwhelming ethical reasons to abandon the randomized prospective clinical. The latter practical difficulties with the trial are also reasons to search for alternatives. Abandoning randomized prospective trials may temporarily decrease the flow and validity of medical knowledge; however, this cannot be the only method of therapeutic research. It is of prime importance that significant resources be directed toward research in methodology to allow more powerful techniques which are consistent with the patient–doctor relationship. Such techniques might include concurrent match-pair analysis where physicians committed to or favoring either one of the two alternative forms of treatment treat their patients in that fashion. The patients can still be staged and evaluated by impartial physicians and all known prognostic variables recorded. In order to further avoid observer bias, the data must be collected by biostatisticians fully knowledgeable in the pitfalls of such analysis. One risk of this is that there might inadvertently be some selection between the two groups, because there are unknown prognostic factors not appropriately distributed between the groups. While this may be true, it is an ethically acceptable technique and confirmatory investigations are perfectly consistent. This is only one suggested alternative; there may be many which not only would be ethically acceptable, but may require fewer patients and have greater statistical power. The criteria for a trial in a patient care setting must include the following:

1. The physician must be allowed to describe the alternatives as he or she understands them and to recommend for each individual what he or she thinks is likely to be the best form of treatment.
2. Information as to outcome of a study, even when this has a chance of being misleading, must be available to the physician.
3. There must be no sacrifice of the patient's prerogatives or of the doctor–patient relationship for the larger good of the community, perhaps not even when this is the patient's wish and after clear exposition of this problem.

Such criteria are not consistent with most randomized clinical trials as currently conceived; however, I believe that they leave much room for innovative and ethically acceptable advances in experimental design. The alternative to the prospective randomized trial must not be uncontrolled anecdotal information but rather the use of new scientific techniques which are ethically acceptable as well as a useful source of new information. We must advance medicine scientifically but within the highest humanistic tradition of the profession.

OF MICE BUT NOT MEN: PROBLEMS OF THE RANDOMIZED CLINICAL TRIAL

Samuel Hellman, Deborah S. Hellman

From *New England Journal of Medicine*, Hellman S, Hellman D, Of mice but not men: Problems of the randomized clinical trial, 1991; 324(22): 1585–1589. Copyright © (1991) Massachusetts Medical Society. Reprinted with permission.

As medicine has become increasingly scientific and less accepting of unsupported opinion or proof by anecdote, the randomized controlled clinical trial has become the standard technique for changing diagnostic or therapeutic methods. The use of this technique creates an ethical dilemma.[1,2] Researchers participating in such studies are required to modify their ethical commitments to individual patients and do serious damage to the concept of the physician as a practicing, empathetic professional who is primarily concerned with each patient as an individual. Researchers using a randomized clinical trial can be described as physician-scientists, a term that expresses the tension between the two roles. The physician, by entering into a relationship with an individual patient, assumes certain obligations, including the commitment always to act in the patient's best interests. As Leon Kass has rightly maintained, "the physician must produce unswervingly the virtues of loyalty and fidelity to his patient."[3] Though the ethical requirements of this relationship have been modified by legal obligations to report wounds of a suspicious nature and certain infectious diseases, these obligations in no way conflict with the central ethical obligation to act in the best interests of the patient medically. Instead, certain nonmedical interests of the patient are preempted by other social concerns.

The role of the scientist is quite different. The clinical scientist is concerned with answering questions—i.e., determining the validity of formally constructed hypotheses. Such scientific information, it is presumed, will benefit humanity in general. The clinical scientist's role has been well described by Dr. Anthony Fauci, director of the National Institute of Allergy and Infectious Diseases, who states the goals of the randomized clinical trial in these words: "It's not to deliver therapy. It's to answer a scientific question so that the drug can be available for everybody once you've established safety and efficacy."[4] The demands of such a study can conflict in a number of ways with the physician's duty to minister to patients. The study may create a false dichotomy in the physician's opinions: according to the premise of the randomized clinical trial, the physician may only know or not know whether a proposed course of treatment represents an improvement; no middle position is permitted. What the physician thinks, suspects, believes, or has a hunch about is assigned to the "not knowing" category, because knowing is defined on the basis of an arbitrary but accepted statistical test performed in a randomized clinical trial. Thus, little credence is given to information gained beforehand in other ways or to information accrued during the trial but without the required statistical degree of assurance that a difference is not due to chance. The randomized clinical trial also prevents the treatment technique from being modified on the basis of the growing knowledge of the physicians during their participation in the trial. Moreover, it limits access to the data as they are collected until specific milestones are achieved. This prevents physicians from profiting not only from their individual experience, but also from the collective experience of the other participants.

The randomized clinical trial requires doctors to act simultaneously as physicians and as scientists. This puts them in a difficult and sometimes untenable ethical position. The conflicting moral demands arising from the use of the randomized clinical trial reflect the classic conflict between rights-based moral theories and utilitarian ones. The first of these, which depends on the moral theory of Immanuel Kant (and seen more recently in neo-Kantian philosophers, such as John Rawls[5]), asserts that human beings, by virtue of their unique capacity for rational thought, are bearers of dignity. As such, they ought not to be treated merely as means to an end; rather, they must always be treated as ends in themselves. Utilitarianism, by contrast, defines what is right as the greatest good for the greatest number—that is, as social utility. This view, articulated by Jeremy Bentham and John Stuart Mill, requires that pleasures (understood broadly, to include such pleasures as health and well-being) and pains be added together. The morally correct act is the act that produces the most pleasure and the least pain overall.

A classic objection to the utilitarian position is that according to that theory, the distribution of pleasures and pains is of no moral consequence. This element of the theory severely restricts physicians from being utilitarians, or at least from following the theory's dictates. Physicians must care very deeply about the distribution of pain and pleasure, for they have entered into a relationship with one or a number of individual patients. They cannot be indifferent to whether it is these patients or others that suffer for the general benefit of society. Even though society might gain from the suffering of a few, and even though the doctor might believe that such a benefit is worth a given patient's suffering (i.e., that utilitarianism is right in the particular case), the ethical obligation created by the covenant between doctor and patient requires the doctor to see the interests of the individual patient as primary and compelling. In essence, the doctor–patient relationship requires doctors to see their patients as bearers of rights who cannot be merely used for the greater good of humanity.

As Fauci has suggested,[4] the randomized clinical trial routinely asks physicians to sacrifice the interests of their particular patients for the sake of the study and that of the information that it will make available for the benefit of society. This practice is ethically problematic. Consider first the initial formulation of a trial. In particular, consider the case of a disease for which there is no satisfactory therapy—for example, advanced cancer or the acquired immunodeficiency syndrome (AIDS). A new agent that promises more effectiveness is the subject of the study. The control group must be given either an unsatisfactory treatment or a placebo. Even though the therapeutic value of the new agent is unproved, if physicians think that it has promise, are they acting in the best interests of their patients in allowing them to be randomly assigned to the control group? Is persisting in such an assignment consistent with the specific commitments taken on in the doctor–patient relationship? As a result of interactions with patients with AIDS and their advocates, Merigan[6] recently suggested modifications in the design of clinical trials that attempt to deal with the unsatisfactory treatment given to the control group. The view of such activists has been expressed by Rebecca Pringle Smith of Community Research Initiative in New York: "Even if you have a supply of compliant martyrs, trials must have some ethical validity."[4]

If the physician has no opinion about whether the new treatment is acceptable, then random assignment is ethically acceptable, but such lack of enthusiasm for the new treatment does not augur well for either the patient or the study. Alternatively, the treatment may show promise of beneficial results but also present a risk of undesirable complications. When the physician believes that the severity and likelihood of harm and good are evenly balanced, randomization may be ethically acceptable. If the physician has no preference for either treatment (is in a state of equipoise[7,8]), then randomization is acceptable. If, however, he or she believes that the new treatment may be either more or less successful or more or less toxic, the use of randomization is not consistent with fidelity to the patient.

The argument usually used to justify randomization is that it provides, in essence, a critique of the usefulness of the physician's beliefs and opinions, those that have not yet been validated by a randomized clinical trial. As the argument goes, these not-yet-validated beliefs are as likely to be wrong as right. Although physicians are ethically required to provide their patients with the best available treatment, there simply is no best treatment yet known.

The reply to this argument takes two forms. First, and most important, even if this view of the reliability of a physician's opinions is accurate, the ethical constraints of an individual doctor's relationship with a particular patient require the doctor to provide individual care. Although physicians must take pains to make clear the speculative nature of their views, they cannot withhold these views from the patient. The patient asks from the doctor both knowledge and judgment. The relationship established between them rightfully allows patients to ask for the judgment of their particular physicians, not merely that of the medical profession in general. Second, it may not be true, in fact, that the not-yet-validated beliefs of physicians are as likely to be wrong as right. The greater certainty obtained with a randomized clinical trial is beneficial, but that does not mean that a lesser degree of certainty is without value. Physicians can acquire knowledge through methods other than the randomized clinical trial. Such knowledge, acquired over time and less formally than is required in a randomized clinical trial, may be of great value to a patient.

Even if it is ethically acceptable to begin a study, one often forms an opinion during its course—especially in studies that are impossible to conduct in a truly double-blinded fashion—that makes it ethically problematic to continue. The inability to remain blinded usually occurs in studies of cancer or AIDS, for example, because the therapy is associated by nature with serious side effects. Trials attempt to restrict the physician's access to the data in order to prevent such unblinding. Such restrictions should make physicians eschew the trial, since their ability to act in the patient's best interests will be limited. Even supporters of randomized clinical trials, such as Merigan, agree that interim findings should be presented to patients to ensure that no one receives what seems an inferior treatment.[6] Once physicians have formed a view about the new treatment, can they continue randomization? If random assignment is stopped, the study may be lost and the participation of the previous patients wasted. However, if physicians continue the randomization when they have a definite opinion about the efficacy of the experimental drug, they are not acting in accordance with the requirements of the doctor–patient relationship. Furthermore, as their opinion becomes more firm, stopping the randomization may not be enough. Physicians may be ethically required to treat the patients formerly placed in the control group with the therapy that now seems probably effective. To do so would be faithful to the obligations created by the doctor–patient relationship, but it would destroy the study.

To resolve this dilemma, one might suggest that the patient has abrogated the rights implicit in a doctor–patient relationship by signing an informed-consent form. We argue that such rights cannot be waived or abrogated. They are inalienable. The right to be treated as an individual deserving the physician's best judgment and care, rather than to be used as a means to determine the best treatment for others, is inherent in every person. This right, based on the concept of dignity, cannot be waived.

What of altruism, then? Is it not the patient's right to make a sacrifice for the general good? This question must be considered from both positions—that of the patient and that of the physician. Although patients may decide to waive this right, it is not consistent with the role of a physician to ask that they do so. In asking, the doctor acts as a scientist instead. The physician's role here is to propose what he or she believes is best medically for the specific patient, not to suggest participation in a study from which the patient cannot gain. Because the opportunity to help future patients is of potential value to a patient, some would say physicians should not deny it. Although this point has merit, it offers so many opportunities for abuse that we are extremely uncomfortable about accepting it. The responsibilities of physicians are much clearer; they are to minister to the current patient.

Moreover, even if patients could waive this right, it is questionable whether those with terminal illness would be truly able to give voluntary informed consent. Such patients are extremely dependent on both their physicians and the healthcare system. Aware of this dependence, physicians must not ask for consent, for in such cases the very asking breaches the doctor–patient relationship. Anxious to please their physicians, patients may have difficulty refusing to participate in the trial the physicians describe. The patients may perceive their refusal as damaging to the relationship, whether or not it is so. Such perceptions of coercion affect the decision. Informed-consent forms are difficult to understand, especially for patients under the stress of serious illness for which there is no satisfactory treatment. The forms are usually lengthy, somewhat legalistic, complicated, and confusing, and they hardly bespeak the compassion expected of the medical profession. It is important to remember that those who have studied the doctor–patient relationship have emphasized its empathetic nature.

[The] relationship between doctor and patient partakes of a peculiar intimacy. It presupposes on the part of the physician not only knowledge of his fellow men but sympathy. . . . This aspect of the practice of medicine has been designated as the art; yet I wonder whether it should not, most properly, be called the essence.[9]

How is such a view of the relationship consonant with random assignment and informed consent? The Physician's Oath of the World Medical Association affirms the primacy of the deontologic view of patients' rights: "Concern for the interests of the subject must always prevail over the interests of science and society."[19]

Furthermore, a single study is often not considered sufficient. Before a new form of therapy is generally accepted, confirmatory trials must be conducted. How can one conduct such trials ethically unless one is convinced that the first trial was in error? The ethical problems we have discussed are only exacerbated when a completed randomized clinical trial indicates that a given treatment is preferable. Even if the physician believes the initial trial was in error, the physician must indicate to the patient the full results of that trial.

The most common reply to the ethical arguments has been that the alternative is to return to the physician's intuition, to anecdotes, or to both as the basis of medical opinion. We all accept the dangers of such a practice. The argument states that we must therefore accept randomized, controlled clinical trials regardless of their ethical problems because of the great social benefit they make possible, and we salve our conscience with the knowledge that informed consent has been given. This returns us to the conflict between patients' rights and social utility. Some would argue that this tension can be resolved by placing a relative value on each. If the patient's right that is being compromised is not a fundamental right and the social gain is very great, then the study might be justified. When the right is fundamental, however, no amount of social gain, or almost none, will justify its sacrifice. Consider, for example, the experiments on humans done by physicians under the Nazi regime. All would agree that these are unacceptable regardless of the value of the scientific information gained. Some people go so far as to say that no use should be made of the results of those experiments because of the clearly unethical manner in which the data were collected. This extreme example may not seem relevant, but we believe that in its hyperbole it clarifies the fallacy of a utilitarian approach to the physician's relationship with the patient. To consider the utilitarian gain is consistent neither with the physician's role nor with the patient's rights.

It is fallacious to suggest that only the randomized clinical trial can provide valid information or that all information acquired by this technique is valid. Such experimental methods are intended to reduce error and bias and therefore reduce the uncertainty of the result. Uncertainty cannot be eliminated, however. The scientific method is based on increasing probabilities and increasingly refined approximations of truth.[11] Although the randomized clinical trial contributes to these ends, it is neither unique nor perfect. Other techniques may also be useful.[12]

Randomized trials often place physicians in the ethically intolerable position of choosing between the good of the patient and that of society. We urge that such situations be avoided and that other techniques of acquiring clinical information be adopted. For example, concerning trials of treatments for AIDS, Byar et al.[13] have said that "some traditional approaches to the clinical-trials process may be unnecessarily rigid and unsuitable for this disease." In this case, AIDS is not what is so different; rather, the difference is in the presence of AIDS activists, articulate spokespersons for the ethical problems created by the application of the randomized clinical trial to terminal illnesses. Such arguments are equally applicable to advanced cancer and other serious illnesses. Byar et al. agree that there are even circumstances in which uncontrolled clinical trials may be justified: when there is no effective treatment to use as a control, when the prognosis is uniformly poor, and when there is a reasonable expectation of benefit without excessive toxicity. These conditions are usually found in clinical trials of advanced cancer.

The purpose of the randomized clinical trial is to avoid the problems of observer bias and patient selection. It seems to us that techniques might be developed to deal with these issues in other ways. Randomized clinical trials deal with them in a cumbersome and heavy-handed manner, by requiring large numbers of patients in the hope that random assignment will balance the heterogeneous distribution of patients into the different groups. By observing known characteristics of patients, such as age and sex, and distributing them equally between groups, it is thought that unknown factors important in determining outcomes will also be distributed equally. Surely, other techniques can be developed to deal with both observer bias and patient selection. Prospective studies without randomization, but with the evaluation of patients by uninvolved third parties, should remove observer bias. Similar methods have been suggested by Royall.[12] Prospective matched-pair analysis, in which patients are treated in a manner consistent with their physician's views, ought to help ensure equivalence between the groups and thus mitigate the effect of patient selection, at least with regard to known covariates. With regard to unknown covariates, the security would rest, as in randomized trials, in the enrollment of large numbers of patients and in confirmatory studies. This method would not pose ethical difficulties, since patients would receive the treatment recommended by their physician. They would be included in the study by independent observers matching patients with respect to known characteristics, a process that would not affect patient care and that could be performed independently any number of times.

This brief discussion of alternatives to randomized clinical trials is sketchy and incomplete. We wish only to point out that there may be satisfactory alternatives, not to describe and evaluate them completely. Even if randomized clinical trials were much better than any alternative, however, the ethical dilemmas they present may put their use at variance with the primary obligations of the physician. In this regard, Angell cautions, "If this commitment to the patient is attenuated, even for so good a cause as benefits to future patients, the implicit assumptions of the doctor–patient relationship are violated."[14] The risk of such attenuation by the randomized trial is great. The AIDS activists have brought this dramatically to the attention of the academic medical community. Techniques appropriate to the laboratory may not be applicable to humans. We must develop and use alternative methods for acquiring clinical knowledge.

REFERENCES

1. Hellman S. Randomized clinical trials and the doctor-patient relationship: an ethical dilemma. *Cancer Clin Trials* 1979;2:189–93.
2. Idem. A doctor's dilemma: the doctor-patient relationship in clinical investigation. In: Proceedings of the Fourth National Conference on Human Values and Cancer. New York, March 15–17, 1984; New York: American Cancer Society. 1984:144–6.

3. Kass LR. Toward a more natural science: biology and human affairs. New York: Free Press, 1985:196.
4. Palca J. AIDS drug trials enter new age. *Science* 1989;246:19–21.
5. Rawls J. A theory of justice. Cambridge, MA: Belknap Press of Harvard University Press. 1971:183–92, 446–52.
6. Merigan TC. You can teach an old dog new tricks – how AIDS trials are pioneering new strategies. *N Engl J Med* 1990;323:1341–3.
7. Freedman B. Equipoise and the ethics of clinical research. *N Engl J Med* 1987; 317:141–5.
8. Singer PA, Lantos JD, Whitington PF, Broelsch CE, Siegler M. Equipoise and the ethics of segmental liver transplantation. *Clin Res* 1988;36:539–45.
9. Longcope WT. Methods and medicine. *Bull Johns Hopkins Hosp* 1932;50:4–20.
10. Report on medical ethics. *World Med Assoc Bull* 1949;1:109,111.
11. Popper K. The problem of induction. In; Miller D, ed. Popper selections. Princeton, N.J.: Princeton University Press, 1985:101–17.
12. Royall RM. Ethics and statistics in randomized clinical trials. *Stat Sci* 1991;6(1):52–62.
13. Byar DP, Schoenfeld DA, Green SB, et al. Design considerations for AIDS trials. *N Engl J Med* 1990;323:1343–8.
14. Angell M. Patient's preferences in randomized clinical trials. *N Engl J Med* 1984; 310:1385–7.

ETHICS OF RANDOMIZED CLINICAL TRIALS

Reprinted with permission. © 2016 American Society of Clinical Oncology. All rights reserved.

Emanuel EJ, Patterson WB, eds. *Journal of Clinical Oncology* 1998;16(1): 365–371.

Case Presentation

A 29-year-old white woman discovered a mass in her left breast in January 1995, which her gynecologist thought was a cyst. She had minimal risk factors for breast cancer: menarche was at age 12; she had no family history of breast cancer in her mother or sister; and she was gravida 2, para 2, aborta 2. Past medical history showed a psychiatric hospitalization at age 11 and irritable bowel syndrome. She was on no medications and she did not use alcohol.

The impression of a cyst was confirmed by ultrasound and biopsy was deferred. However, in April 1995, the patient returned with a small mass. A mammogram was negative. Aspiration disclosed cells suspicious for cancer, and biopsy showed a 1.5-cm invasive ductal carcinoma, poorly differentiated, with some necrosis, lymphatic invasion, and tumor close to the surgical margin.

With no evidence of metastases, in May 1995, the patient underwent re-excision of the mass and auxiliary lymph node dissection. Pathology showed a small focus of residual invasive ductal carcinoma within 0.2 cm of the deep margin. There was extensive lymphatic vessel invasion and two of 13 lymph nodes were involved with tumor. Estrogen-receptor assay (ER) was positive at 76 and progesterone-receptor assay (PR) was positive at 97.

The patient, a computer administrator, is newly married to a man who has four children ages 10 to 16 by a previous marriage. She is very interested in preserving her fertility, because she wants to have children.

At the first meeting, I spent approximately 90 minutes with the patient and her husband, explaining the nature of her breast cancer and summarizing the data justifying the use of chemotherapy in premenopausal women. I indicated that the real question for her was not whether to get chemotherapy, but rather what type of chemotherapy she should receive. Using a typed sheet, I reviewed standard cyclophosphamide, methotrexate, fluorouracil (CMF) chemotherapy and its side effects.

I then reviewed with them a typed checklist of prognostic factors that indicated there were several adverse factors in her case—a poorly differentiated tumor with two positive lymph nodes and extensive lymphatic vessel invasion.

I stated that given her age, many oncologists would urge more aggressive treatment than standard CMF chemotherapy and indicated that if she were inclined to consider more aggressive treatment, we had a protocol for this involving cyclophosphamide, doxorubicin, and paclitaxel. I explained the rationale for more intense therapy, but also that at this point in research, there was no proof that more intense therapy was more effective in reducing the risk of breast cancer recurrence. She and her husband did want to consider more aggressive chemotherapy, but also to discuss fertility issues. We discussed the rate of early menopause with chemotherapy that involved alkylating agents, the relationship of infertility rates to age, and the risks of pregnancy after breast cancer. We then spoke in detail about more intense chemotherapy. I showed the patient and her husband the flow diagram of the trial and the rationale for adding paclitaxel to cyclophosphamide and doxorubicin. We also spoke about the side effects of treatment, emphasizing that it had more significant side effects than CMF. The husband posed most of the questions and often spoke in the patient's name. After 90 minutes of discussion, I said they should think about the options and in a week we would talk on the phone and plan the start of therapy.

I asked the clinic nurse practitioner to call the patient and make her services available, believing that it would be helpful to have her involved. On Friday afternoon of that week, the nurse practitioner called the patient to check in with her and asked if the patient had any questions about the protocol. The patient seemed quite confused, asking if the nurse practitioner was referring to some kind of "experimental treatment." The nurse practitioner tried to explain the rationale for conducting a clinical trial. The patient seemed shocked by the idea of considering an experimental treatment.

At 9:00 PM that evening, the patient's husband called, upset, to say that neither he nor the patient had realized that the more aggressive chemotherapy was part of a randomized trial until told by the nurse practitioner. I apologized for not making it clear and explained again the trial and randomization. The husband said that the patient would not be randomized, but that they wanted her to get the cyclophosphamide, doxorubicin, and paclitaxel chemotherapy. I indicated that I could not give her that chemotherapy off protocol, although I could give CMF or cyclophosphamide plus doxorubicin. He insisted that if the more intense therapy was best, that is what they wanted his wife to have. I explained that oncologists had reason to think that cyclophosphamide, doxorubicin, and paclitaxel might be better for breast cancer patients, but that we had no scientific proof and that the trial was an attempt to get the proof. Without the proof, I could not give them that chemotherapy off protocol. He insisted that since I suggested it and since the Dana-Farber Cancer Institute (DFCI) was offering the cyclophosphamide, doxorubicin, and paclitaxel chemotherapy as part of a trial, it must be better and that his wife should get it. We discussed the rationale for randomized trials and the difference between suspecting that something is better and proving it. The husband re-emphasized that his wife would not participate in a randomized trial, but that they wanted the most intense therapy and what I considered the best chemotherapy. After an hour of discussion, I suggested they return to the DFCI for another visit to discuss these issues in person.

The following Monday, we discussed chemotherapy options, including randomized trials and giving protocol drug combinations off protocol. I explained in detail several other chemotherapy options for the patient and her husband, including cyclophosphamide plus doxorubicin and the Milan group's sequential doxorubicin/CMF regimen. After more than 1 hour of further discussion, they left to think over the options. I would like our nurse practitioner to describe her earlier phone call.

Nurse Practitioner: The patient was very anxious. My reason for calling was to try to assuage her anxiety, to answer her questions about the chemotherapy, and to discuss particulars of the trial. What struck me was her "shock" that we were considering "experimental therapy" for her and that we were going to be "experimenting" on her. I spoke to the patient, probably for 45 minutes to address these concerns.

Questioner: As chairman of the Human Subjects Protection Committee, I don't like the word "experimental." I always use the word "research" instead. I hope that you did not use the word "experimental."

Nurse Practitioner: I used the words "protocol" and "clinical trial." It was the patient's perception that it was "experimental." She used that terminology.

Questioner: As physicians, we must be lucid to the patient and make sure that the patient understands what treatment he or she will receive. If the term "clinical trial" does not mean anything to the patient, then as physicians we do have a responsibility to explain clearly what a "trial" is and in what sense it is experimental therapy and research. It should be noted that the consent form uses the word "research."

Presenter: At the initial office visit, I usually do not provide the consent form. I prefer to explain to the patient the rationale for why we would consider enrolling him or her in a "clinical trial."

When I met with the patient and her husband after the telephone call, what they were clearly most upset about was randomization. They were upset that they would not know or be able to choose which arm the patient would be on. I explained that all of the six arms were either equal to or more intensive than standard cyclophosphamide and doxorubicin chemotherapy. This point was of no interest to the patient and her husband; what they were concerned about was that they be able to choose which therapy she would receive.

Questioner: How did you respond to the husband when he asked why you cannot give the patient the more intense therapy off protocol?

Presenter: I explained that . . . there are reasons to suspect that the more intense therapy will lead to longer survival but that there is no proof. In the absence of proof, physicians rely on standard therapies, including CMF and cyclophosphamide plus doxorubicin. I also mentioned the recent results of the Milan sequential regimen as another alternative. Finally, I noted that more intense therapies could be worse, because they were more toxic, with greater side effects, and may not be more effective in prolonging survival.

Discussion

Samuel Hellman, MD, Discussant

A. N. Pritzker Distinguished Service Professor, Department of Radiation and Cellular Oncology, The University of Chicago, Chicago, IL

While I am a clinical investigator, I do not like randomized controlled clinical trials. Often, they violate the physician–patient relationship, force investigators to use patients instead of treating them as individuals. As physicians, we act as an agent of the patient and also as an agent of society. The problem with randomized trials is that they may force us to put society before very sick patients. While patients do not have rights *to* specific forms of healthcare, but patients surely have rights *in* health care. Patients should be entitled to six things from their physicians: (1) personal care, (2) honesty, (3) fidelity, (4) loyalty, (5) protection, and (6) respect. Patients are entitled to personal care, by which I mean individualized care. We tend to lump patients together to do studies, but in fact, patients are not all the same and should not be treated as if they were interchangeable. Second, patients are entitled to honesty; there should be no deception. The doctor should be candid and the institution should be truthful. Third, patients should be able to expect fidelity. Physicians should be faithful to their obligations as physicians. Both patient and physician should enter the relationship understanding that obligation the same way. Fourth, they should be able to expect loyalty. Physicians should be faithful to the interest of that patient. Fifth, the physician should respect and protect the patient's vulnerability. Patients are not the equal of the physician in the physician–patient relationship. The patient is sick, without all necessary information, scared, and therefore vulnerable. In contrast, the whole institution stands behind the physician. So the ill person comes to an uncomfortable place, with limited supports, authority, and power. The physician, therefore, has a special responsibility not to abuse the patient's vulnerability and to protect the patient's interests. Finally, physicians should respect the patient's autonomy. The patient has the right to decide what should and should not be done. He or she does not have the right to make you do it, but the right to choose. These six duties of the physician to the patient should not be controversial. I believe they constitute the ideal that has guided physicians throughout history. We can assess how well they are achieved in this case and more generally in any situation in which any patient is asked to participate in a randomized clinical trial.

The physician clearly considered this patient's individual circumstances, the fact that she is at higher risk for recurrence because her breast cancer is poorly differentiated, has close margins, extensive lymphatic invasion, and has two of 13 lymph nodes involved. All of those things indicate that it is an aggressive tumor.

What about the patient? At 29 she's very young to have breast cancer. She has a psychiatric history and evidence of irritable bowel syndrome. During the cardiac examination she banged her legs against the table in her anxiety. She has a new marriage and a husband who is very assertive, who speaks for her, and who dominates the conversation. She is very interested in having children. Most importantly, as indicated during the presentation, why did this patient come to the DFCI? It's stated a number of times that she came for advice.

Since it's a doctor–patient relationship, what do we know about the doctor, at least as regards this patient? We know that the doctor considers this patient to have a bad prognosis because he says the real question is not whether chemotherapy, but what kind and how aggressive? He reminds the patient that she has a poorly differentiated cancer, positive lymph nodes, extensive lymphatic involvement, and is very young. All of these are in his description. He summarizes by saying that many oncologists would therefore tend to urge more aggressive treatment. To me, that's advice.

He also says there's no proof of benefit from more aggressive treatment. And then we learn that the randomization question was not appreciated. The patient decides to have the more aggressive therapy, but the physician states (and this is an interesting phrase) that he "could not" give her the more aggressive treatment that is described in the protocol "off protocol," which, of course, means without randomization. We might reflect a little about the word "could" versus the word "would."

"Could not" means he's unable. "Would not" means he chooses not to. If he is unable, truly unable to do it, does he include in his advice ways in which she might avail herself of that treatment? Another point I don't want to fail to mention is that the only legitimate justification for a patient to be randomized, in my judgment, is that the patient chooses to be altruistic. The patient does something for society. There is a role for altruism, but the doctor needs to worry about the potential for coercion, because this person is dependent and therefore vulnerable.

How do you avoid coercion? One, you separate the doctor who's doing the trial from the caring physician. They both act in their particular roles, but the roles are different. Two, you recognize the patient's vulnerable state. Three, as directly relates to this patient, you avoid trial participation as the only way to get the desired treatment.

Has this patient been accorded her rights in healthcare? Let's go through my earlier list and do a report card. First, with regard to personal care, I think partially, yes, the doctor clearly recognized the individuality of this patient.

But, paradoxically after recognizing this, he suggests putting her into a group with all other patients lumped together for randomization. And what I believe is the cause of their difficulty, while he recognizes individuality, his prescription for this is to homogenize and treat her like any one of a number of patients.

Has he been honest? Yes, I believe he's been honest. I think he gets an A or maybe an A plus. What about fidelity, that is, his obligation as a physician? I believe the issue here, and also regarding my point of loyalty, involves the choice of "could" and "would." That to me is at the heart of whether he has been loyal to his physician obligations and whether he has been faithful to the patient. Both, it seems to me, are weakened by the statement that he is unable to give the intense chemotherapy "off protocol."

What about respect for vulnerability? He has been sensitive to it in the many times he has visited with the patient and the careful descriptions and the care. Those are all good. But in the end, he's not respecting her vulnerability and giving what he wants and she wants. He should act as her agent in providing what he feels—but is not proven—and what she desires, even if to do this she will not be in the trial. This obligation to her personal care is his responsibility as a physician and, I believe, takes precedence over his responsibility as a scientist.

Weatherall[1] quotes Lewis Thomas describing the different qualities required of the practitioner as compared with the medical scientist as follows: "Self confidence is by general consent one of the essentials of the practice of medicine, for it breeds confidence, faith and hope. Diffidence, by equally general consent, is an essential quality of investigation, for it builds inquiry. Here then are chief characteristics, each necessary in its own sphere, each unsuited to the other. . . ." Sir David Weatherall, a noted physician and medical scientist, the Regius Professor of Medicine at Oxford, agrees. He suggests that the "sick need an air of confidence at the bed-side: their recovery may not be hastened by if's and but's and by explanations of the current state of scientific ignorance about their disease." Neither Lewis nor Weatherall derogates the importance of clinical investigation and the scientific method, but rather they recognize that clinical care and scientific investigation are different and require different skills and attitudes. I would suggest that combining them in the same setting confuses both the patient and the doctor and serves neither the goals of medicine nor of science well.

What about autonomy? I believe the patient's autonomy is not being respected. She is unable to act on an informed judgment arrived at after a discussion with her physician. Her judgment accords with his recommendation, which is for aggressive treatment. I know that we haven't proven that the aggressive treatment is better, but even if this new experimental treatment turns out to be worse, it is still a question of how the doctor has dealt with the patient. Even if there's no proof that more intensive therapy will be more effective, did the patient come for proof? No, the patient came for advice. What do you really mean when you say you know something versus when you are ignorant? Are there intermediary positions? You may have a hunch. You may have strong views. Accepting that you're wrong many times when you have hunches and strong views, is it not honest and loyal to the patient to share those hunches and opinions with the patient, prefacing it that these are, in fact, just hunches and opinions?

Does one accept statistical proof from a randomized trial as proof, even when you believe that trial to be flawed or against all your intuition? Even if you don't think it's flawed, is it automatically proved? I would argue that doctors act in a Bayesian manner. You incorporate previous knowledge into your opinion of the trial design, execution, and results, to form a new opinion. The result is not binary—not "I don't know" and "I absolutely know"—but an opinion that has all shades of gray in it. I would argue that's what you're supposed to share with the patient. Scientific proof in this case is not available.

The next issue to consider is the setting of interaction. When you go in to the doctor's office off Beacon Street, with a shingle out front, you go in expecting certain things.

You think that doctor has only one purpose with regard to you. He or she is supposed to be taking care of you. When you come into the DFCI, you discover a complicated place, where there is clearly a mission of discovering new knowledge. Is that other role really understood by the patient? Patients see the white coats, the little rubber tubes hanging around the neck, the diplomas may be on the wall next to the blood pressure cuffs. It looks to them like a doctor's office. Not a scientist's office, a doctor's office. This structure may connote a relationship similar to relationships with physicians in the past. I wonder if we are using that notion of a doctor's office and not separating it sufficiently from the office of a scientist so that patients are intentionally made to be just a little bit unclear. They come to see a doctor and they end up seeing a clinical investigator, a scientist. I think setting is an ethical issue.

I want to make a point about randomized trials when the prognosis is poor, although this case is not a perfect case for it. Her prognosis is intermediate. I don't think it is as bad as we see it many times since she only has two positive lymph nodes. I wonder whether it's really justified for us to offer randomized trials to patients whose outcome is known to be terrible. This was not a problem until AIDS came along. When zidovudline (AZT) was being tested, it was very clear to me that it was extraordinarily difficult to do a trial in which there was a control group. We didn't know whether AZT was working, but we knew the natural history of AIDS. Even accepting that AZT might have made the disease worse, it is very difficult to assign such a patient to a "no-treatment" group.

I leave with you the thought that there are situations for which you cannot do trials. Don't these include seriously ill patients for whom, you believe, it's very predictable what is going to occur? This does not fit the patient under consideration, but I didn't want to leave this out.

My final word on altruism. Is it fair to ask a seriously ill patient to consider an altruistic decision at the risk of denying her what she believes to be the best treatment? But why deny her what she believes to be the best therapy when the reason she believes it is because of her discussion with you? She didn't come in with that belief. Is that fair? Is altruism in that case legitimate?

> *Questioner:* If paclitaxel is not approved by the Food and Drug Administration for use in this combination of drugs, is it legitimate to offer it "off protocol" or "off label?"
>
> *Dr. Hellman:* You've never used a drug "off label?"
>
> *Questioner:* If something went wrong I could be sued for having done it, so to be very careful we explain that to patients. As a second question, when you have a discussion about various therapies, you can include a whole gamut. Are you obligated to offer a potentially very toxic, but perhaps effective unproven

> remedy? What are the limits in what options you are obligated to discuss with the patient?
>
> *Dr. Hellman:* I think you have to share your opinions with the patient. It's not a matter of the patient making the decision from a menu with many choices. You have to give the patient your informed judgment. In this particular case history, her doctor's informed judgment was in favor of the most aggressive therapy. That's clearly what she understood from his discussions. After extensive discussion with her, she came out and said, "I got it. What the doctor thinks I should do is take very aggressive treatment."

He didn't say to her, "You ought to have a bone marrow transplant," or even bring it up in the spectrum of options because he didn't feel he should. I agree with him. He should give his best advice, which was aggressive chemotherapy. Since he liked the notion of the particular aggressive treatment that's in this protocol, he offered the protocol to the patient.

You don't have to say what you don't believe. But patient autonomy doesn't mean you give up your responsibility. In a very nice article Emanuel[2] describes the different roles of physicians. In one role the physician is just the information bearer, but I believe the physician needs to give much more—a judgment. If you don't think it's appropriate to give a bone marrow transplant, you don't mention it.

> *Questioner:* When we're rendering our opinion don't we have the responsibility to give all the possible alternatives and what we think about those alternatives? I don't see how you can selectively omit some, but not others.
>
> *Dr. Hellman:* In regard to bone marrow transplant, you can handle this one like a good doctor. You cannot mention it if you think it's so outrageous it's not worth mentioning, or you can mention it and damn with faint praise, pointing out that, in her case, it's not appropriate, it's far too toxic, and the outcome data don't impress you as being worth the mortality risk associated

with it. Or you can decide that it's beyond the pale. You don't mention everything all the time.

You mention some spectrum that you think is appropriate for that patient. We might differ on whether bone marrow transplant is included in that. But if you do mention it, you mention it with the caveats you feel are appropriate.

Coming back to the question of whether it's ethical to randomize when you truly don't know which treatment is preferable. Absolutely. If you don't believe one treatment is better than the other, but that the circumstances are in clinical equipoise, where the risks of harm and the risks of good are in balance, then you have the right and maybe even the obligation to offer randomization. I have no problem with the offering of randomization in those circumstances. I have a problem with the patient saying, "I don't want to be randomized because, as I heard it, I'm not in equipoise. I want treatment 'A.'" If you've ever seen a child's teeter totter, you know it's hard to stay in equipoise to be balanced. You get a few patients on a protocol and they get toxicity. Your view about toxicity changes. A few patients have miraculous responses, not in a blinded setting where you can't tell, but in settings in which you can tell, and your equipoise starts to slip away. Equipoise is a big discussion on its own but it isn't pertinent to this case. This case is not about the doctor's ability to offer randomization. I'm not questioning that, but rather what happens when the patient says, "I heard it and I want treatment A." Then he says, "I can't give it," when, in fact, I wonder whether he can't or won't.

> *Questioner:* Wouldn't it be unethical to ask patients to participate in a randomized trial, but if they don't want to, to give them the experimental therapy? That seems to set a precedent that would be unethical, at least in this institution.
>
> *Dr. Hellman:* The exact opposite might be more true. The only chance that an AZT randomized trial had of being ethical was to have said, "Look, this is a brand new drug. It causes harm. It could cause good. We really don't know. We are in equipoise.

We aren't going to find out without a trial. But it's a heavy load to ask of you. So if you want to take your chances with it, we'll give it to you. We would prefer you to be in the trial, but that's for our gain and for future gain and for altruism. If you want it, who are we to say you can't have it?" I believe, in fact, that's what you have to do with the seriously ill.

Questioner: If we don't know whether it is more toxic, how can we say there'll be no harm in taking it?

Dr. Hellman: This fear of doing harm misinterprets Hippocrates, who is translated as follows: "As to diseases make a habit of two things—to help, or at least to do no harm."[3] He never said, "Do no harm," he said, "Above all, if you can't do good, at least do no harm." I object to that quotation being taken out of context. The notion was first to do good and only when you can't do good, at least do no harm. Here you offer the possibility that you might do good, but you tell the patients you don't know. That's why you want them in the trial, because the treatment could make things worse. But you give them their "out." In fact, that's what happened in the AZT trial; the investigators got the AZT on the street and because it was a blinded study, nobody knew who was getting what. Some of the patients took twice as much dose because they didn't know they had AZT before.

Questioner: Because our society has very limited resources, people are theoretically going to be only allowed to have standard therapy. You can't come to my office and ask for paclitaxel. You can't come and ask for a bone marrow transplant. We already live in a society that says, "No, you must take CMF, unless you want to go into the experimental study." How do you respond?

Dr. Hellman: I don't believe it's as bleak as that. I'm an optimist. I take care of cancer patients. If you believe what you said, then the fabric of the doctor–patient relationship, as we know it, has been torn. That is a point about which I have written.[4]

Questioner: Do you leave open the possibility that at an institution like DFCI we will offer a research protocol such as the one offered to this patient, in order to find out whether adding paclitaxel does, in fact, improve the outcome?

Dr Hellman: I don't have any problem with that. I have a problem when the patient says, "Look. I'm convinced. I'm so convinced I don't want to run the risk of not getting the paclitaxel." Then you're coercing her into the trial if you say, "The only way you can get the paclitaxel is to participate in the trial."

Questioner: If you're giving paclitaxel "off protocol" based upon your perception of the patient's clinical situation, and if you have a randomized protocol with a more intensive arm with paclitaxel, you're biasing the trial.

Dr. Hellman: I don't think you're biasing the trial with regard to the answer, but you're surely taking a group of patients you think are in worse shape out of the trial.

Questioner: If you always offer the experimental arm of the program off protocol, how many people, realistically, would bother to participate in a trial? It seems to me, that if you directly or indirectly impart to the patient during a discussion information that makes her feel a certain way about the benefits of one regimen versus another, you're never really going to have enough patients to complete the necessary studies.

Dr. Hellman: I have three responses to that. First, the way you ask the question suggests to me that you're using the gain of putting patients into the trial as a justification for not fulfilling your obligation as a physician. That's exactly what I meant by the conflict of being a double agent. You have two conflicting values. You're saying to me, "With this patient I feel a little more obligation to science, and I don't really think I'm doing a disservice to the patient because I don't really know which treatment is better." Pushing this patient into the trial for science is really important but it's a utilitarian argument. In so doing, you have limited the contract as that patient understands the contract to be, that her interests are the paramount ones.

We are in the classical ethical dilemma of "right-based ethics," the view that says people have certain rights and regardless of how good it is for society, we must not abuse those rights.

There are conflicts between the utilitarian goal and the rights goal. If this were straightforward we wouldn't be having this discussion. That is a tension in our society. What I'm saying is that when you act as a doctor to a patient, your ethics should be rights-based. When you act as a clinical investigator, the ethic is utilitarian. That's why you're in a conundrum at DFCI. If you are a clinical investigator, make sure that the setting is one where people are not coming for personal care, they are coming for investigation. If you control the setting, you reduce the ambiguity of the encounter. But you have to be careful that you don't masquerade and act deceptively when you wear your white coat and people call you "doc."

> *Questioner*: Do you feel that the doctor in this case really is personally convinced that one arm of this protocol is better than another?
>
> *Dr. Hellman*: I think the message that got across to that patient after an extended discussion was, yes.
>
> *Questioner*: During the past 20 years, the treatment of primary breast cancer has changed as a result of prospective randomized trials. Those trials were more resisted by doctors than by the patients, who didn't want to be mutilated by a radical mastectomy. So, progress was made in breast cancer management because of a clinical trial. Everything that you're saying makes a lot of sense, but the point really boils down to how the doctor presents the situation to a patient. It has nothing to do whether he's really a clinical investigator at DFCI or anywhere. What he leaks out can be dangerous if it shows his bias. The higher-dose arm was immediately picked up on by the patient as the forbidden fruit, and that was a mistake. Perhaps it was presented as,

"You'll be no worse off than what we would consider standard therapy, but we're trying to see whether or not giving more is better." Yet we really don't know that at all.

Dr. Hellman: Your comments include a number of the relevant points, including enforced altruism, and an endorsement of the utility of randomized trials. I agree completely with the utility of trials. Having said that, I think they are a problem and that we can't always use as we currently use them.[5] I believe we have to try to come up with alternatives that achieve what we want, but don't put us into these dilemmas quite so easily. It is a conundrum.

REFERENCES

1. Weatherall D: *Science and the Quiet Art*. New York, NY, Norton, 1995, p 51.
2. Emanuel EJ, Emanuel LL: Four models of the physician-patient relationship. *JAMA* 267: 2221–2226, 1992.
3. Hippocrates: *Epidemics*, book 1, chapter 11, in Kaplan, Justin (ed.): *Bartlett's Familiar Quotations*. Boston, MA, Little Brown, 1992, p 71.
4. Hellman S: The patient and the public good. *Nat Med* 1: 400–402, 1995.
5. Hellman S, Hellman DS: Of mice but not men: Problems of the randomized clinical trial. *N Engl J Med* 324: 1585–1589, 1991.

THE PATIENT AND THE PUBLIC GOOD

This article was first published in *Nature Medicine* 1995;1(5): 400–402.

The prevailing view is that a physician can simultaneously husband economic resources to control health care costs and fulfill a doctor's traditional responsibility to put the patient first. I disagree.

These are extraordinary times in medicine. There is both a revolution in the biology relevant to medicine and a revolution in the delivery of health care. We must translate laboratory discoveries into clinical practice, and we must do so in an increasingly cost-conscious environment. Faced with this challenge, physicians appear willing to modify the traditional doctor–patient relationship. The tension between clinical research and patient care is not new, but it has increased in intensity as we try to incorporate the new biology into patient care in a cost-effective way. It has been argued that research must take precedence if we are to use the advances in biology properly and if we are to efficiently allocate health care resources. Not only will clinical investigation have to assess the medical value of the new discoveries, but it will have to determine whether the advance is worth the cost. The emphasis on controlling costs takes us farther from the traditional physician role to where, in many managed care arrangements, the physician must both take care of the patient and husband the limited resources of the group, either for use for other patients or to provide profit for the plan and the physician. How can this be done in the context of the traditional doctor–patient relationship?

As a part of the doctor–patient relationship, physicians fashion a treatment plan to the needs of each patient. As the physician learns more about each patient and the details of his or her illness, the opportunities for crafting individual patient care increase. The advances in molecular medicine will allow us to know a great deal more about the disease state in each individual patient. Already current advances in oncology offer opportunities to characterize individual patients and their tumors with molecular and genetic information, distinguishing them from others, even within current staging classifications. Molecular medicine will provide many tools for this individualization of the extent, type, and virulence of the disease as well as for characterization of the host in whom the disease is resident. Each constellation of signs, symptoms, disease extent, past medical history, concomitant illness, and molecular markers of disease proclivities will affect the desirability of specific plans of management. This same phenomenon will be true in most diseases other than cancer. Because clinical investigation requires collecting patients into groups, whereas medical practice tailors treatment to individuals, these distinctions will make the role of the clinical investigator doing randomized trials more difficult.

Although it relies on altruism and informed consent, the primary ethical basis for doing randomized trials has been developed by Benjamin Freedman of McGill University who promulgates the concept of "clinical equipoise." This state exists when there is genuine uncertainty within the expert medical community with regard to the alternatives applied in a trial. Most important, the concept applies to the views of the medical community as a whole but not necessarily to the individual physician–investigator for an individual patient. Patient-centered care implicit in the current relationship between doctor and patient requires that patients are seen as individuals rather than as members of a group with similar characteristics. Trials require combining patients into categories while the tenets of patient-centered care stress personal consideration. A related conflict is emerging as managed care is used to control health costs. Can one provide individual care and at the same time be responsible for controlling costs? Peter Toon from St. Bartholomew's Hospital in London argues that the individual physician, in particular the gatekeeper in a managed care setting, can fulfill responsibilities to an individual patient and to the husbanding of scarce public resources, both within the doctor–patient relationship.[1] I disagree!

The lessons of clinical investigation can illuminate the difficulties in containing health care costs in the context of individual patient care. To demonstrate the frequent incompatibility of randomized clinical trials and patient-centered care, let us consider a patient with breast cancer who might be considered a candidate for a randomized clinical trial of therapeutic alternatives directed at either local or systemic disease. The considerations can be separated into three groups: (1) the tumor, (2) the patient, and (3) the physician.

The Tumor

In order to get sufficient numbers of patients into the trial, most studies consolidate patients into what are hoped to be relatively homogeneous groups. This is necessary if there are to be sufficient patients in each arm of a study for statistical analysis. For example, all stage one patients might be randomized. Stage one breast cancer includes tumors of all sizes less than 2 centimeters that have not spread to lymph nodes. However, there are data that indicate that 2 centimeters is an arbitrary cut-off in a continuum in which patients with smaller tumors do better than those having larger tumors even within stage one. Breast tumors can now be subjected to a variety of tests that appear to offer some prognostic significance. These include ploidy, proliferative activity, the relative expression of a variety of oncogenes, tumor suppressor genes, growth factors and their receptors, as well as tumor vascularity, nuclear and cytologic grade, and histological characteristics. Already these are proving to be both of prognostic importance and a useful guide to therapy. Although some of these factors may be confounding variables, it is possible to develop a profile for each patient's tumor. As the number of useful molecular markers increases, so will the ability to characterize each tumor. This emphasizes the individuality of each patient's lesion and suggests that it may not be possible to assure equipoise among medical experts for each tumor although they may feel comfortable in doing so for patients with stage one tumors as a group. Further, even if it is possible for the medical experts, the physician caring for the patient may feel quite differently about each patient within the group depending on such prognostic indicators.

Women and Breast Cancer

There are anatomic differences in patients that might affect the potential benefit of treatment. Past medical history and current health status will be different for each person. Molecular medicine will further quantify the status of important host organ function. Some preexisting conditions may proscribe a patient from the trial, but in almost all studies, patients are included with a spectrum of health states that affect the physician's view of which arm of the study may be more appropriate for the individual patient. As medical advances allow for greater knowledge of the individual, they will also serve as a guide to the most desirable therapy.

There are also differences in attitudes, wishes, and emotional states of individual patients. For example, how does a patient feel about breast preservation? Does her body image require the presence of the breast or, alternatively, is she fearful of occult disease lurking within the breast and would she prefer that it be removed? How do the burdens of daily radiation treatment affect her life? Similarly, how does she feel about reconstructive surgery? What are the patient's social circumstances? Do these affect her choice of treatments?

The Physician

There are also many differences among physicians. How enthusiastic is the physician for an answer to the trial? What is his or her view of the severity of the disease? Is the physician risk-prone or risk-averse with regard to the treatment of suspected micrometastatic disease? What is the effect of previous education and training on the physician? What about differing community standards? What has the physician learned in following prior patients in the trial? All of these will affect the physician's view of the trial. What should the physician do with his or her a priori opinions? One of the founders of controlled trials, Sir Bradford Hill, says, "If the doctor ... thinks even in the absence of any evidence that for the patient's benefit he ought to give one treatment rather than the other, then that patient should not be admitted to the trial. Only if, in his state of ignorance, he believes the treatment given to be a matter of indifference can he accept a random distribution of patients to the different groups."[2]

Patient-Centered Care

This example highlights the conflict between the ethical basis of trials and the requirements of patient-centered care. Freedman's notion that clinical equipoise "is satisfied if there is genuine uncertainty within the expert medical community—not necessarily on the part of the individual investigator—about the preferred treatment"[3] is in conflict with the view of many investigators. Michael Baum, a leading British surgical oncologist, in discussing breast cancer trials states,[4] "To mount national trials there has to be first of all a professional equipoise where roughly equal numbers of the profession favor either the standard treatment or the novel treatment. For a physician to enter a patient into the trial a personal equipoise must exist." This balance must exist for each patient, and the patient's preferences must be considered. This is very difficult to do when treatment is determined by random assignment.

Patient-centered care requires much more than a consensus of the medical community. We must learn about the particular patient and her disease and she must be an active participant in deciding on the best course of action. This is not "clinical equipoise." Only rarely is a balance between alternative therapies ever reached for an individual patient. Even when it is, it may be a different balance than that reached for another patient, and grouping them together may obfuscate rather than clarify. Individual patients may have different views as to the utility of different functional or cosmetic end results. McNeil and colleagues in Boston demonstrated that loss of the larynx was viewed differently when comparing firefighters with management executives and within each group there was great heterogeneity, emphasizing the range of values individual patients place on different clinical alternatives.

The Public Good and Physician Responsibility

But what of the public good? This brings us to some of the vexing questions facing medicine today. Inherent in all proposed health care reform is control of the rising costs of medical care due in large measure to the advances in diagnosis and treatment that result from technical and scientific innovation. Many of these have potential benefit but at a considerable cost. There are powerful pressures to control the rate of rise of medical expenditures by limiting the use of such techniques. There is no problem when the procedure is of no value. The bind comes with those procedures that offer possible benefit but are very expensive. Charles Fried of the Harvard Law School, in discussing what he calls the "economic model," worries that the obligation of personal care inherent in the relationship between physician and patient would be replaced by "the physician as agent of an efficient health-care delivery system." Although physicians should participate as medical experts in judgments as to the allocation of limited resources, the issues of societal cost should not enter into a doctor's decision when caring for an individual patient. Similarly, the patient cared for by the clinical investigator must believe that the physician will not compromise her care to perform the experiment.

Questions of the public good are a responsibility of society as a whole. Physicians should participate in public discussions and decision-making about the allocation of health care resources, but in a different way. The physician can participate as a citizen, expressing views about the distribution of scarce societal resources and the value of various health outcomes. Physicians may also participate in the public discussion of health care issues as experts, providing information about the efficacy of various treatments, but the physician ought not to be given the responsibility of making important societal decisions in the context of individual patient relationships. Not only does this involve the transference of an important public policy choice to small group of individuals, but more important, it requires the physician to base treatment recommendations for an individual patient on general public policy grounds, which will compromise the character of the doctor–patient relationship.

Today financial imperatives appear to dominate medical care considerations. Simply stated, the view is that during these revolutionary times economics must preempt the niceties of the personal nature of the doctor–patient relationship. Most desirable are those arrangements that satisfy both, but, it is suggested, we cannot afford to lose either the randomized clinical trial as a method of acquiring new knowledge or the cost-benefit analysis applied to the individual patient needed for expenditure control, at least until satisfactory alternatives are found. While however altruistically intended, I believe this notion is misguided. We lose much more than we gain if we damage the primacy of individual patient care, for this is based on the inalienable rights of human beings. These are not rights *to* health care but rather rights *in* health care. The patient is not entitled to any medical treatment, no matter how expensive; rather, the patient is entitled to be treated in a particular manner by his or her physician. Society can make choices in which it balances the needs of some individuals against the needs of others. Based on this balancing, society can determine the level of health care coverage available, and physicians must work within these limits. However, the ethical requirements of the doctor-patient relationship, as we now understand it, preclude the doctor from doing society's work of balancing patient and societal needs. The relationship established between the doctor and the patient is one of trust and loyalty. In fact, respect for the value of such relationships explains why maintaining the ability to choose one's doctor figured so centrally in the recent health care debate in the United States.

The doctor-patient relationship requires the fidelity of the doctor to the patient. We must not let the current transformation of health care compromise this ideal. The patient comes to the doctor in a vulnerable state—made so by illness, fear, and lack of knowledge. In order to treat a vulnerable person with concern and respect, one must look out for that person's interests. Therefore the doctor treats the patient with the appropriate respect for both the patient's vulnerability and her autonomy by becoming an agent for the patient. Moreover, it is because the patient knows that the doctor is her doctor that the patient is able to relieve herself of some of the anxiety caused by illness. If the patient is unable to repose this trust in her physician (because she knows that the physician is busy balancing this patient's needs against community needs) she will lose her ally and friend and the doctor will have lost an important instrument to relieve suffering and minister to patients.

If we are to serve the individual patient and society, we must first agree on certain principles and then, within the constraints imposed by them, develop techniques to achieve our goals. There are two such principles that, if agreed upon, will allow enhancement of the public good in the context of patient-centered care. First, individual patients should not be used as a means to achieve even a societally desired end, if in so doing the individual right to personal medical care is compromised. Second, there are two roles for the physician, and they must not be confused. As an agent of society the physician must consider the greater good and be involved in the development of guidelines, directives, and limitations on practice. At the same time, we must fight against unreasonable limits on medical care. This is very important as we consider the best use of restricted resources. Once such regulations are promulgated by society, we as physicians are obligated to adhere to them. On the other hand, within those limits we are expected to act in the best interests of each patient. The responsibilities of physicians to society as a whole must be separated from our obligation to individual patients. These two different responsibilities must be undertaken in different settings with clear understanding by the physician, the patient, and society as to which role is being played. Although clinical investigation and limiting health care expenditures are essential, we should not allow them to change the traditional relationship of the physician to the patient. For clinical investigation this means limiting the use of the randomized clinical trial and requiring that when it is used an individual equipoise exists for each patient. It also means separating the role of personal physician from that of the clinical investigator. These two roles residing in the same physician create conflicting goals, which have the potential to undermine the primacy of the patient. Randomized trials are already cumbersome and administratively burdened. These restrictions will make randomized trials even more difficult to perform. This does not suggest a return to non-scientific subjective methods of research but emphasizes the need to search for alternatives to random allocation that recognize the individual variables in each clinical circumstance. For the physician concerned with controlling health care expenditures, this means insulating the doctor from considering societal costs when advising or treating any individual patient. While decisions about the efficient use of resources may provide limits on management options, concern about health plan expense should not enter into an individual patient-management decision.

Medicine in its essence deals with a relationship between an individual doctor and a particular patient. Clinical investigation and controlling health expenditures concern society as a whole. The physician may engage in both but it would be a most unfortunate unintended consequence if altruistic concerns for the public good undermined the assurance of optimal personal treatment promulgated in patient-centered care. Revolutionary times require greater diligence in assuring the primacy of the patient in the relationship with the caring physician.

REFERENCES

1. Toon PD. Justice for gatekeepers. *Lancet* **343**, 585–587 (1994).
2. Hill AB. Medical ethics and controlled trials. *Br Med J* **1**, 1043–1049 (1963).
3. Freedman B. Equipose and the ethics of clinical research. *N Engl J Med* **317**, 141–145 (1987).
4. Baum M, Zilkha K, & Houghton J. Ethics of clinical research: Lessons for the future. *Br Med J* **299**, 251–253 (1989).

ON FIRST LOOKING INTO KUTCHER'S *CONTESTED MEDICINE*: ETHICAL TENSIONS IN CLINICAL RESEARCH

Copyright © 2010 Johns Hopkins University Press. This article was first published in *Perspectives in Biology and Medicine* 2010;53(2):304–314. Reprinted with permission by Johns Hopkins University Press.

Abstract

Contested Medicine examines the experiments done at the University of Cincinnati by Eugene Saenger and his colleagues during the 1960s, a time of great fear that the Cold War between the United States and the Soviet Union would become a hot war using nuclear weapons. These studies were to provide the Department of Defense information relevant to the consequences of exposure of military personnel to ionizing radiation in such circumstances. Kutcher, a radiation physicist turned historian of science, is especially well prepared to put these studies into the context of the evolving bioethics of the time. He reviews the essential ethical reviews, beginning with the Nuremberg Code and extending to those of the Advisory Committee on Human Radiation Experiments appointed by President Clinton. These evolving ethical standards provide a cautionary note to today's methods of clinical experimentation in search of proper evidence-based medicine. There has been an ascendance of the priority of patient rights over societal good except in increasingly limited special circumstances. Some of what was considered good and necessary science in the 1960s and 1970s is no longer considered proper. Similarly, future ethical norms may well find current trial methodology to be flawed.

I read this book with the greatest of interest since it involves a number of issues central to my medical career. As a radiation oncologist I have taken care of patients with cancer, done clinical and laboratory research related to cancer, as well as studied and applied whole-body radiation in the treatment of malignant disease. I have also written on the ethical complexities of human experimentation. All of these subjects are central to *Contested Medicine*. Further, its author Gerald Kutcher is well known to me by virtue of our professional interests and overlapping professional careers. Professor Kutcher was the head of Clinical Physics at Memorial Sloan-Kettering Cancer Center when I was the physician-in-chief of that institution. The second convergence of interests of both Kutcher and me were the ethical concerns accompanying the conflicting goals of clinical researchers: individual patient care and gaining scientific knowledge. Since the research discussed in *Contested Medicine* is a splendid context for discussing the competing priorities of clinical research and its practitioners, these competing priorities will be a major component of this essay.

Kutcher received his BS and PhD in Physics from the City University of New York. He then did postdoctoral training in medical physics, leading to a faculty position in the Department of Medical Physics at Memorial Sloan-Kettering Cancer Center, rising to be the chief of the Clinical Physics Service as well as a full member and professor of Physics in Radiology at Cornell University Medical College. He subsequently moved to Columbia University College of Physicians and Surgeons as professor of Medical Physics and vice chairman of the Department of Radiation Oncology, serving in that role from 2001 to 2004, when his career took a remarkable and fascinating change of direction.

The final two decades of the last century was an exciting time for a professional involved in improving the treatment of cancer with increasingly precise and targeted devices as well as newly emerging molecular biologically based drugs. Professor Kutcher was among a small group of physicists and physicians at the forefront of intensity modulated radiation therapy, a method for vastly improved targeting of radiation, for which he was recognized internationally. Despite the demanding challenge that these efforts entailed, they provided him the opportunity to reflect on the larger social, historical, and ethical issues involved in cancer and radiation research. This prompted a radical and, as far as I am aware, a unique career change requiring quite different expertise in a new academic discipline. He embarked on this pursuit by entering a new field of inquiry while partially supporting himself doing medical physics. While at the University of Cambridge studying for his PhD in the History and Philosophy of Science, he spent a week each month at the University of Leuven in Belgium to help them improve their efforts in radiation oncology. This was arranged with Professor Emmanuel van de Schueren, to whose memory *Contested Medicine* is dedicated. Professor van de Schueren was one of the leading European radiation oncologists at that time, with wide-ranging intellectual interests. He supported Kutcher in his studies at Cambridge by using Kutcher's expertise to complement the medical physics program in the University of Leuven. Thus, this was a period of transition from a distinguished career in medical physics to a new one in the history of science and medicine.

Kutcher took as the subject of his PhD dissertation and the basis for *Contested Medicine* the experimental treatments using whole-body radiation applied to cancer patients at the University of Cincinnati by Eugene Saenger and his colleagues beginning in 1960 and lasting for over a decade (Saenger 1967; Saenger et al. 1973). Much of the support of this research was from the Department of Defense. Its goals were to study the biological effects of total body irradiation (TBI) in order for the military to understand the consequences of radiation exposure of soldiers during the possible tactical use of nuclear weapons. This was at the apogee of the Cold War, when nuclear weapons were considered likely to be used in both strategic and tactical circumstances. The Soviet Union exploded its first atomic bomb in 1949, and a hydrogen bomb in 1955. Saenger, a nuclear medicine physician at the University of Cincinnati, enlisted his radiation oncology colleagues to collaborate in these experiments when treating patients with disseminated cancer using TBI. While not common, such treatments were also in use in other institutions as an alternative to chemotherapy—then in the early days of its utilization—or when such treatment was no longer effective. Memorial Hospital in New York City had significant experience with the therapeutic use of TBI, and it was from this institution that a radiation therapist had recently joined the Cincinnati staff. The newly installed cobalt-60 machine could be adapted for such a use. A 1973 report of the Cincinnati experiments described 88 patients treated with TBI in these studies. Saenger was particularly interested in the development of a biological dosimeter that could be used to determine the level of radiation received by a soldier. This was studied in the TBI-treated patients receiving different doses of radiation.

Peer review evolved gradually at the University of Cincinnati as it did in most American academic centers, but it was stimulated by the US Public Health Service requirement of peer review of clinical experimentation in 1966. The Faculty Committee on Research, begun in 1964, was given this responsibility at the university. There followed a lengthy iterative interaction between the committee and the investigators concerning the experimental protocols that continued until the early 1970s. All during these discussions the research continued. At first, informed consent was considered to be implied by the general consent form used in patient admission, although the form made no specific mention of research. This apparently was made more specific by 1969, since a research consent form was described in a research proposal submitted at that time.

Social and Ethical Context

After World War II the gross breaches of ethics perpetrated by the Nazi doctors came to light during the Nuremberg tribunals of 1945–46. These resulted in the Nuremberg Code, which defined standards for doing medical research on humans in an ethical fashion. Central to the Code was the voluntary informed consent of the subject. This meant that the subject should be fully informed, must be able to comprehend the study and its consequences and be able to freely decline participation. These requirements necessary for informed consent were intended to eliminate children, the mentally impaired, and prisoners as study subjects. Yet despite the publication of the Code in 1947, much medical research in the United States was in violation of these principles, and it remained so until Henry Beecher's remarkable report, "Ethics and Clinical Research," which was published in the *New England Journal of Medicine* in 1966. Beecher described 22 published studies that seemed to him to be in gross violation of medical ethics. While the individual studies were not specifically referenced in the *NEJM* paper, David Rothman lists them in *Strangers at the Bedside* (1991; Appendix A, p. 263).

Many of these reports were from among the most respected and prestigious institutions and investigators and were published in major medical journals. These comprised studies of antibiotic uses, including those in which known effective therapy was withheld; the effect of thymectomy on skin-graft survival; and the determination of cardiac and hepatic physiology using catheter techniques and other invasive methods. In some studies, terminally ill elderly patients or prisoners were injected with live cancer cells. Being published in leading journals gave these studies a veneer of propriety as being in keeping with acceptable medical research practice. Even after Beecher's review, many of the major experimentalists involved received prestigious academic appointments and awards; a particularly egregious example was the study investigating the viral transmission of hepatitis by intentionally spreading the disease among inmates of an institution for the care of mentally retarded children and adults.

Despite the Beecher report, many leaders of academic medicine defended the criticized studies and their authors. By the standards of the time, these were innovative, important studies quite within the mainstream of medicine. Indeed, in 1983, more than a decade after the Saenger studies were concluded and 17 years after the Beecher report, the hepatitis transmission study—performed contemporaneously with those of TBI at the University of Cincinnati—won for its lead investigator the Lasker Prize, the most prestigious American medical research award.

After the Beecher report, the next revelation to shock the medical community—and even more importantly the public at large—was the description of the infamous Tuskegee study, in which black men with syphilis were left untreated in order to study the natural history of the disease at a time when effective antibiotic treatment was well known. Obviously, the outrage reflected not only the violation of patient rights, informed consent, and unacceptable medical practice, but it was most blatantly racist. There followed the Belmont Report, the result of the National Commission for the Protection of Human Subjects of Biomedical and

Behavioral Research in 1979, issued well after the body of Saenger's work was completed.

Back in 1966, the US Public Health Service required institutional peer review of clinical research submitted for governmental support, and a faculty committee of the University of Cincinnati did review the TBI research. Much later, President Clinton ordered more specific evaluation of studies in which ionizing radiation was involved. The report of the Advisory Committee on Human Radiation Experiments (ACHRE) considered all such studies conducted between 1944 and 1979. This report considered patients irradiated therapeutically, exposure of troops to radiation intentionally following an atomic explosion, exposure of populations of citizens living close to atomic testing sites, and other radiation exposures both intentional and inadvertent. The ACHRE report does not firmly condemn Saenger and his colleagues. Voluminous material was supplied to the committee, and agreement on whether and when the studies were investigational and when they were therapeutic was actively discussed and debated. *Contested Medicine* describes these and many other efforts to develop appropriate principles for ethical research using humans as subjects and relates these in time to the Saenger studies.

There is an added dimension to the conflicting goals in these studies of radiation exposure: urgent threats to the country, in this case by the threat of nuclear war, which may require that ethical behavior be superseded in such perilous circumstances for the greater good of the country and its citizens. A similar accepted practice might be the limitations of freedom required by quarantine to prevent serious epidemic spread of disease to the population at large. This compulsory separation of people possibly exposed to infectious organisms began in Venice in the Middle Ages and since has been an internationally accepted limitation of the rights of citizens, as well as immigrants primarily but not exclusively endeavoring to enter a country. The tension between the rights of individuals and the needs of society can be formalized by conflicting philosophic doctrines: rights-based (deontological) versus utilitarian (Hellman and Hellman 1991).

Immanuel Kant and the neo-Kantian philosophers such as John Rawls assert that individuals are bearers of dignity and as such ought not to be treated as means to an end but rather as ends in themselves. Equally accepted as a philosophic principle is utilitarianism, which describes as right that action with the maximum social utility. As presented by Jeremy Bentham and John Stuart Mill, this means in aggregate the greatest good to the greatest number, or that which achieves the most pleasure (including health) and the least pain. Most importantly, it does not consider of moral consequence the distribution of the pleasures or pain. For a physician caring for an individual patient that distribution is all-important, since by virtue of the doctor–patient relationship the physician must consider the patient's needs to be paramount. This is how the doctor conforms to the requirements of fidelity and loyalty to the patient (Kass 1985). The doctor–patient relationship requires that the patient be a bearer of rights, and as such the patient cannot be used for the greater good of society if it in any way compromises his or her care. Even if the patient wishes to volunteer for a research study, one might question whether the physician is violating his or her primary loyalty to the patient by offering such participation in the experiment. Thus there appear to be two ethical standards relevant to the rights of human beings used for scientific study by physicians: those of society, as evidenced by the previously described Nuremberg, Belmont, and ACHRE reports, and the responsibilities of the doctor to the patient, promulgated first formally by Hippocrates and after Nuremberg as the Helsinki Declaration. As exceptions, society limits the individual's right of patient priority in the doctor–patient relationship by expressly limiting or requiring certain physician behavior in order to assure a greater common good. Examples of this are the requirements of reporting certain illnesses and wounds of a suspicious nature, regardless of the possibility that this reporting may have deleterious consequences for the patient. But these exceptions, by being explicitly recognized as such, affirm the individual patient priority in all other medical circumstances.

Professional Willfulness

Physicians' willful blindness to circumstances or consequences of their behavior may be seen either in accordance with or in violation of the priority of patient rights. An interesting case was recently decided by a US District Court, reviewed by the US Circuit Court for the Fourth Circuit, and retried, resulting in conviction of the doctor, concerning the doctrine of willful blindness (Hellman 2009a, 2009b). The doctor was found guilty of violating the Controlled Substance Act because he prescribed narcotics in high doses to patients who claimed to be in pain. The Court believed the doctor should have known that these patients were reselling the drugs. The Court held that the physician's trust in the patient and his primary professional responsibility to the patient are insufficient justification for the doctor to prescribe narcotics under the Controlled Substance Act. Larger societal interests as mandated in the Act constrict the relationship.

I suggest that in the practice of medicine—especially in clinical investigation—there appear to be other variations of such willful behavior used by physicians to abrogate some of the constraints of the physician responsibility to the patient. For example, there is what I refer to as "willful ignorance," which I believe is necessary in order to justify the entering of patients into randomized clinical trials. Here the physician-scientist accepts the dichotomizing of knowledge. Either something is known, as determined by formal clinical experiments, or the physician has no knowledge regarding the utility of the different arms of a trial and thus can offer entrance to trial to the patient because the doctor can have no valid preference for any of the trial alternatives (Freedman 1987). Ignored here are the physician's previous clinical experience or other methods of creating a preference for a specific therapeutic alternative. While the doctor may be in equipoise regarding the differing trial arms for a group of patients in aggregate, it is far less likely that she or he will have no preference for the particular patient with a specific constellation of medical and social circumstances. Further, there are crucial differences between evidence, belief, and action. While the evidence may not be compelling in determining what the data show and what the doctor should believe, it still may be sufficient to determine what the preferred course of treatment might be (Hellman 2002). There is also some willful ignorance in the failure to recognize the differing motives or goals of the doctor as a scientist in the pursuit of the trial, and those of the physician in caring for the patient. The physician-scientist, while caring for the patient, also values scientifically proper performance of clinical trials and the resulting knowledge. For the academic, such successful clinical research furthers his or her academic career. These examples of conflicting responsibilities to the patient, one's career advancement, the profession, and society demonstrate the various tensions between the rights-based and utilitarian philosophies, as well as the conflicting goals of the physician.

Finally, in medical practice as well as research, there seems to be "willful indifference." In response to concerns of excessive paternalism by doctors, physicians sometime present a number of therapeutic alternatives with their advantages, limitations, and possible untoward effects, but without offering a specific recommendation. The patient recognizes this by asking some variation of the crucial question: "What would you do if you (or any of your relatives) were in my circumstances?" I am reminded of an acquaintance who was taken to the emergency room in severe pain following rupture of his Achilles tendon. He described being offered two alternative treatments: immediate surgery or conservative management. The advantages and disadvantages were presented to the patient, and he was asked to make a decision. He then asked the crucial "what would you do" question, to which the physician merely repeated the alternatives. This is willful indifference in order to avoid a most difficult part of patient care: recommending a course of action. There is also much willful indifference to be found in current performance of clinical research in the quest for evidence-based medicine. For example, doctors seem willfully indifferent to the complicated nature of the informed consent form, and they seem not to recognize the patient's fear of alienating the physician by not acquiescing to participate in a research protocol. Doctors also may seem to be indifferent to the emotional state of the patient at the time of signing the consent form, appearing indifferent to the coercion inherent in a trial, when access to a new therapy is dependent on the patient's participation in the study. As long as an acceptable consent form is signed, he or she is willfully indifferent to the circumstances surrounding the patient at the signing. The doctor appears to be willfully unaware of the trust placed on him or her by the patient when offering participation in a trial.

Patients count on their doctors' loyalty and fidelity and expect them to be truthful and candid, and to act primarily in their best interests. It is expected that these responsibilities to the patient will be paramount to the physician's personal gain, general societal benefit, or the acquisition of knowledge (Hellman 1995). Even in 1966, Beecher recognized the fallacy of informed consent and the essential responsibility of the doctor. He cautioned: "If suitably approached, patients will accede, on the basis of trust, to about any request their physician may make. . . . A far more dependable safeguard than consent is the presence of a truly *responsible* investigator" (p. 368). Some form of one or more of these "willful" behaviors are to be found in much clinical experimentation, as exemplified by the cases reported by Beecher as well as the Saenger studies described and analyzed in *Contested Science*. These represent the intentional avoidance of the potential or real conflicts between the pursuit of the experiment and the best interests of the patient.

Compelling Societal Need

One might argue that the Saenger studies can be considered acceptable because of the great threat of radiation exposure to warriors and even civilians if the Cold War became a hot one, requiring a better understanding of the medical consequences of radiation exposure. This overarching societal need might be thought to trump individual patient's rights in a fashion similar to the acceptance of forced quarantine. Perhaps these conflicting considerations were responsible for the ACHRE's failure to condemn the Cincinnati experiments.

A particular question for these Cold War radiation studies is whether there are instances of societal need so great that this need takes precedence over the primacy of the patient in the relationship between doctor and patient. As a society, we appear to have set limits on the primacy of patient rights. Utilitarian concerns can limit these rights when society's needs are great enough. Battlefield triage is an accepted method of maximally utilizing limited facilities, but it clearly limits the rights of some patients. Society specifically mandates such modification of the doctor–patient relationship in the case of quarantine, reporting certain diseases, and gunshot wounds. Do the Cincinnati studies escape criticism because of such overriding societal need? Less compelling societal benefit arguments were made in defense of the studies of hepatitis virus transmission performed on inmates at Willowbrook, a state institution for mentally retarded children and adults that was referred to in the Beecher report. Here it was averred that the study offered great societal good and that the institutional setting would result in viral transmission anyway. This thesis was eventually rejected by the medical community, but this change in attitude did not come easily, nor was it universally accepted. These studies were done contemporaneously with the Cincinnati studies, as were many of the others described by Beecher. By 1973 reports of these and other examples of patients or inmates being used in medical experiments raised such concern that Senators Mondale and Kennedy caused Congress to establish a national commission to deal with medical ethical principles. This resulted in the Belmont Report of 1979. These reports and many other considerations of the ethics of experimenting on human beings are from the vantage point of the general public and to some extent of the putative patient.

But there are further considerations for the doctor when involved in individual patient care, which further constrict physician behavior. Unless explicitly limited by society, the primary responsibility of the doctor is to the patient, not to society at large. While in the past general societal benefit was sufficient reason to modify the patient priority, recently this preference seems to have evolved to reassert the doctor's primary responsibility to the patient. This is evidenced by the changing attitudes to the experiments described by Beecher and perhaps to the TBI studies. Willful ignorance or indifference is inconsistent with fidelity and loyalty to the patient.

Relevance for Today

Contested Medicine is an interesting, thorough, and thoughtful consideration of the Cincinnati experiments. These studies received widespread attention by the public and academic medical community especially after articles in the *Washington Post*. I had read reports of the research and had heard Saenger speak, and thought I knew the story well. Kutcher's book provides much new information about the history of the Cincinnati project, its dual financial support by the military and the NIH, and the various review bodies both within the University of Cincinnati and in the larger community. The book is quite nuanced and provides the social and historical contest to the studies and the evolving bioethics of the time.

Benthamite utilitarianism conflicting with deontology in clinical research is a recurring issue when considering experiments using human beings during the evolving bioethics of the latter half of the twentieth century. What makes this book especially valuable is the rich context provided for the studies, as well as the case study method used in the analysis. We see different evaluations of the experimental treatment and their ethical status, ranging from those of a junior faculty committee to those of the university administration, the military, the American College of Radiology, the National Institutes of Health, Congress, and newspapers, culminating with the Advisory Committee on Human Radiation Experiments appointed by President Clinton in 1994. The evaluations change depending on evolving norms, the apparent likelihood of the use of radiation as a weapon of war, and the nature of the reviewing body. The book provides a sophisticated appreciation of these factors and is an excellent addition to our understanding of those important times.

Individual rights were foremost in the minds and actions of Thomas Jefferson, the author of the Declaration of Independence, and the framers of the Constitution of the United States of America. The Bill of Rights promulgated by James Madison highlights the importance of individual rights. The Supreme Court's thinking with regard to the first of these rights may be a useful parallel to the tensions between individual patient rights and the potential societal benefit seen in clinical research. Freedom of speech is strongly asserted in the First Amendment, but the Court has subsequently limited this right by indicating that such behavior as falsely shouting "fire" in a crowded theater is not protected as free speech. Similarly, today "hate speech" is prohibited. But in a First Amendment case, even the conservative Justice Frankfurter warned the court to avoid "the passions of the day." Thus while we do accept some limitations on our rights, these are to be uncommon and only applicable in unusual and threatening circumstances for society. Such an abrogation of free speech by the "clear and present danger" criteria used to limit speech against the draft in World War I, while accepted at the time, has been criticized more recently as too limiting, and it might be analogous to the World War II efforts of Saenger and his group studying TBI. Whether and in what circumstances such exceptions to individual rights are valid, the clear trend in bioethics is to enhance and assure patient's rights.

This story should also be read as a cautionary tale. If we continue in the fashion of the last half-century, what seems appropriate today may not be deemed so by the evolving medical ethics of our successors. This admonition may pertain to the vigorous promulgation of formal prospective, controlled clinical investigations as the paramount arbiter of medical knowledge, which may encourage implicitly or even explicitly denigration of information gained by other means. Many randomized trials, especially those using untreated controls with serious or potentially fatal circumstances, may become suspect. Such was the assertion in the early drug therapy studies of HIV/AIDS. Patient advocate Rebecca Pringle Smith cautioned in 1989, "Even if you have a supply of compliant martyrs, trials must have some ethical validity." Our current emphasis on prospective randomized controlled clinical trials, while having as a goal increasing knowledge and thus better care for all, does not have the compelling national need seen in the Cold War at the time of the Cincinnati studies. Restricting access to new treatments only to patients willing to participate in trials may be an effective inducement to participation, but will such coercion be considered acceptable by future generations? Beecher, Tuskegee, and Cincinnati as described and evaluated in *Contested Medicine* urge us to develop research methodologies with less tension between their possible social utility and individual patient rights. Willful indifference to the current discord obscures but does not abrogate the issue. This book—like the Keats poem "On First Looking into Chapman's Homer" as paraphrased in the title of this essay—may provide a vantage point for viewing the future.

REFERENCES

Beecher HK. 1966. Ethics and clinical research. *N Engl J Med* 274:367–372.
Freedman B. 1987. Equipoise and the ethics of clinical research. *N Engl J Med* 317: 141–145.
Hellman DS. 2002. Evidence, belief, and action: The failure of equipoise to resolve the ethical tension in the randomized clinical trial. *J Law Med Ethics* 30:375–380.
Hellman DS. 2009a. Prosecuting doctors for trusting patients. *George Mason Law Rev* 16: 701–745.
Hellman DS. 2009b. Willfully blind for good reason. *Crim Law Philos* 3:301–316.
Hellman S. 1995. The patient and the public good. *Nature Med* 1:400–402.
Hellman S, and DS Hellman. 1991. Of mice but not men: Problems of the randomized clinical trial. *N Engl J Med* 325:1585–1591.
Kass LR. 1985. *Toward a more natural science: Biology and human affairs.* New York: Free Press.
Palca J. 1989. AIDS drug trials enter a new age. *Science* 246:19–21.
Rothman DJ. 1991. *Strangers at the bedside.* New York: Basic Books.
Saenger E. 1967. Effects of total-partial body therapeutic radiation in man. In *Proceedings of the First International Symposium on the Biological Interpretation of Dose from Accelerator Produced Radiation*, ed. R. Wallace. Washington, DC: US Atomic Energy Commission.
Saenger E, et al. 1973. Whole body and partial body radiotherapy of advanced cancer. *Amer J Roentg Radiat Ther* 117:670–685.

General Readings

Fried C. 1974. *Medical experimentation.* Amsterdam: North-Holland.
Royall R. 1997. *Statistical evidence: A likelihood paradigm.* London: Chapman & Hall.
Stone GR. 2004. *Perilous times.* New York: Norton.

MANAGED CARE AND THE DOCTOR–PATIENT RELATIONSHIP: A MÉNAGE À TROIS

1997 unpublished

An apocryphal print shop is reported to have a sign next to the order counter offering

> **Quality, Cost, Speed**
> **Choose Only Two!!**

This sign makes apparent the tension associated with trying to achieve high quality at low cost and at maximum speed. Today, there is a similar tense triad in medical care as we attempt to achieve superior, economical medical care that is equitably distributed. The Clinton administration's proposal "The President's Health Security Plan" emphasized equity and cost control, but many people worried about the maintenance of high quality. That plan has not come to fruition; rather, we have seen an explosion in private managed care. As such it is responsive to the marketplace with cost control being the main objective. According to Jordan Cohen, president of the Association of American Medical Colleges, speaking at The University of Chicago, "rather than managed care this is managed cost."

Managed care produces a second uncomfortable triad: a *ménage à trois* of patient, doctor, and managed care organization quite different from the traditional bilateral doctor–patient relationship. The conflicts associated with both triads need to be addressed. We must attend to the difficulties of controlling cost, maintaining quality, and fairly distributing health care and we must be wary of the effect of interposing the managed care organization into the relationship between patient and doctor. Many individual physicians as well as professional medical groups have registered concern as to how the doctor–patient relationship is affected by managed care. In this new way to practice medicine, the responsibility for husbanding limited resources often resides in the treating physician, producing an unfortunate change in the way in which doctors and patients view each other.

The community should also reject the notion that the medical profession should be the rationing agency rather than the larger society. I understand that the word "rationing" has unfortunate connotations, but it must be accepted as necessary, however disagreeable. Surely these difficult decisions must be informed by community values and rationing allocations made according to these principles. The application of the principles and even the principles themselves may differ for different communities. Physicians will be needed as expert consultants, but the decisions regarding high-cost low-yield diagnostic procedures, investments in expensive procedures for the elderly, palliative care, and many other issues require community, not medical, judgment. It is only such community-determined principles delineating the rights and responsibilities of individuals that can ensure that difficult rationing decisions are consonant with societal values. Further, preserving the valuable doctor-patient relationship requires separating the primary responsibility of the individual physician to the patient being cared for from the responsibility for controlling health care costs. Bedside rationing is bad for the doctor, the patient, and the community.

There is a consensus that medical spending cannot continue as it has in the past. Managed care appears more likely than fee-for-service medicine with a cost-based reimbursement system to control costs and to limit over-utilization and over-charging. In the past because the practice of medicine was relatively unconstrained by cost considerations, therapeutic efficacy—the capacity to produce a desired effect—was valued regardless of expense. In contrast, the competition between various managed care providers emphasizes efficiency—efficacy as a function of cost—rather than efficacy alone. While this may result in limiting medical utilization, it raises concerns as to the choices, extent, and most importantly, the relevant criteria used to determine the efficient use of resources. Society must provide guidelines that balance efficacy and efficiency to achieve satisfactory quality, quantity, and distribution of health care. The physician in dealing with an individual patient must then provide a program that maximizes that individual patient's benefits within these socially-defined limits.

Personal Care

The physician in the doctor–patient relationship is expected to provide personal care requiring that the patient is seen as an individual, not as a member of a group of patients with similar characteristics. The care should be fashioned to meet the individual determinants of that patient's illness, other medical conditions, attitudes, beliefs, and preferences. If, in the managed care organization, the physician is also asked to husband the group's resources, either by the group limiting the pool of funds available for the care of a panel of patients or by rewarding or penalizing the physician according to the extent of resource utilization, then the physician can no longer be concerned only with maximizing that patient's benefits. Furthermore, treatment guidelines for groups of patients with similar traits currently being promulgated as a method to ensure good care may discourage personal care tailored to the individual. Justice Charles Fried, then of the Harvard Law School and now of the Massachusetts Supreme Judicial Court, worried more than 20 years ago that the personal care inherent in the doctor–patient relationship would be replaced by "the physician as agent of an efficient health care delivery system."[1] That concern seems even more pressing today.

Not only does the physician act as double agent when responsible to serve both the patient's best interests and parsimony, he or she is also, in part, a secret agent. The doctor's duties to the managed care organization include constraining cost, a duty largely hidden or at least unknown to the patient. There have always been societal restrictions limiting the physician from being completely the patient's agent even in the traditional relationship. Examples of this are the required reporting of certain diseases or wounds caused in a suspicious fashion. These exceptions are limited and explicit, providing boundaries within which the physician is expected to serve only the patient's best interests. The traditional fidelity of doctor to patient is also modified when patients participate in clinical investigation. Clear, explicit, and regulated procedures have been developed to assure that patient's participation is voluntary and that the patient understands the proposed study. It does not appear that there is similar informed consent given by the patient to the modification of physician loyalty often inherent in the managed care doctor–patient relationship. There are "gag" rules in some plans that specifically prohibit the physician from revealing the general financial arrangements, all the treatment options, and the particular pecuniary implications associated with treatment decisions. Even if the patient accedes to a modified doctor–patient relationship in managed care, the physician should have great difficulty in participating in a situation that requires such divided loyalties. This conflict is the basis of much of the physician concern with practicing in many managed care settings. The basis of medicine as a profession requires that the physician's efforts are devoted to serve the patient's best interests. This is not to suggest that in fee-for-service medicine the physician's behavior is not potentially affected by financial considerations. In the past both patients and doctors understood that the more physicians did, the more they were rewarded. The patient and the profession expected the doctor to ignore these pecuniary considerations and act only in the patient's best interest. In contrast, having physicians responsible for the financial success of the managed care organization, husbanding limited resources in the context of individual patient care, results in a new trilateral arrangement whose premise is quite different from that currently understood.

Health Care Rights

During the health care debates associated with "The President's Health Security Plan" there appeared to be agreement that some minimum level of care should be accessible to all people as a basic right. Currently, there is no plan and there is less security. Access to health care for all Americans should be a compelling community concern. This general right to health care is not served by the current competing managed care organizations. Instead, individual providers attempt to restrict access in order to maximize the profitability of the plan, for example, the use of preexisting conditions as a reason to deny medical insurance. The very fact that coverage is employment dependent and therefore is limited to a person able to work (and his or her family) is a form of selection. Such plans assume no responsibility for the uninsured; rather they favor coverage for the healthiest participants. If universal access is a shared community value, it must be implemented by the community; the marketplace will not arrive at this without direction.

Not only does society appear to endorse a basic right *to* some level of health care, but the community also supports the view, I believe, that individuals have certain rights *in* health care as well. In particular, it expects personal care from doctors—treatment fitting the particular patient's clinical circumstances, attitudes, and preferences. The patient expects the physician to be truthful and loyal without any competing obligations. The patient, by virtue of being more vulnerable, relies on the doctor to protect his or her interests. Since patient autonomy is also an important value, the physician is needed to prepare the patient to make fully informed choices among alternatives. In the managed care context, the physician's duty to the patient is often in conflict with his or her responsibility to the group in husbanding resources. In addition, "gag" rules or other confidential arrangements restrict the candor expected of the physician by the patient. Limiting diagnostic or therapeutic alternatives may make economic sense and may also be more efficient but does not necessarily protect the patient's best interest and will surely restrict the patient's right to make choices.

Untangling the Physician

To deal with this *ménage à trois* we must separate the various roles of the physician explicitly and without confusion. Physicians should provide their expertise, but it is the community rather than the medical profession that should make decisions regarding medical resource allocation. In formulating these policies, doctors can serve a useful role. The physician has specialized knowledge about the potential value and dangers of the various diagnostic and therapeutic procedures. Physicians should accept their responsibility to help limit the rising costs of medicine, and it is also important that they protect patients, both present and future, from unreasonable restrictions on care. This must be done by the participation of physicians and their professional organizations in helping society develop the strategies, criteria, and guidelines for the utilization of limited resources. In order for this to occur, doctors—individually and organizationally—must embrace the need to control health care expenditures. However, it is as members of professional groups and as members of the larger society that physicians act as distributors and monitors of health care expenditures. These important utilitarian public health activities are concerned with maximizing the public good within acceptable budgetary constraints but without concern for how each individual is affected. In contrast, a physician to an individual patient must be concerned with that patient. The doctor must continue to provide personal care designed to best meet the needs of that individual. The physician must in no way be inhibited from treating the patient with dignity as an individual, and the patient must command fully the loyalty and honesty of the physician. This means that "gag" rules and linking of physician rewards and penalties to the economic consequences of his or her behavior must be eliminated. Contracts containing "no-cause" non-renewal clauses should be forbidden. The physician should be judged by the quality of care provided. Measurement of this professional performance must include objective measures of outcome and consistency with management guidelines, but it also should consider how the treatment coincided with the individual patient's circumstances and preferences. We must be assured that appropriate alternatives are presented and that the patient's autonomy is preserved in making decisions. Deviation from treatment guidelines must not only be accepted but embraced, if reasonably justified. For the physician this means devotion to personal care without being capricious in patient management.

Community Values, Not the Marketplace

If the physician were the customer in that apocryphal print shop that allowed only two choices from equity, quality, and cost, he or she would most likely choose equity and quality since this would provide the patients with the best care and make it available to all. While this is the most comfortable choice for the physician, it will escalate costs the mos. The community has indicated that health care expenditures are growing too rapidly and must be controlled. Determining the proper distribution of limited resources is the responsibility of an informed society. It requires forging a consensus on how such decisions should be made and the principles on which such decisions must be based. Oregon's list of Medicare-covered procedures was just a small taste of what lies ahead.

While there are many who feel that government regulation is a blunt instrument poorly suited to solve our problems, already there are regulatory endeavors assuring some minimum level of quality of health care. Both Congress and the President have inveighed against "drive-by" deliveries and outpatient mastectomies. State legislators from at least nine states are expected to introduce the Managed Care Consumer Protection Act in their state legislatures. That title itself questions whether managed care organizations share community values. Being at The University of Chicago has made me quite aware of the value of the free market as an efficient provider. While the marketplace may have such credentials, it is necessarily neither wise nor just. It need not respond to the values of society other than as reflected in their economic consequences. The decisions needed to control health care expenditures require more than efficiency and economics. Health care choices should be the result of a societal consensus as to the extent and method of resource allocation based on shared values that include universal access and provide for individual rights in health care. At present, both are at risk.

REFERENCE

1. Fried C. Rights and Health Care: Beyond Equity and Efficiency. *N Engl J Med* 1975;293:241–245.

FIN DE SIÈCLE MEDICINE: AVOIDING THE UNINTENDED CONSEQUENCES OF HEALTH CARE REFORM

Republished with permission of Brookings Institution Press, from "Fin de siècle medicine. Avoiding the unintended consequences of health care reform," Samuel Hellman, *Brookings Review* volume 12, edition 2, 1994; permission conveyed through Copyright Clearance Center, Inc.

Fin de siècle. Literally, the end of the century. By implication, a time of change and transition, a time to take stock of accomplishments and consider future directions. The sense of imminent change attendant on the turning of a century is particularly palpable in the field of medicine as a result of the political consensus that the US health care system must be reformed, that limits must be placed on American medicine.

The twentieth century has seen great changes in the practice of medicine. First and foremost has been an increase in medical capabilities as medicine and medical education have become increasingly scientific. Technological advances have transformed patient evaluation and therapies. At the turn of the last century, diagnosis was the problem. Today, the ability to diagnose far outpaces the ability to devise effective therapy. Perhaps the most graphic example of the change is the use of x-rays. In December 1895 the German physicist Wilhelm Roentgen presented the world with its first x-ray, a vision of Mrs. Roentgen's hand on a photographic plate. Today, computed tomography (CT) and magnetic resonance imaging have made diagnosis increasingly a matter of technology. Most recently the great advance has been the biological revolution, whose application to medicine is still in its infancy.

The view of the physician has also changed. Medicine has become less pastoral. It is less a calling. The physician is expected to be much more the technical expert. Both patient and physician clearly perceive a financial component to medicine. Specialization has become the rule, with a resulting decrease in primary care physicians. The old view of the caring, empathetic, paternal physician acting in the best interest of the patient, often making unilateral decisions about what was best for the patient, has yielded to the current view of the technical expert who is to involve the patient in decision-making and be a consultant rather than a loyal guide and supporter through the travail of illness.

What further changes will health care reform make in the practice of medicine? Reform, as we all know, has been stimulated primarily by the rising costs of medicine, perhaps most disturbingly, the rate of rise of these expenditures. My colleague at The University of Chicago, Mark Siegler, captures Americans' sense of the profligacy of their health care system by recalling Jack Kent Cooke's explanation of why he fired George Allen as coach of the Washington Redskins football team: "I gave Allen an unlimited budget," snorted Cook, "and he exceeded it." But while much of President Clinton's "Health Security Act" is focused on costs, its proposed solutions will greatly affect medical practice and our expectations of it.

Make no mistake, I strongly favor reform of our health care system. I do not suffer from "mural dyslexia": I can read the writing on the wall. The changes proposed by the president, attacking not only excessive costs but also the grave problem of lack of access to medical care, are all well intended. But in what the president characterizes as the biggest social program enacted since Social Security, the likelihood for unintended consequences is great. Rather than wait to deal with those consequences, we should engage now in a public dialogue about the benefits and shortcomings of our current health care practices so that the changes we make foster and preserve what we value and correct what we do not. Furthermore, making our system more efficient will reduce costs, but it will not affect the rate of increase in health care expenditures. Accomplishing that will require some form of rationing. And that surely requires widespread public discussion—to make sure finance-driven reform does not lead us in wrong directions.

I see potential risks in two areas: first, research and innovation; and, second, the traditional doctor–patient relationship.

Medical Innovation

Many of the treatments medicine offers today are what I would describe as "halfway technology." Although they clearly have beneficial results, they do not solve the medical problem—as, for example, treating a bacterial infection with effective, nontoxic antibiotics solves *that* problem. Examples of halfway technology, to name but a few, are renal dialysis, most cancer treatment today, coronary artery bypass surgery, and the use of insulin to treat diabetes. All have clear benefits. No doubt patients are better for having received them. But all leave much to be desired. And all are very expensive—because of the equipment and personnel involved, because the treatment often produces morbidity, because it often does not cure but only changes the pace of illness. Despite these limitations we value them greatly, for without them much of what is beneficial in medical treatment would be lost for our patients.

When I began my residency in 1960, Hodgkin's Disease was fatal for about 75% of its victims, usually young adults who suffered greatly during their illness. Today, with the advent of halfway technology in the form of precise high-energy linear accelerators and multidrug chemotherapy, as well as much better diagnostic techniques, the situation has reversed. Now 75% of patients are cured. Nevertheless, the treatment is still halfway technology, unsatisfactory because it produces many undesirable early and late side effects and is time consuming, expensive, and not universally effective. What will health care reform do to such expensive, effective, but not optimal treatments? I fear it will try to husband limited resources by constraining these procedures and by trying to make them as efficient as possible—ultimately stifling innovation and discouraging efforts to improve the treatment, while preserving the status quo in medicine.

The primary site for clinical innovation is the academic health center. But investigations carried on in these centers are often not considered to be research, whose support should come from the major funding agencies such as the National Institutes of Health, but rather technical improvements, to be funded by patient care revenues. Naturally, these investigations, plus the cost of extensive medical teaching programs for medical students, residents, and postgraduate fellows, push the cost of care in the academic center far beyond that in the community hospital. Although the president's plan provides funding for these centers, it primarily replaces monies now provided as Medicare Indirect Medical Education Payments, which recognize some of the costs of residents and medical students, rather than supporting investigation. The only clinical investigations slated for support in the president's plan are those that evaluate the outcomes of current medical practices and improve the delivery of care. Preserving medical innovation as a vital mission of the academic medical center will require a clearly designated mechanism of support.

Both innovation and its site of performance are thus vulnerable to a system driven primarily by a cost-control mandate. Already, in the Minneapolis–St. Paul region, the University of Minnesota has been omitted from integrated health insurance plans in favor of community hospitals, which, unencumbered by innovation and training costs, can perform the same services more cheaply. The president's plan requires that health plans have contractual relations with academic centers for treatment of rare diseases and for specialized procedures, but fiscal prudence will encourage restricting these arrangements as much as possible, still leaving academic centers at risk. In arranging for the reform of the financing of health care, society must be clear about the value it accords continued research and innovation and whether it regards them as goals of importance at least equal to controlling costs.

The Biological Revolution

Related is a concern that we will no longer encourage commercial efforts to bring to clinical medicine the fruits of the biological revolution. The proliferation of small biotechnology companies developing new therapeutics such as human growth hormone and growth factors that control blood cell production provides evidence of a new field in which the United States is the world leader. A market that values cost control more than increased spending for improvement in health care is not likely to continue the expansion of biotechnology, at least as directed toward eventual medical use. Some observers are already concerned about the slow commercial development of growth factors that have enormous clinical value in the healing of wounds.

The public has yet to realize the dimensions and implication of the biological revolution on which we have embarked. Some observers have compared it with the revolution in physics triggered by the development of quantum mechanics. In some ways, and without much hyperbole, a more apt comparison might be with the industrial revolution—for the biological revolution will transform our daily living. But how will the biological revolution be affected by health care reform? Once begun, the revolution cannot be stopped. But it can certainly be slowed or redirected.

The new biology has already begun to present us with vexing ethical questions, most obviously those concerning the beginning and end of life. More questions will come, many hinging on considerations of individual versus societal good and raising the specter of rationing. It is simplistic and wrong to say that these difficult problems are caused by science and can be avoided by no longer supporting research. The genie is out of the bottle. What we must do is encourage public dialogue on how to use the results of scientific discovery. Societal value judgments must underlie any discussion of the rationing of health care required by cost containment.

Doctors and Patients

The nature of the doctor–patient relationship has already been changed by the scientific advances of medicine during the twentieth century. How will it change further under the pressure to reform health care to control costs?

Traditionally the medical profession has been primarily concerned with healing, with the family doctor caring directly for his patients with unswerving loyalty—reducing suffering, curing if possible, and comforting always. The increase in specialization and scientific medicine in this century has challenged this romantic view of the physician and has generated a nostalgic longing for general practitioners—who, we tend to forget, had far fewer effective therapies to offer than today's specialists do.

Dovetailing with this wish for a return to the simpler age of the nonspecialist is the conviction of health care reformers that expanding the role and number of primary care physicians would be a major force for cost control. We are already moving, under pressure to lower medical costs, toward "managed care," with primary care physicians assigned the role of "gatekeepers." Will the president's plan increase the switch to managed care, and if so, is that what we want?

Will the increased importance of the primary care physician as opposed to the specialist, for example, reduce the use and availability of halfway technology? Will the new forms of practice diminish further the relationship between patient and doctor? Perhaps more disturbingly, will concerns for cost and societal utility undermine the confidence of the patient that the physician is acting in his or her best interests? Increasingly, physicians will be members of organizations whose primary mission will be providing acceptable care at the lowest price—admittedly a laudable goal for the system. But what are the implications for the physician–patient relationship? Both the traditional view of the caring doctor and the more recent one of the technical expert are based on the belief that the physician will act in the patient's best interest. Will this belief be eroded in a managed care system, especially as physicians are rewarded or penalized based on expenses incurred as a result of their efforts on the patient's behalf? A recent report in the *Los Angeles Times* describes the development of for-profit "super groups" of physicians, formed in preparation for health care reform legislation, in which generalists will benefit financially by handling patients and procedures themselves rather than referring them to specialists. Rather than a warm, empathetic general practitioner, will health care reform offer us instead a busy physician responsible both for husbanding limited resources and for being the patient's advocate? I fear the conflicting responsibilities will undermine the essence of the doctor–patient relationship: the assurance of the physician's primary loyalty to the patient.

Reform and National Values

To conclude, I worry that the emphasis of health care reformers on correcting problems of cost may inadvertently damage some aspects of the current system that we value greatly. We must also accept that control of the rate of rise in health care costs will require some form of rationing. Public discussion of all these issues is essential. Rather than finding later that we must undo the unintended consequences of reform, we must guide the reform process to be consistent with our values.

Do we as a nation believe that we should slow down the engine of medical innovation? This engine is traditionally thought to be in the university, but it is also in industry, where many of the technologic and biologic advances found in the laboratory are brought to fruition. What of the opportunities provided by the biological revolution? Reducing medical innovation and discovery will have consequences for our position as the leader in biomedical research and the quality of our very best medicine.

The changes in the social context of medical care also suggest a changing social contract, one in which the relationship between the doctor and the patient will be much more constrained by considerations of the common good. The physician may be asked to be less an agent of the individual patient, to assume divided obligations and responsibilities. While we must develop societal consensus regarding cost control, we should not undermine the individual doctor–patient relationship and the shared understanding of the physician's primary loyalty and fidelity to the patient.

PREMISE, PROMISE, PARADIGM, AND PROPHESY

This article was first published in *Nature Clinical Practice Oncology* 2005;2(7):325.

While the inductive method of scientific research is powerful in disproving hypotheses, it cannot prove them. Repeated efforts failing to disprove a theory tend to reinforce our sense of the validity of the hypothesis. If the hypothesis is associated with added benefits to its proponents then a conditional premise may become a paradigm, or occasionally a dogma. Two examples from breast cancer research are Halsted's contiguous-spread model and the systemic-dissemination model championed by Fisher. Halsted's central premise was that cancer spread centrifugally from the primary tumor to regional lymph nodes, and only afterwards to distant sites. This led to treatments designed to eradicate the tumor at the primary site in conjunction with draining regional lymph nodes becoming the paradigm for all cancer treatment. This model was reinforced by its attractiveness to surgeons, because it rewarded technical proficiency and made the surgeon the center of cancer management.

Surgeons who had the temerity to question this premise, such as Geoffrey Keynes in the UK and later Bernard Fisher in the US, were considered heretics. The Halsted model failed to explain distant tumor metastases in patients for whom local regional tumor ablation was successful. Thus, the systemic model emerged, which described tumors of two types: local only or systemic. If the former, then only local treatment is needed, but if the latter, dissemination occurs before clinical detection, and cure depends on effective systemic therapy. Acceptance of the systemic model was aided and abetted by the resulting central position of the medical oncologist in cancer care. We now appreciate that both hypotheses have limitations and that cancer should be considered a spectrum of disease proclivities, ranging from those whose disease will remain localized to those that appear to have disseminated disease before clinical detection; most breast cancers have a malignant capacity somewhere in between.

Much enthusiasm exists for "targeted" pharmaceuticals that are expected to be very effective for certain tumors with specific molecular characteristics, while exhibiting limited toxicity. Gleevec® (imatinib) in chronic myelogenous leukemia is considered to be the prototype of these. While it is still too early to have strong opinions as to the validity and robustness of targeted drugs in other tumors, it is not too early to caution against their enthusiastic and uncritical acceptance. Targeted agents are attractive, and the promise for future designer drugs is enhanced by the advent of the molecular era and modern drug formulation. This can lead to hyperbolic prophesy, such as that attributed by Gina Kolata to Nobelist James Dewey Watson a few years ago, in heralding the transforming power of antiangiogenic treatment on the front page of the *New York Times*. I read recently in that same newspaper that the success of Herceptin® (trastuzumab), targeted to *HER2* overexpression in certain breast cancers, and Avastin® (bevacizumab), an antiangiogeneic drug, caused a 50% rise in the stock price of their manufacturer, Genentech, in only a matter of weeks. While it is recognized that group opinion and naive enthusiasm are hallmarks of stock market participants, such behavior can have serious consequences in medical science. The results are promising but we must be careful not to over-promise our patients, the public, or ourselves. How these results will change the treatment paradigm is still uncertain. We may wish for them to herald an attractive new paradigm, but wishing that something were so does not make it so, but rather deceives us and confounds our thinking. Acceptance of the conditional nature of the scientific method should lead to humility as well as a healthy skepticism when confronting excessive promises. We should leave that to stock market enthusiasts.

LEARNING WHILE CARING: MEDICINE'S EPISTEMOLOGY

Reprinted with permission. © (2014) American Society of Clinical Oncology. All rights reserved. Hellman, S. *J Clin Oncol.* 32(25):2804–8.

Abstract

An essential epistemic consideration is the conditional nature of medical knowledge. This uncertainty must be understood when acquiring new knowledge or designing treatments. We must value all sources of information, neither discarding those deemed lower on the current value scale, nor slavishly accepting randomized clinical trials or their meta-analyses as the fount of all knowledge. Generally, the tension between clinical investigation and individual care can be framed in a utilitarian versus deontologic or rights-based philosophy. The utilitarian is clearly appropriate to public health considerations, but what is learned for public health may not necessarily be in the best interest of an individual patient. In utilitarianism, the distribution of goods—in this case, health—is not important; rather, it is the amount of total good gained that is to be maximized. Too often we assume that survival or cure is a sufficient metric, with no similar quantitative measure of other factors. This often leads to the so-called best treatment being not what the patient wants. All personal care requires consideration of both the helpful and harmful consequences of treatment in the context of individual patient comorbidity, preferences, and fears. Knowledge of patients in general is not what is required; rather, it is how to apply the information to the particular patient that is the heart of medical practice. Each patient's episode of illness is the consequence of a unique interaction of that individual with the disease. Good patient care considers the disease and its management in the context of each patient's values.

Introduction

Physicians have a responsibility to continue their professional education while they practice medicine. Learning while caring for patients must be consistent with their responsibilities as physicians as well as with patient's health care rights. Epistemology, the study of knowledge and justified belief, is especially relevant to how physicians learn and apply this knowledge to the individual patient. This essay considers some of these methods of learning and the nature of that knowledge. Because my interest is in oncology, the examples used are from that field, but I am confident that similar ones could be found in many other fields of medicine dealing with serious illness.

The medical profession accepts that although intensive preparation is essential, much of what is taught in medical school needs to be discarded, corrected, or modified throughout the physician's career. New knowledge changes our understanding of disease and its management, and lifelong learning is essential to continue to practice properly. Continuing evolution of knowledge is meant to modify that acquired during one's medical education and postgraduate training. Medicine is a program of lifelong learning, but for the practitioner, this must be acquired while caring for patients. New medical knowledge comes from reading the literature, both print and electronic, and from presentations at professional meetings. It comes from the teachings of leaders in the profession; it comes from clinical experience in the aggregate as well as from individual patients. All of these sources may provide some new evidence or concept leading to improved knowledge so as to treat future patients more skillfully. Medicine is a learned profession, but perhaps more important, it is a learning profession.

An essential epistemic consideration is the conditional nature of medical knowledge. It is not binary. We are neither completely ignorant nor reasonably certain. In reality, our knowledge is conditional, is often approximate, and varies over a wide spectrum of confidence. Karl Popper[1] tells us that the inductive method may give us an increasingly more satisfactory approximation of truth, but knowledge derived inductively is always conditional and subject to being disproved. The conditional nature and thus the uncertainty of medical knowledge must be understood when either acquiring new knowledge or designing patient treatment.

Information Hierarchy

During the last few decades, there has been a new emphasis on the valuation of medical information resulting in a hierarchy of the quality of medical evidence. This critical assessment of the evidence used to change medical practice has led to evidence-based medicine, an epistemologic consideration of the quality of medical knowledge. In general, the National Institute for Health and Care Excellence (NICE) in the United Kingdom and similar US agencies have developed hierarchies of medical knowledge, with randomized clinical trials and their aggregating meta-analyses as the most estimable evidence, and case reports, individual experience, and expert opinions as the least satisfactory methods of attaining knowledge. Although there have been some disagreements with the notion that randomized controlled trials or that meta-analyses of such trials should produce necessarily better data than well-designed observational trials, their priority seems well accepted. We should be careful to regard all sources of information as worthwhile, neither discarding those considered to be lower on the current value scale, nor slavishly accepting randomized clinical trials or their meta-analyses as the fount of all knowledge. All information may be useful if critically appraised. A poorly conceived or performed study high in the hierarchy is less meritorious than a well-done, less fashionable study. Whatever the relative value of the different sources of information, they all contribute to the physician's knowledge. How these multiple sources are combined is the heart of interpretation, some of which may be tacit rather than explicit. Polonyi[2] believes that these actions are not just deduced from the information, but rather, when combined with tacit knowledge, they provide more knowledge than the explicit information alone. Although related, the acquisition of knowledge is different from clinical judgment and knowledge gained from personal care; this essay is about learning in the context of clinical practice and research. Clinical judgment uses this knowledge combined with experience and the clinical circumstances. Personal care modifies this judgment with consideration of the patient's wishes, as well as other clinical and social circumstances. Forming clinical judgment, Quirk[3] emphasizes, involves intuition and metacognition; the former is rapid and unconscious, whereas the latter is deliberate and conscious. However, this knowledge of patients in general is not what is required for practice; rather, it is how to apply the information to the particular patient that is the heart of medical practice.

The Past

"Those who cannot remember the past are condemned to repeat it," Santayana admonishes us.[4] Nowhere is this truer than in medicine. Past experience, both of the individual physician and of others, as reported in the literature or in person, can be an important guide. Clinical experience, individually and even more importantly when collected, can be a rich resource for the physician and educator. Unfortunately, there are many pitfalls having to do with patient selection criteria and observer bias. One physician's selection criteria may result in favorable outcomes, but the clinical judgment in his or her selection is often not apparent in published reports or lectures. Despite its limitation, learning from one's own clinical experience is often the most powerful educational instrument used.

Information about past patients can also be considered at a later time, as new techniques become available. Such "old wine in new bottles" may provide extraordinarily valuable information: for example, applying new molecular techniques to archival pathologic material and then correlating them with prognosis and the results of the treatment applied. Such studies are especially important because of the limitation of prospective trials of diseases with a long natural history.

Randomized Clinical Trials

Because this technique, with its aggregating meta-analyses, is considered the most important and reliable source of medical information, we should consider some of the problems with the method. Although I have discussed elsewhere my concerns with the potential ethical conflict imposed by this study design—between the patient's rights in health care and the professional obligations of the physician on the one hand, and the potential societal benefit of the knowledge gained on the other[5]—there are some epistemic limitations to this method as well. The more we subdivide patients into smaller and presumably more homogeneous groups, the more cumbersome the randomization and the more patients required in the experiment. With the increasing use of molecular tools to discriminate smaller, more homogeneous subgroups, there will be more groups, but many fewer patients in any particular group. Conversely, the more we lump patients into larger heterogeneous groups, the more unlikely the results will be applicable to individual patients and the less appropriate the knowledge gained will be for individual patient care. Randomized trials often require large numbers of patients to detect a statistically significant difference, resulting in a logistic hurdle that is often solved by multi-institutional collaboration. Unfortunately, this adds to the heterogeneity of patient groups and increases concerns about the uniform application of the study design. One highly valued solution to the problem of insufficient power of individual trials has been the use of the meta-analysis, but this only exaggerates the problem by aggregating patients into large, heterogeneous groups.

Meta-analysis also depends on the premise that various studies can be considered together if they have a common variable: that is, being randomized. This is only true if the same theory of disease underlies the hypothesis being tested; otherwise, the results can be quite confusing. The individual studies in a meta-analysis may have the same variable but compare different classes of patients, often while asking different questions. For example, there have been extensive meta-analyses of the use of postoperative radiation therapy for breast cancer. In these meta-analyses, both patients who received systemic adjuvant therapy and those who did not are often combined because, in both types of studies, the administration of radiation therapy is the randomized variable. However, the studies in which all patients receive adjuvant systemic therapy and are then randomly assigned to postoperative radiation therapy are testing a hypothesis based on a different theory of disease spread than those studies of patients not receiving systemic agents. In the latter case, the question being asked is whether the destruction of persistent subclinical disease in the breast, chest wall, and lymph node areas is important because it is the source of subsequent metastases. Although in the case of the uniform use of adjuvant systemic therapy, randomizing postoperative radiation therapy is testing whether such systemic treatment, by eliminating previously disseminated occult metastases, allows regional irradiation to effectively eliminate residual tumor as an important source of subsequent metastases. In this case, regional irradiation may be unimportant without effective adjuvant treatment because of the extent of microscopic metastases disseminated before the regional irradiation. Such a notion posits that only when systemic agents destroy these preexisting disseminated tumor cells does the ablation of regional disease have an impact on metastatic spread and, ultimately, on survival. Thus, these studies could be positive, whereas those studies not using adjuvant systemic therapy are negative. Such differing results in studies with the same variable being examined would not be inconsistent. The reverse might also hold true: that is, regional irradiation might only be important when adjuvant systemic treatment is not administered. Finally, both of these may be true but for different patients. Combining both types of studies will obscure the evaluation of the study results. This is an example of flawed meta-analysis. Frei et al.[6] also question the early use of randomized clinical trials before the treatment to be studied has been optimized. They refer to studies of neoadjuvant or combined chemotherapy with surgery or irradiation in the treatment of head and neck epithelial neoplasms. Such early trials using lower doses of drugs may be negative and, when included in a meta-analysis, may cause a negative result when proper treatment truly is beneficial.

There are problems with the use of prospective randomized trials when the outcome can only be determined after a long period of time. Randomized trials to determine the appropriate treatment of early prostate cancer are unlikely to be helpful, because it will take such a long time for differences to be determined that the treatment techniques will have significantly changed, resulting in the study results having only limited application. Alternative study designs such as analysis of patients matched by known relevant characteristics may be especially useful. If an independent party does the matching, observer bias is minimized. The limitation is, of course, that there are hidden relevant factors that are not evenly distributed between or among the study groups. The ability to repeat these studies without ethical concerns may reduce this problem. No study design is perfect. All require confirmation, but the advantage of this design is that it can be done either prospectively or retrospectively. Retrospective analyses may have more problems with selection bias, but they can be done repeatedly to different data sets to confirm other studies without incurring any ethical difficulties. They are also useful when the disease has a long natural history, and intermediate markers are not available. Any prospective trial is a poor tool in these circumstances.

Underlying the randomized clinical trial is the a priori acceptance that it is the null hypothesis that must be disproved to accept a change in practice. The null hypothesis serves the study by reducing the likelihood of false-positive results, but it does so at the expense of increasing the possibility of false negatives. This may be useful in some circumstances, but it may not always be the desired bias, especially when there is no satisfactory therapy for a fatal disease or when related information suggests that a real difference between groups is more likely than no difference. In serious illness, where the consequences of the current treatments are uniformly bad, rather than fear the adoption of a therapy that is ineffective, we should be more concerned with the premature abandonment of a therapy that might have some value. Rather than minimizing the likelihood of a false positive resulting in acceptance of an ineffective treatment, we may want to ensure that no false negatives result in discarding potentially valuable therapy. The balance between these two ways of forming the question—minimizing false positives versus minimizing false negatives—also depends on previously acquired knowledge and the consequences of the two strategies. When there is little reason to suspect an intervention to be valuable, and the costs both financial and in morbidity are great, then one should begin with the null hypothesis and reduce false positives. But if the costs of falsely accepting the value of an intervention are small, or prior information suggests the intervention to be valuable, then the proper hypothesis to be tested is that the intervention is of value, and it is this that must be disproved. Bayesian statistical analyses are designed for incorporating previous knowledge, but medical reports seldom use them. An example of the questionable acceptance of the null hypothesis is its use in assessing the value of mammography in young women. One might argue that although there is some disagreement, many studies demonstrate that screening mammography reduces breast cancer death by 25% to 30% in women age 50 to 70 years, and therefore, this benefit is likely to be obtained in younger women as well. This bias does not reject the possibility that the technique has no value in this group, but rather, it determines what the hypothesis to be tested should be. Framing the question this way changes the burden of proof dramatically, because the study must be designed to reject there being a meaningful difference rather than requiring that the difference be proven. Selecting the proper hypothesis to be tested also depends on the purpose of the study. In the case of mammography for the 40- to 50-year-old woman, adoption of this technique for population-based screening might require disproving the null hypothesis, because the financial consequences of widespread mammographic screening as a public policy would be large. Furthermore, because the incidence of breast cancer is much lower in women in this age group, screening will be less productive, will result in more false positives with the attendant unnecessary additional diagnostic studies, and ultimately may benefit fewer women. This conclusion is pertinent to general public health considerations. However, the application of mammographic screening for the individual young woman might be more properly informed by the a priori assumption of there being a similar benefit as seen in older women. This is especially so because the disease is more aggressive in young women, rendering early diagnosis to be of more potential value. Not only does the application of the knowledge differ when used for the individual patient as compared with public policy, but the assumptions in the testing are also different.

Generally, the tension between clinical investigation and individual care can be framed in a utilitarian versus deontologic or rights-based philosophy. The utilitarian is clearly appropriate to public health considerations, but what is learned for public health may not necessarily be in the best interest of an individual patient. In utilitarianism, the distribution of the goods—in this case, health—is not important, but rather, it is the amount of total good gained that is to be maximized. In contrast, for the physician caring for the individual patient, the distribution of goods is all important because the patient's rights in health care must be the physician's primary concern. We can see the dichotomy clearly in considering mammography in younger women. Although the cost–benefit analysis appropriate for a utilitarian view of a screening procedure might show it to be too expensive for the life-years gained when adopted as a population screening program, individual physicians might still decide to use that screening technique to offer the patient as much benefit as possible. This has led to the widespread use of mammography in patients between age 40 and 50 years, despite there being no uniform public policy for recommending population screening in this age group.

Technology

The rapid advances in technology and biotechnology are continually revising the current state of medicine. Arguably, the major medical advances made in the latter half of the twentieth century are a result of the increased ability to diagnose disease as a consequence of major saltations in diagnostic imaging and laboratory medicine. Not only do these modalities provide determinative diagnostic information, they also provide tools to assess the extent of disease, thus influencing the design of the treatment. The pace of improved technology and emerging biotechnology provides a challenge in determining their clinical usefulness. A suggested framework for doing this while caring for patients is to separate proximate and ultimate utility. By proximate utility, I mean does the method do what it is designed to achieve? For example, does computed tomography diagnose pancreatic cancer better and at an earlier stage than clinical examination? Estimating ultimate utility requires determining whether such earlier diagnosis will improve treatment outcome. The former is easily ascertained, but the latter is far more complicated. Ultimate utility is only determined in an iterative fashion, which may depend on continuing improvements in diagnostic technology leading to new therapy or even to making previously ineffective treatment useful when its effectiveness depends on the extent of disease. Because the determination of ultimate utility is an evolving process that will take time, I suggest that we accept evidence of proximate utility as sufficient to begin to determine clinical utility. Requiring effectiveness too soon may result in abandoning what might have been an important clinical advance. Unfortunately, there is little benefit in the early diagnosis of pancreatic cancer, but to abandon technology able to provide its earlier diagnosis would reduce the likelihood of developing innovative therapy for such early-stage disease. Although ultimate utility is the goal, this should not denigrate surrogate markers—often measures of proximate utility—because these may better serve to directly measure the effectiveness of the early detection and tumor evaluation technologies. Only after this utility is established can the new method be tested for clinical usefulness. Plain chest radiographs have not been shown to be useful for lung cancer screening, but there are data supporting the use of modern computed tomography for that purpose. The limited benefits of surgery for lung cancer detected by conventional means seem to be markedly increased by the early detection provided by currently available, rapidly acquired helical computed tomography. A representative biotechnologic advance is the ability to test for breast cancer susceptibility genes. *BRCA1* and *BRCA2* have proximate utility by determining risk and developing strategies to reduce this risk through removal of targeted organs, but we are still searching for their ultimate utility: the reversal of the action of the mutation to decrease cancer risk without mastectomy and oophorectomy.

This may come with the development of specific treatments designed to address these mutations or their protein products. Learning in medicine about the uses of technology and biotechnology needs proof of proximate utility and then the freedom to innovate for ultimate utility.

Personal Care

To pursue our obligation to personal care we must first consider the individual patient's goals.[7] The physician needs to determine the relative importance to the patient of the achievement of each of these goals. For example, how important is cure of the disease as compared with relief of the symptoms? How distressing is the morbidity produced by the disease or potentially by the treatment contemplated? How does the patient value various bodily functions and appearances that may be affected by either the disease or the treatment? This constellation of relative values is individual to each patient and likely to vary greatly among patients. Furthermore, because of the differences in patient comorbidity, goals of treatment, and individual values, it is not possible to have a treatment algorithm specific for the care of patients other than in the most generalized form. Combining patients into groups restricted or coerced by insurance rules, investigational protocols, or algorithms for care and assigning a common treatment may be contrary to personal care. When considering the patient with breast cancer, although it is quite easy to place the patient into appropriate stage grouping, and although there may be treatment recommendations for each stage in general, these are regularly modified, not only by how the particular patient fits into the stage. Montgomery[8] considers the problem of particularizing in determining clinical judgment, but particularizing must also involve the patient's desires and comorbidity. Because there are many goals of treatment, survival—the most commonly used measure of success in cancer management—is not sufficient for determining what is best for the individual patient, nor is it necessarily the best parameter for selecting a patient care program or for evaluating clinical results. The evaluative criteria must incorporate quality-of-life considerations and patient values in individualizing patient care. All too often we assume that survival or cure is a sufficient metric, with no similar quantitative measure of other factors. This often leads to the so-called best treatment being not what the patient wants. These issues are illustrated in studies of patient treatment preferences comparing early versus long-term survival in patients of different ages treated by radiation therapy or surgery for lung cancer[9] and the willingness of some patients to accept a reduced likelihood of cure for better voice preservation.

All personal care requires consideration of both the helpful and harmful consequences of treatment in the context of individual patient comorbidity, preferences, and fears. In practice, we must consider the quality of life, the patient's risk-taking preferences, and how the imposition of treatment and continued management will affect the patient's life. To understand a person with an illness, one must do so considering the whole organism, not only a molecular aberration or even a diseased organ system. Social and societal considerations are essential to understanding a patient's illness and designing appropriate care. For example, useful speech is of such value that to some people it is worth sacrificing some likelihood of survival from laryngeal cancer. Most interestingly, this varies among and within social groups, as was shown by a study comparing management executives with firefighters.[10] The former are willing to sacrifice more survival likelihood to retain useful speech, but in both groups, there was extensive individual variation. Each patient's episode of illness is the consequence of a unique interaction of that individual with the disease. Good patient care considers the disease and its management in the context of each patient's desires, wishes, and values. Relying on information limited to disease control or survival without considering the patient's goals is not personal care, nor is it in the best interest of the patient. Aristotle[11] reminds us that learning in general must be modified to be useful for the particular: "Nor is prudence a knowledge only of general principles, but it must also know the particulars; for what are practical and action are always about the particulars."

REFERENCES

1. Popper K (1985). *Popper Selections: The Problem of Induction*, ed Miller D (Princeton University Press, Princeton, NJ), pp. 101–117.
2. Polonyi P (1966). *The Tacit Dimension* (University of Chicago Press, Chicago, IL).
3. Quirk M (2006). *Intuition and Metacognition in Medical Education* (Springer, New York, NY).
4. Santayana G (1905). *Life of Reason, Reason in Common Sense* (Scribners, New York, NY).
5. Hellman S, Hellman DS (1991). Of mice but not men: problems of the randomized clinical trial. *N Engl J Med* 325:1585–1591.
6. Frei E 3rd, Clark JR, Fallon BG (1986). Guidelines, regulations, and clinical research. *J Clin Oncol* 4:1026–1030.
7. Hellman S (1995). The patient and the public good. *Nat Med* 1:400–402.
8. Montgomery K (2006). *How Doctors Think* (Oxford University Press, New York, NY).
9. McNeil BJ, Weichselbaum R, Pauker SG (1978). Fallacy of the five-year survival in lung cancer. *N Engl J Med* 299:1397–401.
10. McNeil BJ, Weichselbaum R, Pauker SG (1981). Speech and survival: Tradeoffs between quality and quantity of life in laryngeal cancer. *N Engl J Med* 305:982–987.
11. Aristotle. *Nicomachean Ethics:* Book I, Chapter 2, pp. 1094a28–1094b5.

2

Academic Medicine

COMMENTARY

This chapter begins with an address given to graduating medical students in 1999. While it obviously follows some of the ritual of commencement addresses, it tries to place medicine in the context of a university while also indentifying some of the aspects of patient care beyond the biological sciences. It emphasizes the breadth of the knowledge necessary for a doctor to fulfill his or her role in the differing contexts of individual patient care, public health, and medical research. The chapter then considers how a medical school fits into a university, using a brief invited response I made to the then president of The University of Chicago, Don Randel, in a symposium entitled "The University of the Future." Mentioned during this discussion was Alexander von Humboldt (1769–1859), an indefatigable explorer and polymath whose discoveries and theories of the interconnectedness of the natural world provided the basis for much of the subsequent science to follow in the next century. Darwin, Thoreau, Emerson, Muir, and Rachel Carson all owe a debt to this most astounding man. His name should be familiar to almost everyone since it appears on so many geographic locations. A sample: Humboldt's Current, various parks, mountains, towns, rivers, waterfalls, capes, and glaciers. More than 400 species of plants and animals bear his name. In addition to those monumental contributions, he is also relevant for the company he kept, including but not limited to Goethe and Schiller, his German intellectual colleagues; Lord Byron, who mentions him in "Don Juan"; Mary Shelley, whose Frankenstein's monster desires to escape to the South America that Humboldt explored and described; such diverse but exalted Western Hemisphere leaders as Simón Bolivar, Thomas Jefferson, and Dolley and James Madison. But it is not for these acquaintances that I bring him to this discussion, but for the many intellectual friends and colleagues with whom he interacted during his lengthy stays in Paris, the center of intellectual life during the first half of the nineteenth century. A partial list relevant to the position of medicine and medical leaders in these intellectual soirées and meetings includes the anatomist Baron Georges Cuvier; René Laennec, the most distinguished French physician of the time and inventor of the stethoscope; and Thomas Hodgkin, whom I will describe more fully later in this volume when I present him as one of my two professional heroes. Hodgkin (of the eponymous disease) was particularly impressed with Humboldt, whom he met at these meetings, describing him as "the hero of my youth." I recommend the excellent new biography of von Humboldt by Andrea Wulf, *The Invention of Nature*, to any who would like to learn more about this fascinating man. All of this digression is to demonstrate the significant participation of leading medical figures in the intellectual life at that time. Medicine was a major intellectual and scientific endeavor of that time and was well represented in the leading universities.

The place of a modern medical school in a university is unusual because of its necessary involvement in the practice of medicine with at least one hospital and often more, its large faculty, and even larger budget. Nevertheless, I argue that it is essential for medicine to be within the university intellectually and, even better, physically located as closely as possible to the other parts of the institution. This is discussed and amplified in "The Intellectual Quarantine of American Medicine." Alternatively, some of the unusual if not unique experiences of the leader of this medical enterprise within the university are fodder for the hopefully humorous but not completely fanciful description of the dean's life depicted in the fourth essay, "Tales of the Unnatural." While this is a light-hearted take, it is based on the real problems of governance in academic medical centers.

There is great genius in combining medicine and biology into a single division of the university as does The University of Chicago. It is the correct continuum of thought, research, and application. It provides wonderful integrated teaching opportunities and collaborative research ventures. It caused me to project an evolutionary perspective on biology and medicine in general, and cancer in particular. Some of these considerations of the role of medicine in a university and the imposing of current biological thought to medical thinking and research have enriched my thinking, research, and writing greatly. One such example of the relevance of evolution to cancer development is included in the essays that follow. It is very useful to consider why certain biological pathways and programs exist normally and are appropriated by the malignant process. Considering why and how they evolve helps understanding, as well as providing opportunities for tumor prevention and treatment. The most recent example is the ability of tumors to co-opt "brakes on the immune system" that evolved to prevent autoimmunity and stop immune responses when they are no longer needed, to inhibit the body's ability to reject cancers. Most exciting are the effectiveness of new agents to abrogate this inhibition of immunity to allow host natural immunity to destroy the tumor, or other immune treatment to be effective in destroying cancers.

The University of Chicago is collaborative, and it is a community as well, and so faculty are concerned with individual buildings and programs not only within but also outside their respective divisions. I remember well Provost Gerhard Casper—later to become the President of Stanford University—informing me of a problem associated with the planned construction of a new BSD building with integrated undergraduate, graduate, and medical school teaching and research space in a single structure. Apparently some members of the Physical Sciences and Social Sciences divisions were concerned about the location and function of the proposed structure. Having experienced Harvard's "every tub on its own bottom" approach, and since I had presidential and board approval as well as funding, I couldn't understand the problem. The provost reminded me of the nature of our community and suggested a "teach-in," with invitations to all members of the community, in which our purpose, program, and architectural drawings would be presented with ample opportunity for discussion. This was done and the concerns disappeared. The Quadrangle Club is the faculty club, but in addition, Hyde Park residents can also become members. About half of the faculty lives in the neighborhood and about half of Hyde Park residents work at the University, making the community and the University independent but interconnected.

BSD had many academic stars, but to compete at the highest level, the press for retaining them, fostering development of new stars or recruiting them, is relentless. It was my view that it was not possible with our resources to have world-class programs in every field: that rather we should build on our strengths and ensure that they are at the highest level while sustaining the other fields at a satisfactory level. This requires strategy and discipline with regular re-evaluation. As the "Red Queen" observed, one has to run as fast as you can just to stay where you are. The pressure to slow down is great, with "regression to the mean" much more comfortable. This must be resisted! Resting in place ensures that you will fall behind. Reviews not only by peers at the university but also by outside reviewers must be stringent and lead to appropriate responses, pruning when necessary so that others can fully flower and occasionally, to continue the metaphor, new seeds sown or new plants acquired. This can cause strife and uncertainty; making compromises that maintain the existing state of affairs unfortunately often results in mediocrity.

A medical center must teach and do research, but it also must provide care. Our location means that we have an obligation to provide medical care for our community and those neighboring us. Teaching, research, and patient care are our missions. Since our patients often are less able to pay than they would be if we were surrounded by affluent neighborhoods, we could not use maximizing the hospital's financial statement as a measure of our success. Responsible financial behavior was necessary, but neither an appropriate nor sufficient criterion. More important were teaching, research, and providing the best care possible to the community we served. Serving our neighbors could also offer opportunities to study methods, racial disparities in treatment and outcomes, and the economics of health care delivery in such needy communities. The hospital administration and its board sometimes lost sight of the centrality of this mission, making reaching our goals more difficult.

During the efforts of "managed competition" that occurred as a result of the then First Lady Hillary Clinton's efforts, the Joint Center for Radiation Therapy (JCRT) at Harvard became an unfortunate casualty. Competition can be good in some endeavors, but not so in attempting to provide medical care. The demise of the JCRT is detailed in the lamentation provided in the fifth essay, "A Lamentation of the Death of Collaboration." It was never published, but after more than two decades it still retains my angst about this unnecessary destructive event.

In contrast to the difficulties of a dean's life, the life of a faculty member of a medical school can be extremely fulfilling. Irwin Freedberg was a close friend with whom I shared many similar experiences of our professional lives during the beginnings of the applications of the biological revolution to medicine, when the funding of medical research was plentiful. I recounted these heady days in a remembrance of Irwin's career as a part of a published memorial to him (the sixth essay, "Irwin Freedberg and the Changing Times of Academic Medicine"). And finally for this chapter, I end with a brief essay—"Ivar, Michael, and Zvi"—on developing foreign friends, a special treat of academia. Ivar Johanson and I shared a laboratory bench as young post docs in Paul Howard Flanders' lab at Yale that was studying the mechanisms of DNA repair. I was Ivar's first American friend and helped in his initial adjustment, although he was an outgoing, gregarious fellow who interacted easily and well within and beyond the laboratory. He and his wife Toni more than reciprocated when they led Rusty and I in a wonderful tour of southern Norway, the highlight of which was an overnight stay with Toni's parents at their summer home on an island in Oslo Fjord. Michael and Catherine Peckham became good friends at the instigation of Henry Kaplan. I also first met Zvi Fuks and his wife Miriam through the good offices of Henry Kaplan when Zvi was a visitor to Henry's department at Stanford. I greatly treasure these and other international friendships, as I do that with Irene and Irwin Freedberg and many other American friends on a similar journey in Academic Medicine.

MEDICINE: A UNIVERSITY

(1999 unpublished remarks to graduating medical school class at The University of Chicago)

Members of the last class of this millennium, your families and guests. This day is likely to be remembered for the rest of your lives. I remember well that time 40 years ago when I was in your place, but I don't remember the speaker or the message. I hope I do better, but I am realistic.

I am sure that you consider this ceremony to mark your leaving the university to embark on further preparation for your life's career. In this talk I want to suggest to you that medicine itself is a university. Universities aspire to encompass most areas of intellectual activity. One characteristic distinguishing medical schools in the United States from those in most other countries is that our graduates have had an undergraduate education before entering medical or graduate school. There is a reason for this; medicine requires the sciences—but also a general education—because it is the application of the sciences to the human condition.

Let us consider some of the parts of the university, which find their place in medicine. We start with biological sciences, the required essential for modern medicine. Because of the proscription of autopsy, science did not make its appearance until the Renaissance with studies of anatomy, but its real momentum was in the second part of the last century and especially during this century.

It is foolish for me to describe the biologic revolution to you. You are on the front lines of this revolution. This is the golden age of biologic reductionism. While some may feel that all medical problems can be solved by the increasing application of molecular techniques, I believe this to be overstated. The fruits of this revolution will have incredible value to medicine, but they are not sufficient. I am reminded of Professor James Gowans—a distinguished immunologist from Oxford—whose concerns for the limitations of reductionism led him to compare the complicated lymphocyte traffic with that of the automobile. He felt that there is much more to be learned about the nature of automobile traffic than can be gleaned from intensive study of the internal combustion engine. Similarly, complicated organisms and societies must be studied at many levels. The practice of medicine requires utilization of many of the university's other disciplines.

In the philosophy departments, one learns about competing moral theories—each appropriate for different physician roles. The concerns for public health require the adoption of utilitarian values, that is, the greatest good for the greatest number. Patient care requires right's based philosophies, which emphasize the primacy of the individual patient in the practice of medicine.

Sociology too is relevant to our profession. Different cultures have different views about medicine, even in the Western world, and even within Chicago. These cultural views have to do with the goals of medicine, its instruments, and the criteria for evaluating success. Physicians, to be effective, need to understand these different attitudes and expectations.

Medicine is both an art and a science, and it is a humane general education that furthers the art of medicine. Hippocrates describes our goal in patient care: "To fully deliver the diseased from their sufferings and to blunt the violence of their diseases, and not to begin to treat those who are overmastered by their diseases, knowing that in such cases medicine is powerless." This is the essence of clinical judgment—when to be active, how to be active, and when to be restrained. It requires understanding the patient, the disease, and how to craft a management plan that is responsive to the patient's beliefs, values, and cultural heritage. Francis Weld Peabody—a famous Harvard physician—said about the art of medicine that "the secret of the care of the patient is in caring for the patient." This requires more than knowledge of pathophysiology. Samuel Taylor Coleridge condemned physicians' preoccupation only with the human body when he described us "as shallow animals" who "imagined that in the whole system of things there is nothing but gut and body."

The relationship between the physician and the patient is the basis of modern medicine. Foremost, it requires the loyalty of the physician to the individual patient. There must be honesty, guidance, and counsel, while respecting the patient's autonomy. Yet we also have a responsibility to advance the health of the larger public. How we fulfill this larger obligation while maintaining our fidelity to the patient requires careful consideration of the individual circumstances. There is an innate tension between competing values: public welfare and individual best interest. Think of quarantine or issues about when and how to engage in clinical experimentation. All of your university education will be required to prepare for these questions.

George Santayana cautioned that "those who cannot remember the past are condemned to repeat it." Medical history offers many lessons. We study the practices which served the patient poorly in hopes that it will enable us to be more successful in the future.

Theology is also important to medicine. Becoming a doctor is considered a calling by some. There is a strong pastoral nature to the profession. It is for these reasons that society has held the physician in a privileged position. How the future will view the doctor is in your hands.

Manichaeism is a religious philosophy emphasizing the duality of life, with both good and evil inherent and in conflict in all things. In this sense, medicine is Manichaean. Consider that pharmaceuticals can be both poisons as well as medicines. To the ancients, *pharmacos* meant both remedy and poison, similar to the current usage of the word "drug." The knife is a weapon as well as a surgical instrument, depending on how it is used. Radiation has obvious harmful effects as well as beneficial use in both diagnosis and treatment. Medicine attempts to maximize the good while minimizing the bad. Hippocrates admonishes us "to help or at least do no harm." But there is harm inherent in trying to help that cannot be completely eliminated. Understanding the risk, even the necessity, of harm in order to benefit is a difficult part of being a doctor. The proper balance of risk for gain is individual to each patient and depends on our understanding of both the science and the art of medicine as applied to that individual patient.

I need not remind you that the other professional schools in the university, such as law and business, relate directly to medicine. We live in a litigious age—a significant amount of medical expenses and professional time is concerned with both preventing and being involved in legal processes. Not only is there a biologic revolution, there is a lesser revolution in the organization and economics of medical care. There are efforts to control medical costs by rationing. These are both economic and moral issues.

I have tried to convince you that while the roots of medicine are in science, medicine encompasses much more of the teachings of the university. It is important for new physicians after intensive emergence in science to be reminded of their broad undergraduate experience in applying the art of medicine.

I will end this address with a personal anecdote. At a university with which I was formerly associated, I had a medical student working in my laboratory. She was the youngest of three sisters—all children of a very distinguished biologist who is one of the leaders of the biologic revolution. I asked her why she, like her two sisters, went to medical school. She said to me that her father had a great influence on them. Her father was not a physician, but he believed it was especially important that they get a liberal education and that the best liberal education was becoming a doctor.

It is my great pleasure and privilege to welcome you as both students and teachers to medicine's university—for a lifetime of learning.

COMMENTS ON THE PRESENTATION BY PRESIDENT DON RANDEL, THE UNIVERSITY OF CHICAGO SYMPOSIUM, "UNIVERSITY OF THE FUTURE"

(2001 unpublished)

It is a special opportunity to comment on President Randel's paper. In most occupations commenting on your boss's presentation—in public, especially while in his presence—is fraught with risks and should be approached with trepidation, but in our line of work that is not so. A colleague once told me that tenure is never having to say you're sorry. In that spirit I offer my comment in three parts; those things I agreed with in the paper, those things I didn't agree with, and finally things that were never mentioned but that I should like to discuss. This latter may be the longest part of this presentation. Since I am from Biological Sciences Division and the medical school, I will use this vantage point for my presentation.

There is a biologic revolution occurring with enormous amounts of information becoming available. The signal examples of this are the projects both public and private to document the human genome. Fortunately, this university requires of its undergraduates a year of study in the biological sciences. I believe this is especially important for those liberal arts graduates who have no intention of further study or a career in the biological sciences. As a member of the informed public, it seems to me that the important social discussions occurring require a familiarity with the concepts and vocabulary of biology. It is not possible to discuss genetic engineering without some real understanding of what a gene is and isn't.

Within current biology and medicine there is the suggestion that advances are made by discoveries at molecular and sub-molecular levels. This emphasis on reductionism—almost to the exclusion of other levels of knowledge—surely is misplaced. Organisms are complicated, and as a physician I know that there is no more complicated organism than the ill human within the social context of his or her life. This is not to say that reductionism is not of value, but rather that it is not necessarily appropriate for all important biologic and medical knowledge. I once heard James

Gowans, an Oxford immunologist, discuss the traffic of lymphocytes throughout the body; he worried about reductionism by comparing the use of this method to that of studying automobile traffic by only detailed analysis of the internal combustion engine. The physicist Erwin Schrödinger believed that quantum theory—the ultimate in reductionism—was the proper level for studying genetics. Time has proven that to be too basic a level. Universities in general, and this university in particular, are especially prepared for this problem by having academic programs at many levels of organization and for the interdisciplinary investigations determining their relationships. Isolated investigations will continue to be important, but multidisciplinary studies will determine the success of the University of the Future.

The second revolution which is occurring is the digital revolution. There are some disturbing implicit assumptions. Data enthusiasts speak of "the disaggregation of knowledge into data" or "datafication." This also misses the importance of context. John Seeley Brown, in a recent book about the digital revolution and education, suggests that "the way forward is to not look ahead but look around."

The University of the Future then has to provide the advances of reductionism, but also the complex systems promoting their interaction and cross-fertilization. It must embrace the digital revolution but not develop digital tunnel vision. Contextual formulation best occurs in an interdisciplinary atmosphere. It is not amenable to mere datafication. Fortunately, The University of Chicago has a long history of interdisciplinary transfer of concepts and of collaborative study. This, perhaps, is the only university where one can hear the term "transaction costs" in the business school, the law school, the medical school, and the social sciences division.

President Gray was especially eloquent in her discussion of the university and its history. As a physician I would like to emphasize the participation and—dare I—the centrality of medicine in the university by expanding on parts of her presentation. She told us that the University of Bologna is the oldest university. Berengario da Carpi (1460–1530) encouraged dissection and autopsy at that university. The word "autopsy" derives from "to view oneself." Surely, that is one of the major functions of a university.

The second oldest university was the University of Paris. Vesalius (1514–1564) was educated at that university and then went to Padua. His studies at the University of Padua corrected those of Galen. Also to Padua went Caius (pronounced "Keys"; 1510–1573). He returned to Cambridge and refounded his old hall in 1557 as Gonville and Caius College. It was at Cambridge that circulation was discovered by William Harvey. Pharmacy, too, began at Padua, where the first chair in botany, founded in 1533, became the basis for Materia Medica. Descartes regarded medicine as the key to the natural world; he was especially interested in the mind/body problem.

During the Enlightenment the universities of Leiden and Edinburgh were leaders of academic medicine. As the hospital developed relationships to universities, scientific medicine emerged early in the nineteenth century. With the development of scientific medicine, medical epistemology changed. Observation and experiment replaced learning primarily from old texts. The practice of medicine required learning in the context of caring for patients with all the ethical considerations that this imposed. Medicine's epistemology then meant that the pure scientific method had to be modified with concern for the human being as having inalienable rights.

The German university of the nineteenth century provided the model for The University of Chicago. Baron von Humboldt's (1769–1859) wide interest in science and in its relationship to the human condition was a great influence on Thomas Hodgkin, one of the greatest figures in medicine and my personal medical hero. I leave you with the translation of the quotation on Hodgkin's grave from the Roman slave Terence: "Nothing of humanity was foreign to him."

THE INTELLECTUAL QUARANTINE OF AMERICAN MEDICINE

Samuel Hellman, "The Intellectual Quarantine of American Medicine," *Academic Medicine* 1991;66(5):245–248.

Abstract

Powerful forces, which are increasing in number and intensity, are causing unexpected changes in medicine. The biological revolution offers opportunities for intervention of a magnitude unknown previously, while at the same time, society is concerned with the increasing costs of medical care. Access to such care and its equitable distribution are the subject of public debate. All of these are issues for ethical consideration. With so many forces acting, there is the opportunity for both effective change and catastrophe. Medicine must be studied in the whole university, where such forces can be considered in an appropriate scholarly fashion with the perspective of history and the methodology of the many academic disciplines. Multidisciplinary units within the university must be formed to consider the complicated issues and the consequences of suggested courses of action. Surely this is better than the advocacy positions of the various parts of organized medicine, regulatory bodies, or insurance companies. Medicine must return from the often intellectually and geographically separated medical school to the center of the university's intellectual life.

Medicine and its practitioners are undergoing profound changes in direction, purpose, even in definition, without a coherent view as to which, if any, of these new formulations is in society's best interests. Consideration of societal interests requires the study of the many health-related goals, the alternative mechanisms to achieve them, and the consequences of implementing such programs. Such investigation involves the efforts of a panoply of disciplines far more extensive than those found in medical schools.

The forces impinging on medicine are powerful and are various in source and direction. Some of these forces are exciting, the results of new knowledge providing opportunities unavailable before. While we should like to expedite them into practice, they often have ethical, social policy, or financial implications that limit this process. Other changes have developed from ethical, social policy, or financial considerations. These are altering the very fabric of medicine by redefining the physician's role, the nature and institutions of health care, its regulation, and its finances. These changes are so numerous and manifold that it is difficult to determine what their effects will be. That they appear driven by differing and sometimes conflicting goals only adds to the sense of confusion and uneasiness that attends medicine today. They require direction and guidance in order to assure society that the greatest benefits of medicine are made available to the greatest number in the most efficient fashion. Such considerations must be mindful of both today's medicine and tomorrow's.

Quarantine

Most important, however, we must consider whether the intellectual position of academic medicine within the university is appropriate to aid in these considerations. Is the university the correct institution to guide the profession and the culture in which it exists? Surely, the forums for such study and discussion should not be limited to the various professional societies or issue-inspired organizations concerned with the growth and development of different fields, disciplines, or specialties of biology or medicine, nor should they be only in the professional schools. Medical schools separate, insulated, or isolated from the centrality of intellectual thought of the university do not benefit from their participation in the university. Medicine must return to the center of the university so that it can affect and be affected by the forces of current intellectual ferment. It must influence rather than primarily be influenced by the new ideas, concepts, and formulations so central to the intellectual life of the university. This requires extensive intellectual exchange between medicine and the other disciplines, divisions, and schools within the university. All too often universities are organized as a loose confederacy of independent schools with little holding them together. Because medical schools have grown so large they are held at a distance lest they exert undue influence on the remainder of the university. The large budget and faculty associated with the medical schools may be considered too powerful. The university may fear that the large medical faculty will dominate the rest of the university. There is also some elitism that classifies physicians as less intellectually broad or accomplished and, thus, less distinguished than other faculty members. The university administration may fear being overwhelmed by the financial powers of the medical school with its research grants and patient care revenues or, alternatively, disturbed by the potential financial obligations attendant to its large faculties, research laboratories, and health care facilities during times of limited research funds and constraints on health care costs. The result of these contrasting concerns has been to try to distance the medical school intellectually, socially, financially, and often physically from the rest of the university. *U.S. News and World Report* quotes President Rhodes of Cornell as describing the "University of Hell" as one in which there are two medical schools. Such fear, suspicion, and isolation may impede medicine's participation in the central intellectual life of the university. This is harmful for medicine, but it also limits the breadth and meaning of the intellectual activities of the university itself. The institution, as a whole, suffers from the medical center's isolation.

We live during a time of profound expansion of our knowledge of biological processes. Biology has been transmogrified from a descriptive science that is informed slowly through extensive observation to one characterized by great leaps in our knowledge and understanding of many of the basic mechanisms associated with the organization and functions of living things. Powerful new techniques are available to biology, which enable us to acquire knowledge rapidly. This knowledge and the techniques themselves may be applicable to many of society's activities, but most obviously to health. This revolution in biotechnology has been likened to that in physics seen in the 1920s and 1930s associated with quantum mechanics, the results of which are still unfolding. The biological revolution may be even more powerful because it will affect not only our material existence but also the very terms of that existence. Biotechnology companies have been sold at great profit even before bringing any product to market because of the financial community's expectations of the profits and benefits of biotechnology. These products, while exciting, are only the first and most muted harbingers of change.

At the same time that this revolution in biology is occurring, the role and position of the physician in society are being reconsidered. The role of the doctor has been changed in that the physician is now seen more as a highly skilled technical expert whose purposes, motivations, and advice are subject to question, rather than as the paternal wise counselor and healer. The notion of medicine as a higher calling has been greatly diminished. This role previously afforded the physician a special place in society, insulated from many of its more usual methods of control. Thus, economic and legal devices were not commonly used to actively control medical practice. They were present only at the margins to limit the extremes of medical behavior. Physicians usually acted independently with minimal regulation because of the belief that they would be guided by a higher responsibility for the patient. It was expected that physicians would tell the patient and the family what they thought to be in the patient's best interests and would act as the patient's agent in making medical decisions, even those concerning the timing and conditions of death and dying. This has all changed. Physicians are less often independent; even if they are in independent practice, for most serious illness, specialists become involved. No longer are these experts merely consultants whose advice is sought, but rather medical care today is divided among these different specialists, restricting the primary physician's previously central role. With this has come a loss of a single, paternal figure and an increase in technical experts. Physicians and their practices, it is felt, can and should be subject to financial scrutiny, government regulation, and the full extent of tort law. Organized medicine has had difficulty in dealing with these changes. Although physicians' incomes still are quite high, there is discontent within the profession with this revised social role and position. This, as well as the increasing allure of alternative careers, has decreased medical school applicants by more than one-third in the last ten years. These concerns within the profession are demonstrated by the involvement of many professional organizations' becoming mainly involved with protecting the financial position of the profession and with defending medicine and physicians from as much regulation as possible.

However, academic physicians have a different agenda. They are concerned with research funding and the future of medical schools. What is missing is a scholarly consideration of the appropriate place of the physician and of medicine in society. For such a consideration we must rely on the university, for it is here that all the disciplines appropriate to such considerations reside.

Financial Constraints

Ironically, at this time of greater ability to heal and greater promise for better health, there are increasing restrictions on expenditures for health care and research. Many in society believe not only that there must be limits on health care expenditures, but also that we are not getting good value for our health care dollar. We all note with concern the maldistribution of health care and the generally unsatisfactory nature of health insurance. The latter is expensive, not universally available, and linked primarily to employment or Medicare. Both the government and employers are actively considering limits on the services provided; in fact, it is the third-party payers that are making many societal decisions concerning the extent of medical care now available. Payment restrictions determine the choice of treatments, as well as their setting. We need only look at the reduction in the number of hospital beds devoted to ophthalmology to see an example of these efforts. This reduction occurred because, as a condition for reimbursement, certain procedures must now be done without an overnight hospital stay. Oregon is preparing a list of diseases and procedures ordered in priority so that rationing can be done in the face of limited finances. How this listing is determined requires complicated cost–benefit analysis consistent with societal values and priorities. Surely, the university should reflect and debate on these issues. Governmental priorities have also greatly limited medical research funds so that only about one in six approved research applications is now being funded. Not only does this limit current research, but it also discourages potential young physician-scientists from considering research careers. Economic and marketplace considerations are deciding medical policy and practice, as well as the future of the research establishment, rather than fostering consideration of what should be society's goals and objectives.

The new medical capabilities and scientific advances coupled with the reconsideration of the physician's role and financial restrictions have created new, and have accentuated older, ethical and cultural problems. Issues currently considered as a result of biomedical discoveries include genetic engineering, in vitro fertilization, the status of the in vitro conceptus, genetic testing of the unborn, and the pill to terminate pregnancy, to mention but a few. Soon medical science will cause society to consider the implications of prolonging life and of modifying the processes of senescence. Already financial concerns are driving discussions of rationing health care, with a careful scrutiny directed at the expenses associated with the care of the elderly, especially those incurred at the end of life. Such important decisions should not be made solely by those responsible for health care or by those responsible only for its financing. What is required are more encompassing considerations of all the factors influencing health care. These deliberations must be held outside the heated cauldron that is the health care institution. I recognize that everything cannot stop until appropriate consensus is achieved and rationally applied. Both short-term and long-term questions require attention, but without thoughtfully considering the direction and purpose, the enterprise will steer a very erratic course, often ending in an unwanted destination.

Let me illustrate the latter with a discussion of a patient and her care recently held by a group of sincere, well-meaning physicians, nurses, and social workers. This patient had advanced breast cancer for which the team all held that a recently developed therapy offered the most promise. The discussion quickly left the traditional medical considerations and focused largely on the nature of the patient's health insurance and what devices or techniques should be used to assure that this woman received the recommended treatment. They were fearful that, because the innovative treatment was considered experimental by third-party carriers, appropriate coverage would not be available. These health professionals had no personal financial incentive for recommending such treatment, as all were salaried and received no payment from the patient. Their goal was to consider and decide on the best treatment for the patient. Without insurance coverage, the patient could not afford the hospital care provided. The medical issues were easily resolved, and all efforts were devoted to guide this patient and the treatment plan through the complexities of the health insurance system. The purpose of the discussions was not only to reduce the bureaucracy but, most importantly, to subvert the intent of the insurer, whose goals were to limit health care expenditures. These are hardly constructive efforts of health care providers, but they are felt to be necessary today. This is also a time when access to and adequacy of health care competes with the financial imperatives of payer mix, length of stay, and patient census.

Cataloging the various forces and opportunities impinging on medicine today is bewildering. Dealing with each of these issues separately often has unintended effects on others. Nowhere is the "law of unintended consequences" more at work than in manipulating one variable in the complex of medical care in America today. The example just given is a simple case in point. Insurance companies try to limit health care expenditures and use the bureaucratic device of prohibiting experimental treatment, stating that it is unproven. The real reason is not to either prescribe or proscribe medical care but to limit expenditures. Health care workers with a different set of goals—that is, obtaining the best treatment for their patient, regardless of cost—use any method at their disposal to obstruct the intent of the third-party carriers. While both goals may be laudable, in this circumstance they conflict, resulting in each side devoting energy and expense to prevent the other from achieving its goal.

Ending the Quarantine

This example just begins to demonstrate the interrelationship between the different forces involved in medical care today. How can the university help? The university functions well in allowing individual disciplines to isolate issues, dissect them with trenchant analyses, and offer possible solutions. The individual disciplines in the social sciences, humanities, and even the physical sciences must be recruited to address the problems of health care and disease. Sociology, history, economics, philosophy, religion, literature, and statistics, as well as the various disciplines of medicine and biology, should all be involved.

While these problems must be analyzed individually, perhaps the most important thing to be done by the university is to study their interactions, to investigate the implications of actions in one area with respect to an entirely different problem of discipline. For example, actions proposed for economic reasons may have social and ethical considerations. They also may result in consequences contrary to those intended. The university should form organizational units to consider these interrelationships. They must be multidisciplinary, incorporating various skills and disciplines. They should not be new separate units, but rather structures that facilitate interaction by the various disciplines on the issues of health, disease, and medicine. These institutes, centers, inter-institutional committees, task forces, or whatever the particular university's culture dictates must consider the desired societal goals, purposes, and opportunities provided by medicine and biology. Such pluralism and diversity should provide the richness of ideas and analyses necessary for these times. By so doing, not only will society benefit, but medicine and the university will gain.

This brief discussion just begins to touch on the sea change in medicine today. It is even difficult to list the array of changes, both potential and actual, that press on medicine today. The "new biology" with its associated biotechnology and the changing role of the physician, from the primary care physician rendering care and advice to the technical expert serving as a part of a complicated health care team, provide new opportunities for effective treatment. Hospitals provide shorter, more intensive treatment;

physicians and hospitals, with their associated high technology, have become more expensive, resulting in high health care costs that concern all of us. Despite this impressive panoply of opportunities for better health care, the system has a disturbing maldistribution, with little organized preventive medicine. All of these changes have vexing ethical and social policy considerations. At such times there are unique opportunities for scholarly thought and discussion involving much of the university, with the possibility that changes may be directed by such considerations.

Medicine is part of the body of our art, sociology, history, philosophy, and science. As an essential part of our culture, it is included in the fabric of many of the university disciplines. Physicians were involved in much of the intellectual life of times past, for knowledge of medicine was considered essential to an educated person. We must find a way to return medicine from the province of the intellectually and often geographically separated medical school to that of the whole university. This is desirable for medicine, very important for the rest of the university, and essential for society. Although we often decry physicians for the narrowness of their education, we permit without comment students to graduate from our colleges and universities without adequate education in medicine or biology. How can we expect informed debate on such issues as genetic engineering when many involved in the debate do not understand what a gene is? Biology and medicine must be made an essential part of the general education required of an informed public.

Physicians must be broadly educated as well. They must understand what society expects of the profession. Physicians must act as translators of science as it advances and must help society integrate and apply new biomedical knowledge. For this to occur, colleges and universities must better integrate biological science and medicine throughout the university. The medical school cannot be either an independent trade school or a research and teaching institution loosely affiliated with the university. Instead it must be an integral part of the university, returned from across the river or from the center of an urban area far removed from its parent institution. Intellectual quarantine does not serve medicine, the university, or society well.

TALES OF THE UNNATURAL: RETURN FROM THE DEAN(D)

Reproduced with permission from the *Journal of the American Medical Association*, 1998. JAMA. 280(19):1657–1658. Copyright © (1998) American Medical Association. All rights reserved.

It has been 5 years since I stepped down as dean/vice president for a medical center after serving in that position for the same duration and thus having exceeded the 3½-year average tenure for medical school deans since 1980. Allowing this time to pass has provided me an opportunity to develop a more nuanced perspective on the position of leader of an academic medical center. I had been cautioned about accepting a deanship by a number of colleagues including a former dean/VP (for brevity I will use the term *dean* to describe this position). Perhaps the most poignant caution came when one of my colleagues pointed out that the word *dean* is but one letter from *dead*. While the implications of that comment have not been realized, it was a very near thing.

Being a dean has certain surprising characteristics. Most astonishing was my abandonment by academic and professional colleagues. To them I seemed to have ceased to exist. This was exemplified by the wonder in others when I attended professional meetings. If, like me, you were formerly an active clinician, you may find yourself patronized by staff and residents; they assume you are "out of it." And with time you may become so. Patient referrals began to evaporate immediately on my appointment as a dean. My referrals were more from foreign than domestic colleagues. I presume this was because my foreign colleagues were unfamiliar with the stigma of deanship in the United States.

Another characteristic of deanship is the time spent functioning as a psychiatrist. A colleague mentioned that the only difference between a dean and a practicing psychiatrist is that the dean's patients have tenure. This old saw, while amusing, has a distinct kernel of truth. Also on a psychiatric note, there is a positive aspect to becoming a dean: absolute immunity to the development of paranoia, since all feelings of persecution are justified.

As a member of a faculty, as a department chair, even as physician-in-chief at Memorial Sloan-Kettering Cancer Center, I was used to going to meetings, but nothing like this! Meetings, committees, fundraising, soothing of egos, and putting out fires are enormous time sinks. And this does not include private and group psychotherapy.

Statisticians are familiar with the principle of regression to the mean: the tendency for outliers to return to an average position. If as dean you are trying to raise an institution to the highest level possible, you must guard against regression to the mean. I am reminded of Garrison Keillor's description of his hometown as a place where "all the children are above average." This, I suspect, is how most deans feel concerning those areas of potential institutional excellence. The tendency to mediocrity is often demonstrated in accepting easy solutions to problems and in making appointments knowing they are less than superlative but important for practical or political considerations. The other phenomenon associated with regression to the mean is described by the Red Queen, who, in *Alice's Adventures in Wonderland*, responds to Alice's concern that, while she is running, the scenery does not seem to change. The Red Queen answers, "it takes all the running you can do to stay in the same place." In academic medical centers, any slowing of pace puts you behind.

I pass on some lessons I learned as a dean for those who, even after reading this account, still might consider such a position.

It is important not to take credit for your accomplishments. This is not as difficult as it may seem, since most people will resent your taking credit, feeling that the accomplishment was (1) inevitable, (2) trivial, (3) their doing, or (4) at least their idea. There is a converse to this lesson of forced humility: take credit for anything favorable that occurs during your tenure for which you had no responsibility, if only to balance the former.

It is crucial to make decisions. Inaction and vacillation paralyze progress, while an incorrect decision can be corrected. This decisiveness leads to a general policy—while not a rule—that I found particularly effective as dean: the "yes, yes, no" method, to be used during any meeting initiated by a faculty member. At such a meeting I agree to the first two requests but deny the third. This allows decision-making and is particularly helpful since rarely does the supplicant ask the important question first or even second. What he or she really wants is disclosed only late in the meeting, at which time my negative response appears fair and balanced, my having agreed to the first two requests.

There are three types of problems that deans face: personnel, money, and space. All are troublesome, but of these, space is the most arduous. In *Star Trek* space was described as the final frontier. In a different context, space is surely the most vexing issue for a dean. Nature abhors a vacuum but not as much as does a medical faculty.

The Unnatural

My essay's title is apt because of the creatures (and their behavior) inherent in the dean's universe. First there are the vampires. Vampires often emerge from the nobility (Count Dracula). In the academic setting, nobility means chairs, senior professors, and senior university officers. Vampires suck blood in order to survive and sometimes just for pleasure—behavior common in academic medical centers. The "victims" are not restricted to the dean but may include other colleagues, both junior and senior. It is quite difficult to recognize a vampire, since the exsanguination is often camouflaged as an act of love. And it is very difficult to eliminate a vampire: a stake in the heart was required for the Count. Thus the dean must exercise constant vigilance to avoid personal attack, as well as to protect others from the bite that will transform them into vampires.

A second group of creatures present in this unnatural world are ghosts, of which there are three classes. Ghosts of deans past are the fond remembrances of figures whose foibles are lost in the mists of time but whose accomplishments are amplified and used in invidious comparison with the current dean. Similarly there are ghosts of deans future. These are presumed to be saviors without fault, implying that a simple leadership change will to solve the vexing problems of the academic medical center. Perhaps the most important ghost is that of deans present. The dean perceives this ghost differently than do other observers. To the dean this ghost appears as a wise, benevolent leader with clear goals exhibiting outstanding leadership, resulting in numerous accomplishments. Unfortunately, other observers see a much less salutary apparition.

Not only do ghosts and vampires inhabit this universe: there are goblins, creatures causing mischief or evil. The goblins of the academic medical center are even more insidious, since they are not always grotesque; sometimes they are angelic in appearance. They can come from any constituency (faculty, staff, or administration) and any part of the university.

Not only are there bizarre inhabitants; there is also unnatural behavior exhibited by certain denizens of this strange land. The most disturbing social behavior in academic medicine is cannibalism. Mentors often eat their young, considering them a threat to their own position. There is also selective cannibalism, such as picking another's brain, which can be risky behavior when it concerns academic precedence.

Mammals that live in groups often have an alpha male or female with a pack of subservient individuals. Inhabitants of the academic medical center believe that this pyramidal structure is reversed, since they all consider themselves alphas, with the dean and administrators subservient facilitators of their wishes. The very term *administrator* is used in academic institutions so as not to connote the status implied by *executive* in the business world.

Medical schools may contain remnants of past ecosystems and thus may be inhabited by extinct species. Perhaps the most obvious fossils are the persistent reminders of former organizational priorities. These include anachronistic departments, committees, evaluative processes, and traditions embraced by the institution. The more venerable the institution, the more encrusted it is with fossils. There are also dinosaurs in this land: formerly esteemed but now out-of-touch colleagues. Even more anachronistic dinosaurs are those who were not esteemed even in their heyday. The dean must separate these living fossils of eras past from wise senior colleagues whose advice and guidance can be extremely helpful.

The most worrisome inhabitants of this unnatural world are the monsters. The most obvious monster—able to devour large quantities of the dean's time and effort—is the hospital because of its size, finances, and organization. There is an almost inherent conflict between the goals of the hospital administrative leadership and the purposes of academic medicine. Also characteristic is the vague and/or competitive organizational relationship between the hospital CEO and the dean. It is rare that there is an organizational structure with a single leader. Hospitals are downsizing, reducing beds and personnel, with efficiency as a primary objective. There are perceived organizational prescriptives requiring mergers and networks. In addition to these business challenges are special financial pressures on hospitals because they are considered to be the fulcrum for controlling health care costs. The increased emphasis on finances can cause great strain and often displaces the primary purposes of the teaching hospital. While financial viability is needed, maximizing profits is not the primary mission of the academic medical center. Mergers and networks often introduce physicians not formerly involved in or committed to academic goals. Incorporating these physicians into a faculty system puts great stress on the criteria and quality required for academic appointments.

Minor monsters also occupy the academic netherworld. Among these are those empowered amateur members of the hospital board: usually executives or lawyers who believe physicians are incapable of grasping business principles but that they—the board members—are able to understand medicine. Admittedly, while there may be some justification for the former, there is none for the latter. This results in either inappropriate decisions or an extraordinary amount of time and effort expended in order to have the correct course followed. Often board members have little sensitivity to the varied missions of an academic health center, acting as though they were on the board of a purely business entity valued primarily for the financial consequences of any decision without sufficient balance for academic purposes. Donors are a heterogeneous lot, some of whom may be minor monsters. I classify them as minor since unlike vampires, they do not suck blood but rather time and sometimes require the suspension of reason or taste.

Resurrection

The dean's world is bizarre, but escape is possible. I have been fortunate in being able to accede to that most exalted university status, that of a senior member of the faculty. The perks of this position include few, if any, committee assignments, and, most important, sufficient time for scholarship. Unfortunately, while the transition to such a position is possible, it is quite daunting. This difficulty is time-related, the possibility of resurrection being inversely proportional to the time spent as a dean. During an extended incumbency the dean may have forgotten too much, may be unable to keep up because of other pressures and because of the general beating taken by the dean. Returning to active laboratory research is challenging because his or her field has changed so much. Clinical research and clinical care are possible, but the dean must undergo an active program of remediation. The primary impediments are those behaviors, beliefs, and attitudes acquired as a dean. The position is dangerous because it promotes confidence in knowing you are right. It encourages a certain world-weariness proportional to the length of time spent as a dean. Such behavior may lead to excess philosophizing, consulting, joining the staff of professional organizations, or even becoming a foundation executive.

As in most of medicine, prevention is more effective than attempting cure. The preventive medicine associated with the role of dean is to resist temptation of the initial offer of a deanship, even of an initial interview. This may sound simple, but it requires acting against all the instincts of a successful academic physician. These include alpha one behavior, confidence that you can succeed where others have not, and general assurance based on insufficient evidence. Since this is so difficult, a convenient solution may be to demand an organizational structure with a single CEO of the medical center who is also the dean. This has two desirable, possible outcomes: if accepted you may actually be able to accomplish something during your limited tenure on the job, but more likely such a structure will not be offered, allowing you to avoid the state of administrative purgatory.

A LAMENTATION ON THE DEATH OF COLLABORATION

(2002 unpublished)

The primary premise underlying cost containment in medicine today is to depend on competition to produce efficiency while retaining quality. I was recently asked to advise the Brigham and Women's Hospital and the Dana-Farber Cancer Institute about the radiation oncology program in those institutions following the dissolution of the Joint Center for Radiation Therapy (JCRT). This assignment has allowed me to see first hand some of the disturbing unintended consequences of relying on the marketplace to make medicine more efficient.

Background

The concept of a joint center for radiation therapy within the Longwood Avenue hospitals of the Harvard Medical School was developed by Dr. Sydney Lee under the auspices of Dean Robert Ebert with the strong support of Dr. Herbert Abrams, the then recently appointed chairman of radiology. I was recruited in 1968 to develop this collaborative venture, conceived to provide those hospitals collectively with medical and physics faculty, modern equipment, and the support to operate without unnecessarily duplicating personnel or equipment. A vigorous academic program was to complement these efforts. The twin goals of the JCRT collaborative venture were excellence in cancer care and efficient use of resources—goals not dissimilar from those the competitive system is expected to achieve.

The JCRT began as a collaborative venture of the New England Deaconess Hospital, the Beth Israel Hospital, the Boston Hospital for Women, and the Peter Bent Brigham Hospital. Shortly thereafter, the Children's Hospital and the Dana-Farber Cancer Institute joined. The program worked well. Personnel and equipment were acquired by the Center and located at the individual hospitals to serve the common enterprise. Patient treatment was designed, simulated, evaluated, and administered on the equipment best suited for each patient, regardless of the hospital from which the patient had originated. While there was an effort to have patients cared for at the hospital of origin, often patients were treated at other hospitals because of technical requirements. All patients received some services, such as treatment planning, from a central provider within the JCRT member facilities. Because of differences in machine utilization among the hospitals, patients were often treated where facilities were most available so as to ensure timely care. There were mutually agreed-upon treatment protocols and techniques administered throughout the member facilities. The size of the combined effort provided physicians the opportunity to specialize in certain diseases, develop treatment guidelines, and evaluate results. The JCRT became a model for such collaborations in other parts of the country. Basic and clinical research, as well as a residency and fellowship program, flourished at the JCRT under a number of successive leaders.

Current Situation

The revolution in the financing of health care encouraged hospital competition, making the joint center concept precarious. The arrangement was terminated, resulting in two competitive units: one for the Beth Israel and New England Deaconess Hospitals; and the other for Brigham and Women's Hospital, Children's Hospital Medical Center, and Dana-Farber Cancer Institute. It was this latter group that I was asked to advise.

My visit with the staff, residents, and the various hospital leaders was as Dante described: "There sighs, lamentations and loud wailings resounded through the starless air, so that at first it made me weep." The staff and residents lamented the end of the JCRT. For the hospital leaders faced with financial pressures, the hallmarks of an academic program—teaching, training, and research—assumed a lower priority. The hospitals formerly associated with the Joint Center formed two competitive units. Patients are restricted to their institution of origin, sometimes wait-listed at one hospital unit while the other has treatment times available. The treatment planning center recently built at Beth Israel Hospital to be used by patients from all JCRT will be limited to patients from Beth Israel and New England Deaconess Hospitals only, once appropriate facilities can be provided at the Brigham and Women's Hospital, resulting in seemingly needless duplication promulgated by these new competitive arrangements.

The Dana-Farber Cancer Institute has developed a small radiation oncology department that includes a single linear accelerator—hardly enough for comprehensive treatment—so that its patients can be treated in house. This expense buys the Dana-Farber the ability to claim an identifiable radiation therapy program—this, despite the fact that all the rest of the equipment that may be needed for Dana-Farber patients will reside at Brigham and Women's Hospital. There is competition for technologists between the Beth Israel–Deaconess group and that of Brigham and Women's Hospital and Dana Farber Cancer Institute. Two separate physics groups have been formed with almost certain redundancy.

Lessons

While the demise of the JCRT is unfortunate for cancer care in the Longwood area, it is also illustrative of the consequences of the current trends in health care delivery. There is much talk about reducing health care costs through competition, but perhaps we need to rethink the assumption that competition is the preferred mechanism to ensure efficient high-quality health care. The saga of the JCRT should provide an instructive corrective. We learn that competition isn't always the best way to assure either quality or efficiency. On the contrary, in medicine it is often collaboration that can reduce costs and increase quality. The Joint Center was able to accomplish both, and it is unlikely that dissolving it will improve performance. As the fiscal constraints on health care grow, the medical marketplace is under increasing pressure to control cost while maintaining quality. Paradoxically, the resulting competition may reduce both the efficiency and the quality of health care as well as reinforcing inherent chauvinistic tendencies.

The Joint Center for Radiation Therapy is no more, a victim of the currently promulgated medical care paradigm. This focus on competition at the expense of the common good reminds me of Yeats:

> Things fall apart; the center cannot hold;
> Mere anarchy is loosed upon the world.

IRWIN FREEDBERG AND THE CHANGING TIMES OF ACADEMIC MEDICINE

Republished with permission of Elsevier, from "Irwin Freedberg and the Changing Times of Academic Medicine," Samuel Hellman, *Journal of Investigative Dermatology*, volume 126, edition 3, 2006; permission conveyed through Copyright Clearance Center, Inc.

Irwin and I were fortunate to become physicians during the early years of the scientific revelations of the "new biology" that began to inform academic medicine. We both were medical house officers at Beth Israel Hospital in Boston during the latter days of Hermann Blumgart's reign as chair of medicine. Superb clinical medicine prevailed with great emphasis on clinical–pathological correlation, infectious disease, and, most importantly, the observation, quantification, and manipulation of human physiology. These pursuits were the bedrock of academic medicine. But Watson–Crickery was in the air! At Beth Israel Hospital, Blumgart was succeeded by Howard Hiatt, recently returned from participating in the earliest days of the new biology at the Pasteur Institute. Hiatt brought a whole new vision of academic medicine. Irwin left Beth Israel Hospital during the Blumgart era to do his dermatology training at Massachusetts General Hospital and returned to join Hiatt in implementing a new paradigm of academic medicine. I too left for my training and a junior faculty position at Yale. After I returned to Boston, both Irwin and I were engaged in building our respective academic programs in the clinic and the laboratory. Not only was Irwin building dermatology; under Hiatt's leadership he, H. Richard Nesson, Howard Frazier, and others were remaking academic medicine at Beth Israel.

Irwin had spent the academic year 1961–1962 as a postdoctoral fellow in the biochemistry department at Brandeis University and that of 1969–1970 on a Guggenheim Fellowship at the Weizmann Institute in Israel. Both of these experiences equipped him with the tools of modern molecular science. The titles of two papers authored by Irwin and published by the *New England Journal of Medicine* capture these two phases of his academic medical research. The first, published in 1957, "The thyroid gland in pregnancy," was the kind of careful observation and quantification of human physiology that was characteristic of the academic medicine of the time. Irwin was the first author, and his coauthors were Milton Hamolsky (later to chair the Department of Medicine at Brown University) and Irwin's uncle A. Stone Freedberg, a distinguished cardiologist interested in the relationship between thyroid function and the heart. The second paper, "Rashes and ribosomes," authored only by Irwin and published just 10 years later, offered promise of the practical relevance of basic molecular biology to clinical medicine.

We were bursting with energy and enthusiasm for our growing families, these medical and scientific enterprises, and life in general. Though this may not be imaginable today, federal funding for research was plentiful. Good and not so good ideas were funded, and, because funds were plentiful, offbeat but imaginative ideas could be pursued. Those were heady days! Commercial involvements were less common, health-care reimbursements were cost-based, and there was little competitive pressure among hospitals. In fact, inter-hospital collaboration was encouraged. Irwin developed a combined dermatology program for some of the Harvard-affiliated hospitals around the Harvard Medical School, while I developed the Joint Center for Radiation Therapy for these and other hospitals. These programs were collaborative clinical, teaching, training, and research enterprises.

Easy funding, cost-based reimbursements, and, of course, our youth, along with a major saltation in science—the new biology—that resulted in a Kuhnian paradigm shift, made these the best of times. Others in this volume will discuss Irwin's academic contributions, but suffice it to say that he was very successful and drew notice. In 1977 Johns Hopkins convinced Irwin to resign his Harvard professorship in order to become the first chairman of their fledgling dermatology department. He leapt into this endeavor with his accustomed enthusiasm. Then, in 1981, the opportunities offered by chairmanship of the biggest, most distinguished and well-financed department of dermatology, as well as the allure of New York City, attracted Irwin to New York University to lead what is now the Ronald O. Perelman Department of Dermatology and to become the MacKee Professor. He reached the full flower of his academic potential during the almost quarter century of his tenure in that position.

Alas, during that time academic medicine changed and academic leaders faced new and different challenges. Research funding became more difficult, and funds from private and commercial sources became more important. As we both accepted senior positions in medicine in New York City—the heart of commercial and economic America—our dealings with the shakers and movers were extensive and necessary for the fulfillment of our missions. A small vignette to capture that time: I too was planning to leave a Harvard Medical School professorship for new opportunities in *la Grande Pomme* as the physician-in-chief at Memorial Sloan-Kettering Cancer Center. While considering and negotiating in New York, I stopped by to see Irwin and to ask about being a medical leader in that great city. He recollected that, in Boston, when we went to the symphony we saw many familiar faces, and being a professor in a medical school was a desired and respected position. This, he assured me, was also true in Baltimore. But things were different in New York. One rarely saw a familiar face at the opera or the symphony, and to those captains of industry, medical professors were not particularly important or respected. They were, however, collected and/or cultivated by these business leaders, primarily for possible medical advice and care for themselves and their families, colleagues, and employees. This was especially true for plastic surgeons.

Throughout the United States, medical-care concerns changed as well. Institutional competition, managed care, and containment of healthcare costs made academic medical practice much more difficult; all this occurred at the same time as much greater competition for a limited grant pool. Parenthetically, it should be noted that throughout the vicissitudes of funding availability, remarkably, Irwin's National Institutes of Health R01 grant "Epidermal Macromolecular Metabolism" received 40 years of continuous funding until 2001. Despite these challenges to medical leadership, both Irwin and his wife, Irene, flourished in New York professionally and personally. They partook of much that that city has to offer with their usual vigor and enthusiasm. Opera, symphony, theater, temple, friends, and, of course, family all vied for their time and attention. This would appear to be a full life, but it was not sufficient for Irwin, for he had a special feeling for New Hampshire. It was there, at Dartmouth, that he had received his undergraduate education, and Holderness is the site of the family retreat. His *joie de vivre* was fully requited by the lakes and mountains, in summer and winter, boating and swimming in the former and skiing in the latter, all in the company of his family and friends.

Irwin was committed to academic medicine throughout his final illness; he continued to work as long as possible and was busy reviewing book galleys almost to the end. He was very concerned about the state of academic medicine in general and dermatology in particular. He fretted about the increasing commercialism in both and the lure of procedural reimbursement affecting dermatology. At the same time, Irwin was excited about the great promise offered by the new biology to greatly improve medical care. These concerns generally applied to all of academic medicine.

When we began our medical careers we seemed to have boundless energy, invigorated as we were by the new biology and the opportunities it would offer to medicine. We had only limited concerns regarding healthcare financing or the distribution of medical care. Collaboration rather than competition was the norm. In retrospect it seems that times were better then, but that is probably to be expected from those of us in our senior professional years when we look back at our youth. New opportunities, hazards, and diversions require agile reaction and real commitment. This is the only effective response to these interesting times. Irwin possessed these characteristics in abundance. From his great and enthusiastic capacity for work as a caring physician, scientist, and academic leader, to his joyous participation in skiing, swimming, boating, travel, and various cultural activities, Irwin was a man for all seasons, both figuratively and literally. He was also a mensch.

IVAR, MICHAEL, AND ZVI: CELEBRATING THE DIVERSITY OF OUR FRIENDS AND COLLEAGUES

This article was first published in *Nature Clinical Practice Oncology* 2005;2(8):377.

At a recent meeting of the Editorial Advisory Board of *Nature Clinical Practice Oncology* (NCPO), I sat among colleagues from many countries. I was reminded that one of the great but often unstated virtues of an academic medical career in oncology is the opportunity for personal growth afforded by the diverse backgrounds of our partners in improving cancer care and prevention. I grew up in New York City, in what is now somewhat disparagingly referred to as "the outer boroughs"—in my case the Bronx—in a largely first-generation Jewish-American neighborhood. It was not until high school that I encountered Italian-Americans, Irish-Americans, and African-Americans in any number. A small liberal arts college in western Pennsylvania was my first exposure to the (then) dominant American culture: white Anglo-Saxon Protestant. Medical school in upstate New York did not add to the diversity of my peers. It was not until my fellowship at Yale, while working in the lab of a British expatriate, that I befriended someone from outside the United States; I shared a lab bench with Ivar, a Norwegian with rudimentary but rapidly improving English. We soon became friends and remained so until his untimely death. After this laboratory venture in the US, my exposure grew with a fellowship in the United Kingdom, and then expanded almost exponentially, through academic exchanges, joint projects, and meetings. Good friendships developed with Australian, Belgian, British, Dutch, French, German, Israeli, and Italian colleagues. Michael—now Sir Michael—and his family exchanged children with us (of course only temporarily). Zvi, at that time an Israeli radiation oncologist working at Stanford who later became the Professor of Oncology at the Hebrew University in Jerusalem, and then Chairman of Radiation Oncology at Memorial Sloan-Kettering Cancer Center, became, and remains, one of my dearest friends. From visiting Ivar's in-laws on an island in Oslo fjord, to finding 5,000 years of history in Israel, and wide-ranging (often lubricated) political discussions with many of these friends—I found, and continue to find, great pleasure, enrichment, and enlightenment.

We consider ourselves well read, aware of international views and trends in both medicine and world affairs. However, I remember being on a breast-cancer management program sitting between French and Italian colleagues; the Frenchman addressed the Italian in Italian and the Italian responded in French, while intermittently one or the other would translate into English for my benefit. It is an important reminder of our potential parochialism, which should be remedied by international communication, in person, at meetings, and with publications such as NCPO.

Our life's work can be exciting, frustrating, and unfortunately sometimes heart-wrenching, but this expanded worldview is a special (yet often unstated) delight of our efforts. By reminding me of this, I have already gained from my association with NCPO, and my interactions with it have only just begun.

3

Research

COMMENTARY

My research, both basic and clinical, is concerned with understanding cancer, and through that, improving cancer treatment. While my stem cell research may be considered fundamental research, its goal is to understand basic processes so that we can apply this knowledge to improving treatment effectiveness and reducing toxicity. Both of these goals are equally relevant to my clinical research.

My main clinical research began with studying how to combine the three basic forms of cancer therapy at that time: surgery, radiation, and chemotherapy. This was predicated on the notion that each had non-overlapping strengths and toxicities so that it might be possible to take advantage of combining these modalities to have more effective or less morbid treatments. I first studied radiation and chemotherapy in head and neck cancers and then, and far more extensively, in the treatment of Hodgkin Lymphoma—the current preferred usage for Hodgkin's disease though the latter is still often used. I have not performed research in Hodgkin Lymphoma for many years, but I spoke at an international meeting at Memorial Sloan-Kettering Cancer Center (MSKCC) on this topic recently. I had been asked to talk about a favorite figure in medicine, Thomas Hodgkin, but I enjoyed the opportunity to hear what is the current state of such combination treatment of this disease. My fascination with Dr. Hodgkin will be discussed further, later in the volume. I have emphasized the multidisciplinary approach to cancer treatment in two papers: the first, my Presidential Address to the American Society of Clinical Oncology in 1987, focuses on the multiple therapeutic modalities brought to bear on cancer; in the second, the Nobel Symposium Keynote Lecture, I describe the need for physics and technological advances, as well as biological research from molecular to complex systems, and finally research into how tumors grow in the context of normal tissues and host response in the whole organism.

The curative treatment of Hodgkin Lymphoma described by Henry Kaplan and Saul Rosenberg at Stanford using linear accelerator-delivered radiation and by DeVita and colleagues at the National Cancer Institute using a multi-drug chemotherapy cocktail had a profound effect on the approach not only to lymphomas but to many other tumors as well. The multi-drug approach to cancer was pioneered for the treatment of leukemia, but success in tumors of other organs in which the tumors had a primary site in the body with regional lymph node and distant metastases turned out to be much more difficult. At the present time, while causing tumor reduction in size, such anti-proliferative chemotherapy is not very successful in increasing the likelihood of cure, except when given when the metastases are extremely small and not clinically detected or when combined with effective regional treatments such as surgery or radiation. These latter combinations of local and regional therapy and chemotherapy often result in a major advance. Lymphomas seem to be an intermediary between leukemia and these so-called solid tumors. Both radiation and chemotherapy are effective in treating these malignancies of lymphocytes. When to use them individually and when and how to combine them are still the stuff of major clinical experiments and reviews. Similarly, how to combine drugs, surgery, and radiation for solid tumors is still evolving but follows a similar philosophy.

The representative papers of mine to follow in this chapter first speak to the importance of determining the appropriate model or theory of cancer in order to properly fashion treatment. My efforts in emphasizing the importance of the underlying mechanisms of cancer evolution were developed in my studies of breast cancer, but I believe they are relevant for most, if not all, solid tumors. Some of these papers will, by their nature, have medical jargon, but I believe the general reader will grasp the relevant points. My interests in breast cancer began at Yale during my training. This common cancer is the paradigm for many cancers. It is often curable when found early, as the benefit of mammography clearly shows, but even these small tumors occasionally have already spread. The success of treatment decreases as tumors grow. The treatment of early cancer when I started my career was with an aptly named major extirpative operation: radical mastectomy, sometimes with postoperative radiation. The surgery not only removed the breast but also the underlying muscle, causing unfortunate changes in the patient's body image as well as reduced use of the shoulder and arm. Often there was permanent swelling of the arm. Some pioneering surgeons and radiation oncologists in Europe and Canada began to treat with only biopsy or limited tumor removal followed by radiation. The initial results seemed to have a similar likelihood of cure without mastectomy or those undesirable consequences. I was one of the leaders in perfecting this approach and more importantly in advocating this treatment in the United States. There were many vigorous debates during the 1970s and 1980s, requiring much travel, though finally there is now general acceptance of this approach. I was away from home a great deal in order to participate in panels with surgeons committed to the radical mastectomy. No resolution was reached due to these presentations, but my purpose was to convince the audience of both the legitimacy of conservative management of breast cancer and of its effectiveness in destroying the tumor without causing much alteration of the human body. The radical surgeons were often convinced that such treatments were akin to heresy. They foretold dire consequences of my methods that fortunately did not happen, and so with the passage of time, radiation treatment with local tumor removal and breast preservation became the preferred treatment of early stage breast cancer. I use the term "heresy" because radical mastectomy was the dogma, as discussed in one of the papers to follow. I was once invited to a meeting of the Israel Cancer Society at which such devotees were to be attending as representatives of the American Cancer Society, which was a financial supporter of the meeting. Also invited by the

Israeli sponsors was Bernard Fisher, a surgeon who believed that varying local surgical treatment was unimportant. To those ACS representatives, that was heresy, and so they refused to pay for his travel to Israel, while they paid for my trip. While I too advocated conservative management, I presume I was more acceptable because as a radiation oncologist I was not committing heresy, while Dr. Fisher, a surgeon, was. These efforts in popularizing conservative—I prefer "preservative"—breast cancer treatment are not reflected in the papers selected for this collection since they are often technical and do not lend themselves for presentation in this volume, but they do form a considerable part of my scholarly pursuits. They are only mentioned parenthetically in some of the essays.

Dr. Fisher's view emphasized the systemic nature of cancer. To him a tumor either was of a type causing only local growth or, more commonly, was systemic by the time it was found, even if the distant spread was not detected until later in the course of the disease. This conflicted with the conventional view of cancer spreading in an orderly manner from the primary site to regional lymph nodes and then to distant sites. This view of early systemic spread and the fatalistic approach to the value of regional surgery or radiation led Fisher to look for treatments that might destroy these subclinical metastatic deposits. He found that using a drug before such metastases were evident reduced the likelihood of distant metastases. As often happens in science, others were also testing this method of treating before you knew whether cancer metastases were even present in the patient and so giving some patients unneeded potentially harmful therapy in order to eradicate undetected disease in others. Nissen-Meyer in Norway and Bonadonna in Italy reported results similar to Fisher. Early positive findings seemed to confirm the systemic theory of Fisher and were so consistent with this new theory that it too was soon to become dogma. An early indicator of beginning dogmatism was that the National Cancer Institute in 1988 released a two-page document briefly describing these preliminary findings—still not published, and showing a difference in early metastases but no survival advantage as yet—to physicians throughout the United States, urging the widespread adoption of this new "adjuvant therapy." I was and still am critical of such "Clinical Alerts." They reach the press and thus a wide public audience before physicians have an opportunity to study the data. This results in concerned patients expecting considered advice from their doctor before that is possible. Sometimes early results are just that and do not persist. If this were to be the case, then any patient so treated would be exposed to the harmful effects of these adjuvant treatments without any therapeutic gain. As it turned out, adjuvant therapy did improve survival by about 10% and is still widely used, but I remain convinced that allowing the studies to mature and to be published and available for oncologists to study is the proper course.

There is another point to these studies related to the previously described epistemological considerations in confirming theories. These studies of the early administration of chemotherapy following surgery for breast cancer were also initiated in order to reduce any metastases inadvertently released at the time of surgery, an alternative theory to that of early systemic metastases. These positive results do not distinguish between these alternative theories. In fact, Bonadonna and his colleagues reported that further analysis of the timing of metastases supported the notion of reduction of spread caused during surgery. We still do not know which, if any, of these alternative mechanisms of cancer spread are correct—another demonstration of the limitations of the scientific method, as discussed in the first chapter of this book.

The theory promulgated at the end of the nineteenth century by William S. Halsted at Johns Hopkins was of orderly spread of breast cancer from the local tumor in the breast, first locally in the breast and surrounding tissues, then to the lymph nodes close by, and only then to distant sites. This became widely accepted and described as dogma in one of the essays to follow. While these two theories were contrasted, I had a different view that could include parts of both the "systemic" theory and that of Halsted. I believe that cancers evolve in their malignant capacity as they grow. This "spectrum theory" posits that cancer contains a spectrum of states from those capable of only local growth to those that metastasize very widely. This is due to the progressive increase in a tumor's metastatic capacity as it grows— a Darwinian process. Within this spectrum there is a state of oligometastases where there are a limited number of metastases, and these may be cured by regional treatment. Both this theory and oligometastases are discussed in the essays to follow. The work on oligometastases has been done with Ralph Weichselbaum, whose laboratory has also identified molecular correlates for this intermediate state of cancer spread. One may note that the first paper suggesting this entity was published in 1995, and the other paper, "Oligometastases Revisited," in 2011. Even at that date some 16 years later, there was some reluctance in accepting the concept. This appears to have abated with more articles from us and others confirming the concept and the increasing molecular delineations done by Ralph. A former Harvard colleague, then Chairman of Medicine at the Brigham and Women's Hospital, described three phases of medical research that seem applicable to oligometastases: on first learning of a new concept, one wonders, "it is new but is it true?" (in this case, 1995); in the second phase, one feels "it is true but is it important?" (2011); now we appear to be in the third phase, "it is true and it is important but it is not new." So it is in medical science.

Discussing prognosis is an essential requirement of a physician. This is especially important in cancer care. The patient wants to know the unknowable (i.e., the future) but nevertheless she needs what informed guidance she can secure. I find that giving percentages of cure is only of limited value, since for the individual it is binary: cure or disease recurrence. It is better to give a general likelihood of success and emphasize that as the time from treatment without recurrence increases, the chance of recurrence diminishes. This is in contrast to other chronic diseases such as diabetes, coronary artery disease, and most chronic neurological disease where, with increasing time after diagnosis, there is increasing likelihood of disease progression. Another problem with discussing the disease is the very terms "cancer" and "malignant disease." They are associated with many unfortunate images. This is elaborated in Chapter 4, "Perceptions of Cancer."

I am also interested in how tumors evolved. This was greatly stimulated by my not only being Dean of Medicine at The University of Chicago but also Dean of the Biological Sciences Division (BSD). In this latter role, I was responsible for the Department of Evolution and Evolutionary

Biology. Shortly after arriving in Chicago, I recognized the strength of these studies in BSD. Learning from my colleagues involved in modern studies of evolution stimulated me to apply these concepts to the clinical evolution of cancer as described in the spectrum theory. An example of this Darwinian thinking directed to how cancer develops and progresses is included in the essays to follow.

My stem cell research began while I was in training in radiation oncology at Yale. This program included a year of research. I began working in Paul Howard Flanders' lab studying the repair of DNA damage caused by UV radiation to bacteria and their viruses called "bacteriophages." Using such simple organisms and UV was thought to be a way to develop some general principles relevant to more complicated organisms—eventually human beings—as well as to lead to the study of ionizing radiation like X-rays. I enjoyed this opportunity to work in a basic science laboratory for the experience and friendships made—especially with a Norwegian postdoctoral fellow, Ivar Johanson, who is discussed in a small missive included in Chapter 2, "Academic Medicine"—and as a primer for the explosion of molecular biology that occurred between my first year of medical school 1955–1956 and 1963 when I was in this laboratory. Bacteria and bacteriophage were the basic biological material used in those seminal experiments. I took a revelatory bacterial genetics course given by Edward Adelberg, a contributor to some of those experiments. This remedial education has served me well, allowing me to follow some of the major molecular discoveries related to cancer biology. Primary in cancer development is the occurrence of mutations in genes changing their function and activity. Though all cells of an organism contain the same genes, different cells look and perform quite differently; for example, some make muscle while others comprise the nervous system. This is due to different genes being expressed, and this is controlled by a variety of mechanisms still being actively studied. A small example from Nikolai Khodarev and Ralph Weichselbaum's oligometastases studies is that the same control mechanism associated with this appears also to affect genes used during embryological development but not usually expressed in the adult.

This immersion in basic science served me well, but I hungered for an understanding of mammalian biology at a more organized level. I was particularly interested in how continued cell production required for many systems of the body was maintained within a balance between cell birth, cell maturation, and cell death. I chose hematopoiesis, or this activity in the blood-forming system, as my subject for two reasons: first, it is rapidly proliferating like certain cancers, especially leukemia, but this normal blood cell production is extremely well controlled, and understanding how this is accomplished should provide avenues for possibly controlling tumor growth; and second, hematopoiesis is what is most affected by cancer chemotherapy and damage to it results in the most frequent treatment toxicity. The basis for much of rationally designed chemotherapy was (and to some extent still is) that the essential characteristic of cancer is uncontrolled cancer cell proliferation. The model used in most laboratory experiments was rapidly growing mouse leukemia. My belief was different since it was clear that blood cell formation and constant replenishment of the linings of the gastrointestinal system (mouth, esophagus, stomach, small and large intestine) all required continued active proliferation. This was the reason for the toxicity of these drugs and of radiation therapy being due to interference with cell renewal in these normal tissues. Thus rather than studying rapidly proliferating tumors, I studied how normal blood cell proliferation occurred. The key to this, I felt, was the most basic cell from which all blood cells derive: the stem cell. First, I sought to determine whether there was in fact a primitive stem cell that was able to give rise to itself—self-renewal—as well as to both red and white blood cells. I did this by stressing the stem cells by causing bleeding to see whether this demand for more red blood cells would limit white blood cell production. It did, and this was evidence for a common stem cell. I did the reverse experiment as well, to see if bacterial toxins that caused increase in certain demand for white blood cells—granulocytes—would limit red blood cell formation, and this was also the case. At the same time, a new, more direct, measure of stem cells was described by Jim Till and Bun McCulloch in Toronto. They noted that when bone marrow cells were injected into the blood of irradiated mice and allowed to grow, they formed discrete nodules containing primitive and developing blood cells in the spleen. Counting these could be used to assess the number of stem cells injected. Using this powerful new technique allowed me to study the behavior of these stem cells under a variety of circumstances. They were located in the greatest concentration in the bone marrow, and we and others studied whether and how much they circulated in the blood. We also studied whether they were different in young as compared to old mice, how they responded to various chemotherapies and radiation. One especially important finding was that the stem cells do not proliferate rapidly under normal circumstances, but rather only when their number is reduced. The presence of such slowly proliferating normal cells provided a model for similar cells possibly being present in cancer. This has been extensively studied more recently by others with important results still emerging. Most important, because these stem cells are not actively proliferating, drugs that inhibit proliferation while killing the more rapidly dividing cancer cells do not much affect the primitive tumor stem cells. Thus these drugs cause tumors to reduce in size but do not prevent them from regrowing. We also found that, like radiation, there are drugs that do not discriminate between dividing and non-dividing cells. Later we found that we could grow stem cells in cell culture. This gave us another tool to use in studying these fascinating cells. This is a very brief and superficial description of 20 years of work in my laboratory. I am not including any of these research papers; because of the jargon used and the specialized knowledge required, they are not accessible to a general audience. I closed my lab at Harvard when I became the Physician-in-Chief at MSKCC, which required my full-time efforts. While much has changed in our understanding of the stem cells underlying normal tissue and tumors, much of what I studied is still relevant.

REFLECTIONS OF A RADIATION ONCOLOGIST AS PRESIDENT OF THE AMERICAN SOCIETY OF CLINICAL ONCOLOGY

Reprinted with permission. © 1987 American Society of Clinical Oncology. All rights reserved.

Hellman, S. *Journal of Clinical Oncology* 1987;5(12):2051–2054.

It is an honor to have been elected President of this Society and to be given the privilege of addressing you at this time. As the first radiation oncologist, I consider this a special privilege. Similarly, it is a great honor to be the Physician-in-Chief of Memorial Hospital with this particular disciplinary background. It seems appropriate that the subject of my Presidential Address should relate to the interplay of oncologic disciplines.

I have recently returned from Great Britain and had occasion to discuss with colleagues there the history of the specialties and their relationship. As you know, the two countries have developed their oncologic disciplines quite differently. In America, surgical oncology emerged as the first clinical cancer specialty. Appropriately, this emergence was led by my predecessors at Memorial Hospital. One of the first leaders of our institution, William Coley, a cancer surgeon, was asked to treat a young friend of John D. Rockefeller, Jr. It was her illness and eventual demise from the disease that stimulated the interest of the Rockefellers in Memorial and in cancer. This interest resulted in a long and distinguished philanthropic commitment, begun by John D. Rockefeller, Sr., at his son's request, and carried forward by John D. Rockefeller, Jr., who supported cancer research and education long before it was fashionable. This mission has been continued in recent years by John D. Rockefeller, Jr.'s son Laurance Rockefeller, former Chairman of the Board and currently Honorary Chairman of the Board of Memorial Sloan-Kettering Cancer Center.

As many of you know, while William Coley was a surgeon, he recognized the importance of systemic treatment. Having observed "spontaneous" regression of cancers in the presence of certain infections, he began to treat patients with bacterial products. It is only recently that one of the active substances released by Coley's toxins, tumor necrosis factor, has been elucidated by Lloyd Old and his colleagues at our center. Coley was followed by that giant in oncology, James Ewing. Ewing was head of Pathology and the Director of Memorial Hospital. He had a great influence over cancer therapy as practiced at the time, and it is no accident that the Society of Surgical Oncology has developed from what was once called the James Ewing Society. With the availability of improved surgical techniques and a rational basis for surgery, the en bloc dissection, cancer surgery grew at Memorial Hospital, led by such men as Hayes Martin, Alexander Brunschwig, and Frank Adair.

It is interesting to read James Ewing. While he espoused radical surgery, he understood its limitations and was prescient of future advances. He recognized that more conservative surgery could be combined with radiation to improve cure, decrease toxicity, and thus gain the confidence of the patient. With regard to breast cancer, I quote from Ewing in 1931,

> "On the other hand this situation calls for the greatest conservatism on the part of the surgeon. The time is past when every minute cancer or atypical encapsulated adenoma, or suspicious precancerous lesion should lead to radical mastectomy. We may now rely upon radiation with or without partial mastectomy [we would say with tumor excision] to control many of these early localized lesions and to replace operation in many advanced cases. In this way the confidence of the public will be conserved and many more women will be induced to consult their physicians at a favorable time."

Thus more than 50 years ago he espoused techniques of treatment only now coming to be accepted in the local-regional treatment of mammary carcinoma. Moreover, he recognized the importance of proposing therapies that are not only effective but less morbid and more consistent with returning the patient to her prediseased state. These statements predicted that such a treatment alternative will encourage early diagnosis with its attendant opportunities for improved cure.

He also recognized the importance of systemic treatment. With regard to breast cancer, he claimed that "[s]elective radiation is the nearest approach to a rational curative agent, but is available in a limited field only." This points out the problem of occult micrometastasis and the development of instruments designed for their treatment. Such a systemic treatment—cancer chemotherapy—began around the time of the Second World War; among the many who participated in this development, perhaps most important were Sidney Farber in Boston and David Karnofsky and Joe Burchenal at Memorial Sloan-Kettering. It is quite appropriate that our Society has named our most distinguished lectureship the Karnofsky lectureship.

Progress in cancer chemotherapy in the adult, like much of modern cancer therapy, appears to follow advances made in pediatrics. Childhood leukemia was cured with the new chemotherapy due to the pioneering work of Emil Freireich, Emil Frei, James Holland, and Donald Pinkel. Lymphomas were next, the result of the efforts of DeVita and his colleagues. The nonhematopoietic adult tumor first amenable to curative treatment was choriocarcinoma, which like leukemia was rapidly proliferating. This result by Li and Hertz was considered exceptional but perhaps not relevant since the tumor was of fetal origin. Even as early as the 1960s from the studies of M. C. Li and Robert Golbey, it was realized that a small percentage of testis tumors were curable. Subsequently at the M. D. Anderson Hospital, Samuels and coworkers improved on these results, utilizing vinblastine and bleomycin, and then—with the new effective platinum-based chemotherapies—Lawrence Einhorn and his colleagues demonstrated that most patients with metastatic testicular tumors could be cured. Of course, in terms of patients treated, the most ubiquitous application of chemotherapy is as adjuvant therapy, used most successfully in the treatment of breast cancer by Gianni Bonadonna and Bernard Fisher and their colleagues.

Radiation therapy, with its strong link to diagnostic imaging, lagged behind in the United States. Most radiation therapy was done by general radiologists, who, while attempting to do a devoted job, were largely interested in the problems associated with diagnostic imaging. There was a small band of radiation therapists—the American Club of Therapeutic Radiologists—who would gather at the diagnostic radiology meetings, usually in a small room appropriate for their size. This group of remarkable individuals had quite diverse backgrounds. Some were born abroad and most received their training abroad. In fact, Fernando Bloedorn, an early member of this group, once commented with some truth that the international language of radiation therapy was broken English.

There are a number of giants who developed this field: Simeon Cantril, Franz Buschke, Juan del Regato. They were outstanding clinicians who understood the natural history of cancer but were equipped with only limited therapeutic means. They were followed by four who brought the specialty to its modern position. Henry Kaplan, Gilbert Fletcher, Morton Kligerman, and Simon Kramer understood cancer and were able to take advantage of two new developments. Firstly, the modern supervoltage equipment presented a whole new therapeutic armamentarium to be utilized for cancer treatment. They developed careful programs of clinical investigation to explore the application of these new tools in the clinic. Secondly, they understood the importance of the scientific developments in radiation biology and tumor biology and tried to apply these therapeutically. Moreover, it is to these four that I believe we owe the development of training programs for the current leaders of this specialty.

It was into this club that I was initiated in the early 1960s. Over the last two decades things have changed markedly, and from a small club of about 200 members when I joined in 1963, there has grown the American Society of Therapeutic Radiology and Oncology, the lineal descendant which now has over 2,500 members, of whom about 1,000 are also members of the American Society of Clinical Oncology (ASCO).

I started this talk by commenting on how the specialties have developed quite differently in the United States and Great Britain. In the United Kingdom, it was radiation oncology that was developed first and led the oncologic disciplines. Cancer surgery, while practiced, never emerged with the vigor seen in the United States. Until very recently, medical oncology was not separately identified—rather, the administration of chemotherapy was often a part of the activities of the radiation oncologist.

These differences suggest that the relative importance and position of the specialties may in part reflect historical accident, or medical sociology, rather than therapeutic importance or future promise.

In both countries there has been both collaboration and the inevitable friction between the oncologic disciplines. While a certain degree of chauvinism is natural, I fear that in both countries we have sometimes lost track of the primary mission: not to prevail over the other specialty, but to cure cancer with the least morbidity possible. Yet, this is to be understood if not condoned. As disciplines develop, they are, like growing children, unsure of the limits of their strength; they look for greater challenges; they are brash and impetuous. All three disciplines, to carry the analogy, should have reached adult life by now and developed a mature assessment of their limitations as well as their strengths. Indeed, there does appear to be emerging a more integrated approach to disease.

We are oncologists first and only specialists of our disciplines second. We should make the best use of each specialty and work at both improving cure and decreasing toxicity. I am especially pleased to be a co-editor of a multidisciplinary textbook of oncology that attempts to develop such an integrated therapeutic approach. Similarly, we at Memorial Hospital are trying to develop disease-oriented programs of treatment that take into account the contributions of all specialties and limit "trade unionism" to the greatest extent possible.

Of course, there is much to be said for the complementary nature of the disciplines. In some cases, a multidisciplinary approach to a tumor can be considered, which may leave all with an important role in the treatment of the disease. For example, preservative surgery can be applied to remove the radioresistant central nidus of tumor, moderate dose radiation to destroy local and regional subclinical disease, and chemotherapy to destroy occult microscopic disease. This model has allowed cooperation in the treatment of breast cancer, soft-tissue sarcoma, cancer of the anus, and a variety of pediatric tumors. There appear to be further opportunities for this kind of collaboration. A most exciting potential application of this philosophy is in the treatment of bladder cancer. The promising results with aggressive chemotherapy allow its combination with preservative surgery and radiation therapy.

When all three modalities are brought to bear in a meaningful way, collaboration is easy. However, there are times when the specialties are competitive. At these times we must be careful not to lose sight of the patient. For instance, often either radiation or surgery can have a definitive role in the primary treatment and the other specialty may not be needed. This may be the case in the primary treatment of early prostate cancer, and in treatment of cervix cancer and a variety of head and neck tumors. Similarly, radiation therapy and chemotherapy will sometimes appear to be competitive alternatives. An example of this is to be seen in the treatment of some of the lymphomas.

It is worth remembering that our current treatments leave much to be desired. They are all too often associated with significant toxicity and their efficacy is hardly guaranteed. It is, therefore, our goal to change these treatments. It is our business to put ourselves out of business. While this may sound platitudinous, on reflection, it can be quite disquieting. During my tenure as Chairman of the Department of Radiation Therapy at Harvard Medical School, I was often asked by students and resident applicants about the future of radiation therapy as a specialty. They were concerned lest they learn a dying and unneeded art. I am afraid I was not too reassuring. I told them I had full confidence that radiation therapy would become far less important in the treatment of malignant disease. Before leaving the subject, however, I also indicated that I thought the same would be true of cancer surgery as we know it today and for cancer chemotherapy. All three had much that could be improved upon.

With this unsettling news, perhaps the students thought better of their choice of specialties. Perhaps they considered leaving oncology altogether. Had they done so and become cardiologists, however, they would have found diseases for which there were equally rapidly changing therapeutic approaches. I pointed out to them, as I remind you, that we are not primarily chemotherapists, radiation therapists, or cancer surgeons. Rather, we are oncologists using the most effective treatments available today. It is to be hoped that we will be flexible, able to adapt, and learn how to use the most effective treatments available tomorrow.

Our specialty is not, for the most part, any therapeutic discipline but rather oncology itself. Thus it is appropriate for the American Society of Clinical Oncology to be led by a practitioner of any of the therapeutic disciplines, since it is the study of oncology that binds us together, rather than the disciplinary lines that separate us.

Of course, if we are to treat cancer with the techniques available to us, we must learn how to do this well. It is necessary to have radiation oncologists, medical oncologists, and surgical oncologists, but we must not forget our primary concern is with oncology. We must be prepared to change and modify, to discard the old and accept the new—some of which is the result of the biologic revolution now upon us, the fruits of which are beginning to be presented at these meetings. While we are excited about their potential power, we must remember our experience with the other advances. They are unlikely to be panaceas. We will need these lessons of the past to deal with these future treatments.

TECHNOLOGY, BIOLOGY, AND TRAFFIC

Technology, Biology, and Traffic, Samuel Hellman, *Acta Oncologica* (2001), copyright © Acta Oncologica Foundation, reprinted by permission of Taylor & Francis Ltd., www.tandfonline.com, on behalf of Acta Oncologica Foundation.

The purpose of the Nobel Conference 2000 "From the cellular response and DNA damage to biological optimization of radiation therapy" was to consider research extending from biophysics and molecular cell biology to clinical physics in order both to explain and improve treatment of malignant disease by radiation. The fact that I, a physician, was asked to give the Keynote Address testifies to the orientation of the meeting. The conference was convened not only for the discussion of science at many levels, but also in order to focus on improving the treatment of cancer patients. Medicine is an amalgamation of basic science, applied science, and that special relationship between the physician and patient which results in determining the nature of illness and an appropriate plan of management. It is within the context of all three that one should consider radiation therapy. This medical specialty—radiation oncology—is a particular recipient of the advances of technology, the molecular biologic revolution, and the understanding of the complex self-regulating cybernetic system that is the human body faced with a malignant disease. How to evaluate the individual clinical circumstances is benefited by molecular, anatomic, and physiological knowledge of the particular patient and the tumor.

Technology, molecular and cell biology, and an understanding of complex systems all offer opportunities for improvement in radiation treatment, but before discussing these areas, I would like to put the importance of the local treatment of cancer in an appropriate perspective. It is often stated that local-regional treatment of cancer is not a critical factor in the cure of cancer. Although it is important today, it will be supplanted by effective systemic therapies which will eradicate local disease as well as distant metastases, the latter thought to be the dominant cancer problem. This trivializing of the importance of the primary tumor and the regional lymph nodes does not conform to present knowledge of malignant disease. Perez and Brady, in their textbook *Principles and Practice of Radiation Oncology*, review the data from the 1990 American Cancer Society Facts and Figures and estimate that in the United States, of the approximately 440,000 cancer deaths that year, 127,000 were due to local-regional disease alone and that an additional 170,000 were due to both local-regional and distant disease. Collectively, therefore, two-thirds of those patients who died had local-regional tumor as a significant component of their disease, with distant metastasis being the site of disease in only one-third. It is also worth considering the importance of local-regional treatment in those patients with a high probability of occult distant metastases. Two recent studies reported considered whether improved local-regional control was important in breast cancer patients treated with modified radical mastectomy who were treated with adjuvant chemotherapy to destroy occult microscopic disease. In both of these prospective randomized trials the addition of radiation therapy to mastectomy improved local-regional control, as expected, but in addition there was an important improvement in survival. The magnitude of this improvement in survival of about 10 absolute percentage points is equivalent to that found in randomized trials of adjuvant chemotherapy alone. Adjuvant treatment with systemic agents and with local-regional radiation is at least additive. It also suggests that as we develop more effective systemic treatment for subclinical metastases in other types of cancer, locoregional control will become even more important. While we all hope that a single effective therapy will completely eradicate tumor at all locations, until such a panacea is found we must address both distant and local-regional sites of cancer.

It is interesting that the most recently promulgated systemic therapy—which is designed to prevent the angio-genesis induced by cancer—seems to be most effective when combined with local-regional treatment. I conclude that radiation therapy will have an expanded role in cancer treatment for the foreseeable future.

Technology

In our enthusiasm for the truly astounding advances in molecular biology, we may neglect the changes in medicine resulting from technological advances. At the beginning of my medical education the art of medicine was primarily in determining the appropriate diagnosis, with the medical history and physical examination playing the most prominent role. Today, I believe that the diagnosis is largely established by technological means, while medical practice is more concerned with the treatment of the disease. This improvement in diagnosis is due to a variety of laboratory instruments but most importantly to the imaging revolution. Imaging advances are being applied to local treatment and will play an increasingly important role in radiation oncology. Advances in computed tomography applied to the patient in the treatment position will greatly reduce uncertainty, resulting in increased accuracy and reproducibility of treatment.

Magnetic resonance improves tumor imaging greatly and—like computed tomography—its digital format and software allow integration of these images. Magnetic resonance spectroscopy and positron emission tomography enable imaging of the anatomy of tumor physiology both initially and during treatment. Such functional imaging will also allow the identification of occult tumor as well as increasing our accuracy in separating tumor from non-malignant tissue. A major focus of tumor imaging will be accurate estimation of the extent of the tumor. Accurate anatomic identification of all tumor cells might even be possible. Alternatively, one might use imaging methods to determine the concentration of tumor cells within a unit volume of tissue. This I call "tumor density." It can be combined with the probability of tumor cells within a defined volume based on the known proclivities of individual tumors for invasion and metastases. All of these determinations will radically change our understanding of what the treatment volume should be.

Not only is imaging important for locating the tumor and identifying its physiology, but these representations of the tumor can be linked to treatment delivery. Such computer-controlled radiation therapy has been suggested for at least 25 years, but it is only in more recent times that technology has allowed this to have widespread clinical application. Intensity-modulated radiation therapy and tomotherapy are but two current examples of computer-controlled radiation therapy. These approaches require reconsideration of the fundamental paradigm of treatment. This paradigm urges uniform irradiation of tumor while minimizing the dose to the normal tissues. Computer control of treatment with accurate anatomically presented physiologic data and tumor density information offer the opportunity to "paint" the dose in conformity with tumor cell distribution, oxygenation, and other important physiologic characteristics. Reductions in the uncertainty of tumor extent and improvement in treatment precision will allow significant reduction in the target volume.

Feedback and control of the radiation treatment is now being employed utilizing simple gating techniques. However, software has already been developed which could be applied to assure the appropriate radiation delivery while compensating for patient motion or physiologic organ motion. This feedback and control will greatly reduce unnecessary irradiation and will also improve the likelihood of treating the entire tumor to the planned dose. These techniques also depend on an assessment of how to distribute the unwanted radiation administered to traversed normal tissues. Such "dose dumping" depends on understanding the sequelae of organ-specific dose distribution, the biology of which will be discussed later. Improved software should also provide a reconsideration of particle radiation to further restrict radiation to the tumor. Protons are on the immediate horizon and it will be interesting to see whether the theoretic advantage of such particle radiation will have practical consequences in more than very limited circumstances.

Biology

The rapid developments in molecular cell biology are advancing our understanding of the effects of ionizing radiation on biologic material. While this begins with damage to and repair of the genome, it also includes the recently discovered important cytotoxic effects of ionizing radiation on non-genomic structures such as the cell membrane and even a bystander effect resulting in the death of adjacent cells. In association with radiation damage to cells, there is a cascade of cytokines released, which may play a role in further tumor cell kill, as well as contributing to damage to normal tissues.

The importance of oxygen concentration to cellular radiation sensitivity has been noted for more than half of the last century, yet therapy designed to exploit this has been limited. With the anatomic determination of local differences in oxygen concentration within tumors and the availability of new modifiers of the oxygen effect or agents specifically toxic to hypoxic cells, we should finally be able to take advantage of this large effect.

Perhaps the most intensely studied phenomenon in cell biology is the cell cycle and those changes associated with cell birth and cell death. Intimately bound with the cell cycle are those checkpoints at which damage is evaluated and either repaired or the cell committed to programmed cell death. Evaluation of these mechanisms in individual tumors and their manipulation offer the possibility of optimizing and individualizing radiation therapy. The aberrations of the cell cycle checkpoints and of cell kinetics in each individual malignancy will determine appropriate treatment strategies. Determining the importance of apoptosis, as well as how one stimulates or increases terminal differentiation, will offer new therapeutic opportunities.

Tumors require the acquisition of four important phenotypes: growth, invasion, metastases, and angiogenesis. The ability to induce a new blood supply is essential in order for tumors to grow both locally and in distant sites, and so I add angiogenesis to the usual triad of malignant behavior. Tumor angiogenesis provides a new target for therapy. Studies of anti-angiogenic agents are extremely promising in the laboratory and are beginning to be used in the clinic. What perhaps would be most useful would be to combine anti-tumor agents such as radiation with anti-angiogenic agents. Possibly some of the current effectiveness of radiation may be due to its effect on tumor vessels. Cytotoxic agents currently used in cancer treatment, if used with quite different time-dose configurations than those designed for anti-tumor effects, may be quite effective as anti-angiogenic therapy.

The cell cycle, the relative extent of cell birth and cell death, terminal differentiation, as well as angiogenesis, all affect tumor growth. Tumors appear to become more malignant as they progress. This malignant progression may affect not only the likelihood of metastastic spread but may well also affect radiation response. For example, p53 abnormalities increase as a function of the size of a breast cancer. It is well known that p53 is important for the cell cycle checkpoints and for preservation of the apoptotic pathway. We have found that other specific abnormalities associated with growth, invasion, metastasis, and angiogenesis all increase with increasing tumor size or nodal involvement in breast cancer.

In order for radiation or any therapy to be effective, there must be a differential effect on the tumor as compared with the normal tissues. Understanding normal tissue radiation biology is essential to improving the therapeutic efficacy of any treatment. This affects planning the dose distribution both within and outside the target volume. Early-responding and late-responding tissues have different characteristics, which should inform biologically optimized treatment planning. This is especially important with the increasing ability to 'dose paint 'as well to develop appropriate dose-dumping strategies. Permanent implantation of Auger-emitting isotopes should also be considered in this light. These isotopes create problems in homogeneity of dose and dose rate as well as gradual decrease in dose rate associated with the protracted radioactive decay.

Traffic

I have chosen to use the term "traffic" to consider the complexity associated with the establishment of a cancer, its growth, and the response by the normal tissues. I use the term "traffic" because of a comment made by Sir James Gowans, the Oxford immunologist, suggesting that there was little to be learned about automobile traffic from extensive study of the internal combustion engine. He meant, as do I, that while reductionism provides great insights into mechanism, complex systems have to be studied at many levels in order to have an appropriate understanding. The nature of local tumor invasion, preferred pathways of spread, and how these are affected by treatment are all part of such traffic studies.

The traffic considerations associated with the immune system are a special case. The kinetics of tumor cells entering the lymphatic system and how this is affected by radiation should be quite important The growth of tumor in lymph nodes, the kinetics of immune recognition, anti-body-dependent cytotoxicity, and cellular immunity are also likely to be affected in complex ways. Using the increasingly accurate and precise radiation treatment techniques, how much of the regional lymph nodes should be treated? What should the strategy of dose dumping be with regard to irradiating regional lymph nodes? Since these regional nodes are the initial site of the immune response, should they be restricted from the irradiated volume, or is this irrelevant or compensated for by the destruction of nodal metastases? Irradiation of the tumor likely has many effects on the immune response. While tumor-infiltrating lymphocytes will be destroyed, radiation will cause an increase in availability and a modification of tumor antigens. Ionizing radiation is also associated with the production of chaperone proteins. These proteins appear to aid antigen-presenting cells in their function and increase the efficacy of the immune response. Finally, there is the "adjuvant effect" of irradiated tumor cells. How much of it is due to any of these mechanisms is unclear. But what is clear is that there is a great difference between surgical excision of the tumor with little or no antigen remaining, compared with destroying tumors with ionizing radiation.

The most obvious traffic important in cancer is that required for the development of systemic metastases. This process requires access to the blood vessels, egress from the blood vessels, and host organ receptivity. Radiation is likely to have an effect on all of these phenomena in addition to the effects of radiation on the seeding ability of surviving tumor cells. The complexity of the multiple sites and effects of radiation are staggering, but they need to be understood in order to craft the appropriate local-regional treatment plan.

Technological capacity and biological knowledge offer an opportunity to individualize treatment to each host-tumor circumstance. Standard treatment methods will be replaced by such individualization. But in order for this to occur, we must accept and embrace complexity.

KARNOFSKY MEMORIAL LECTURE. NATURAL HISTORY OF SMALL BREAST CANCERS

Reprinted with permission. © 1994 American Society of Clinical Oncology. All rights reserved.

Hellman, S. *Journal of Clinical Oncology* 1994;12(10):2229–2234.

Progress in medicine, like evolution, appears to occur in fits and starts, that is, there appear to be long periods of quiescence and then great bursts of insight into the etiology, natural history, and therapy of particular diseases. With breast cancer, the notion of the disease, its pathogenesis, and its treatment remained relatively static following the formulation of the Halsted paradigm for the disease and the acceptance of radical mastectomy as the logical therapeutic embodiment of this notion of disease spread.[1,2]

Fin de siècle, or end of the century, is used to describe the last decade of the nineteenth century, when this operation was described. It also connotes a time for reflection and taking stock. Since it has been just 100 years since the initial publication on this subject, it is appropriate to consider the state of the paradigm for breast cancer pathogenesis and its therapeutic implications. The acceptance of radical mastectomy was due both to the effectiveness and the attractiveness of the Halsted model. The underlying premise is that breast cancer is an orderly disease that progresses in a contiguous fashion from primary site, by direct extension, through the lymphatics to the lymph nodes, and then to distant metastatic sites. It implies that effective treatment must recognize this orderly, contiguous disease spread. In fact, in his original formulation, Halsted[3] suggested that even spread to the vertebra or to the abdomen was due to translymphatic contiguous extension. Its attractiveness lies in the en bloc approach to surgery, which came to be the guiding principle of cancer surgery. Despite a plateau in the effectiveness of radical mastectomy, it was not until recently that an alternative hypothesis was accepted. That hypothesis suggests that breast cancer is a systemic disease and implies that small tumors are just an early manifestation of such systemic disease, which, if it is to metastasize, has already metastasized. Nodal involvement is not an orderly contiguous extension, but rather a marker of distant disease. Local control, according to this theory, is unimportant to survival. This was first suggested by Geoffrey Keynes,[4] carried forward by George Crile, Jr.,[5] and fully explicated with both laboratory and clinical studies by a former president of the American Society of Clinical Oncology (ASCO) and Karnovsky lecturer, Bernard Fisher,[6] who in that lecture stated "that breast cancer is a systemic disease involving a complex spectrum of host-tumor interactions and that variations in effective local regional treatment are unlikely to effect survival substantially." A third hypothesis considers breast cancer to be a heterogeneous disease that can be thought of as a spectrum of proclivities extending from a disease that remains local throughout its course to one that is systemic when first detectable. This hypothesis suggests that metastases are a function of tumor growth and progression. Lymph node involvement is of prognostic importance not only because it indicates a more malignant tumor biology, but also because persistent disease in the lymph nodes can be the source of distant disease. This model requires that there are meaningful clinical situations in which lymph nodes are involved but there has not yet been any distant disease. Persistent disease, locally or regionally, may give rise to distant metastases and, therefore, in contrast to the systemic theory, locoregional therapy is important. This third, or spectrum, theory suggests that even if, as the systemic theory suggests, tumor cells spread distantly early in the natural history of the disease, metastases do not regularly occur. A most important parameter determining the likelihood of their presentation is tumor size. Therefore, there are significant times in the clinically relevant natural history of the disease when metastases have not occurred, but if tumor is left inadequately treated, metastases will occur.

After this long period of acceptance of the Halsted hypothesis and radical mastectomy as the treatment, we have had, like the rapid changes seen during certain periods of evolution, an abrupt alteration in our conception of this disease. This has been caused by the following three innovations in the diagnosis and treatment of breast cancer: (1) screening mammography, (2) lumpectomy and radiation therapy with breast conservation as an alternative local treatment, and (3) adjuvant chemotherapy as a curative treatment for subclinical disease. All three bear directly on the appropriate paradigm for breast cancer and the use of the Halsted operation. Screening mammography discovers tumors quite different in size with, I suggest, a more favorable biology than those detected clinically, and invites less radical treatment. While lumpectomy plus radiation is based on the Halsted model of disease pathogenesis, it is very different than en bloc surgical extirpation. Adjuvant chemotherapy emphasizes the importance of subclinical disseminated disease.

It is the purpose of this discussion to focus on the small breast cancers that we are seeing increasingly today—the result of active screening programs and a heightened public awareness—to determine which one of these models best fits with clinical experience. The 1990 SEER data indicate that breast cancer incidence is essentially flat except for the increase in stage 1 breast cancer, which has risen from 25% to almost 50% of all invasive breast cancers from 1983 to 1990. Almost certainly, this is the result of screening mammography. If one examines the data for screen-detected breast cancer in two large European studies, that from Nejmegen, Netherlands—a well-performed screening project—and the two-county Swedish trial—a randomized trial[8,9]—one finds that small cancers are the large majority of those observed, even when one excludes the first screen. Such breast cancers are more likely to be node-negative and, as we shall see shortly, if nodes are involved they are likely to be limited in number. This is directly related to tumor size.

The first general question useful in distinguishing among the three hypotheses is at what time in the natural history of breast cancer do distant metastases occur? The systemic disease hypothesis suggests that these occur before clinical detection and argues that local eradication of disease makes little or no difference. The results from screening mammography argue strongly that this is not the case. There appears to be a 30% reduction in deaths due to breast cancer in mammographically screened populations. Again, as an example, let me use the two-county Swedish trial[8] for which the data have now been available for at least 11 years and continue to show a 30% reduction in deaths due to breast cancer. I emphasize breast cancer deaths as an end point, because reduction in this avoids the objections of lead-time bias or length bias to which incidence or survival rates can be subject. I believe the only plausible explanation for this 30% reduction is that, for those 30%, metastases would have occurred between the time of mammographic detection and routine clinical detection. Detection by screening mammogram has allowed effective locoregional treatment before distant spread of sufficient numbers of cells capable of metastatic growth. In my judgment, this is a strong argument against the systemic thesis.

Tubiana et al.[10–12] have studied almost 3,000 patients with breast cancer who were seen at the Institute Gustave-Roussy before the routine use of adjuvant chemotherapy and have shown that metastases in that group is a continuous function of tumor size. For any tumor size, there is an eventual probability of metastases that increases with increasing tumor size. This never reaches 100%. The time to arrive at this plateau is inversely related to tumor size, that is, smaller tumors take longer to demonstrate their metastatic potential than do larger ones. This latter point is especially important when considering small breast cancers. I have taken the liberty of making a table based on a figure in one of their reports.[10] Table 3.1

Table 3.1. CLINICAL APPEARANCE OF METASTASES AS A FUNCTION OF TUMOR SIZE

Class	Diameter (cm)	Estimated Proportion of Initial Metastases (%)	Eventual Metastases (%)	Estimated Initial (%) per Year	No. of Cases
1	$1 \leq 2.5$	3	27	2.5	317
2	$2.5 \leq 3.5$	4	42	5	496
3	$3.5 \leq 4.5$	7	57	7	544
4	$4.5 \leq 5.5$	10	67	9	422
5	$5.5 \leq 6.5$	16	73	12	329
6	$6.5 \leq 7.5$	22	84	15	192
7	$7.5 \leq 8.5$	22	81	15	136
8	≥ 8.5	35	92	22	212

Data from Koscielny et al.[10]

indicates the increased proportion of initial metastases when patients are first seen, as well as the eventual percent of patients who develop metastases as a function of initial tumor size. It also estimates the initial slope of metastases as a function of tumor size. Note the smallest tumors in this study: class 1 tumors that are less than 2.5 cm. Patients with tumors in this class develop metastastic disease at an estimated 2.5% per year, and half of the patients who eventually developed metastases did so by 42 months, as compared with only 4 months for class 8 tumors. This emphasizes the long follow-up duration required for small breast cancers and the limited value of 5-year data, even 5-year disease-free survival data.

What then are the possible natural histories of these increasingly frequent small breast cancers? I define small breast cancers for this discussion as those tumors ≤ 2 cm in size (T1) when first seen regardless of lymph node status. First, some of these may be incidental findings at mammogram of tumors with such benign or indolent natural histories as to have no significant effect on survival. The presence of such lesions is thought to elevate falsely survival calculations of mammographically screened populations. One technique that I find useful to avoid this bias is to consider only cancers found after initial screening. As a clinical issue when patients present to us, we cannot tell whether the tumor detected is one of these indolent and clinically unimportant cancers or not.

The second group would be those that have a localized cancer that, if left to grow, will become disseminated and result in the patient's death. It is this group that must explain the success of screening in reducing breast cancer–related deaths. Also relevant to this group are the effects of locoregional therapy on outcome. If differences are found, they must be due to differences in the persistence of disease in the primary tumor or nodal site resulting in differences in distant metastases. The randomized trial performed in Stockholm of adjuvant radiation following mastectomy bears directly on this point.[13] The study is important since the treatment would be acceptable by today's standards, it was performed before adjuvant chemotherapy (1971 to 1976), and has the required long follow-up duration. This study shows the expected reduction in locoregional recurrences, but it also shows an accompanying decrease in distant metastases and deaths due to breast cancer. The overview analysis of all randomized trials of mastectomy with or without adjuvant radiotherapy has been updated by Cuzick et al.[14] They conclude, "The reduction of breast cancer deaths suggests that radiation therapy may have a value beyond the clearly established improvements obtainable for local control." That statement endorses the notion that distant metastases can be the consequence of persistant local or regional disease and that effective locoregional therapy can reduce their frequency. They point out that the National Surgical Adjuvant Breast and Bowel Project Study B-04, as well as the Stockholm results, shows a significant mortality benefit. B-06 compared lumpectomy with lumpectomy and radiation.[15-17] There was a large difference in local control and, at 5 years, in distant metastases, but this was not true at 8 years. This study included all tumors up to 4 cm. Further study and follow-up evaluation of T1 tumors in this group would be interesting.

One study suggests that treatment of the axillary lymph nodes can affect survival. In the Guy's trial,[18] inadequate radiation treatment of the axilla resulted in more axillary recurrences, and this was associated with a greater incidence of distant metastases and decreased survival.

Thus, we have considered those tumors that are destined to remain localized, those that metastasize as a function of size, and those that possibly disseminate from persistent lymph node disease. Finally, there must be some patients whose tumors have occultly disseminated by the time of diagnosis, since locoregional treatment is not universally effective in preventing metastases, even in those patients who have been rendered free of locoregional disease. It is, of course, the presence of this group that argues for adjuvant systemic therapy. Determination of the relative proportion of such patients when one is considering small breast cancers will inform any therapeutic strategy.

There is also the question of whether tumor progression occurs during the clinically observed portion of the natural history of localized breast cancer. There are two possible effects of tumor size. The first is that metastasic frequency increases directly as a function of tumor size because more cells are available to metastasize. A second possibility is that small tumors are intrinsically less malignant than large ones. The Gustave-Roussy series,[10,11] as well as the results of screening mammography,[7,8] shows an increase in grade as a function of tumor size. This may be due both to tumor progression and to selection of more malignant tumors by their more rapid growth. Thus, the reason that large tumors are more malignant may have to do with their having more cells to seed, by tumor progression with an increase in the malignancy of these cells, and by the more rapid proliferation of more malignant cells.

Analysis of survival data requires consideration of the consequences of different biologic events. Jay Harris and I have discussed this previously.[19-22] I would like to add a further distinction to that discussion. I propose that there are two components of malignancy. These are not necessarily completely independent, but current methods of analysis tend to confound them. For lack of better words, I will call them virulence and metastagenicity. Virulence is the pace or rate of disease growth, dissemination, and clinical manifestation. Metastagenicity is the ultimate likelihood of distant metastases. Fixed-point survival estimates will confuse these when this point occurs before the full expression of metastastic potential. A class of tumors that has a high virulence will demonstrate metastases quickly, even though the eventual likelihood for distant metastases may be no different than another group. An example of this is shown in Table 3.2, which comes from the Chicago experience to be described subsequently. The analysis at the usually accepted 5-year end point shows the expected and statistically significant effect of age on outcome; however, this disappears by 10 years. This, then, is a real difference, but it is in virulence, not

Table 3.2. PERCENTAGE OF T1N0 PATIENTS DYING OF BREAST CANCER AS A FUNCTION OF AGE AT DIAGNOSIS

Age at Diagnosis (Years)	% of Patient Deaths		
	5 Years	10 Years	20 Years
< 50	14	14	20
≥ 50	6	11	19

Data from Quiet et al. see Table 3.3.

metastagenicity. Another possible example is seen in a review of breast cancers ≤ 1 cm or less reported by Stierer et al.,[23] who showed a difference in virulence but not metastagenicity as measured by relapse-free survival when studying the prognostic significance of the number of mitotic figures in these tumors. Using a single point in time such as 5 years will not distinguish between virulence and metastagenicity. This should be especially important in trying to understand the effects of different types of systemic adjuvants. Hormonal manipulation may have quite different effects than chemotherapy. A soon to be published European Organization for Research and Treatment of Cancer (EORTC) trial (Bartelink H, Rubens RD, van der Schueren E, et al., submitted) showed quite different results when analyzed shortly after conclusion as compared with 8 years later. In this trial, which compared hormonal and chemotherapeutic adjuvant treatment for locally advanced breast cancer, the initially statistically significant benefit of chemotherapy disappeared, while the hormonal effect increased in size and significance with longer follow-up durations.

Informed by this formulation of the three alternative hypotheses—Halsted, systemic, and spectrum—and cautioned to observe the complete clinical evolution of small breast cancers, I should like to discuss two series with which I have been personally involved. These are both mature series of patients treated almost exclusively by local and regional methods and monitored for long periods of time. I shall try to ascertain from these data which hypothesis best explains their natural history. In both series, I will be discussing primarily these small tumors. One series comes from Memorial Sloan-Kettering Cancer Center and the other from The University of Chicago. Peter Rosen was the senior author on a study of the long-term survival of patients with T1N0 and T1N1 breast cancer who presented at Memorial Hospital from 1965 to 1970 and were analyzed 18 years later.[24] More recently, Coral Quiet (Quiet CA, Ferguson DJ, Weichselbaum RR, et al., submitted) has reviewed a series of patients with breast cancer, largely operated on and followed by Donald Ferguson, who were seen from 1927 to 1984 with a mean follow-up duration of 14 years and a maximum of 44 years. The node-negative patients were presented at the American Society of Clinical Oncology (ASCO) meeting last year and the node-positive patients are being presented this year. I shall first consider those patients without involved axillary lymph nodes. For those patients whose tumors were less than 1 cm without positive axillary lymph nodes in the Memorial Hospital series, 12% developed recurrence of their breast cancer, that is, for 88% of such patients locoregional treatment was effective. For those patients with tumors between 1 and 2 cm, 26% developed recurrence. Brinkley and Haybittle[25] have suggested a statistical definition of cure to be that proportion of the treated group that has the same survival as an age-adjusted peer population. For those patients with tumors ≤ 1 cm, 88% appeared to be cured and this appears to occur somewhere around 10 years. In those patients with larger T1 tumors, the curves do not become parallel until close to 15 years. The data from The University of Chicago series do not show this difference within T1 tumors, but the aggregate T1 results are similar. Seventy-nine percent of such patients are cured of their breast cancers. In this series, both the median time for recurrence and the time in which it takes 10% of the patients to relapse are inversely related to tumor size. Small tumors take a longer time to recur than do large tumors, and a 5-year end point will not capture many of the recurrences: in this series, almost half of the deaths occur after 5 years. This is consistent with the Tubiana-Koscielny data.[10,11] The results from screening also document the important relationship of size to survival. Tabar et al.[9] show a difference within T1 tumors, as well as the high curability of such tumors as compared with larger lesions. Surely, these high disease-free survival data in the Memorial and Chicago experience before systemic adjuvant therapy argue strongly that stage 1 breast cancer is usually only a locoregional process. This is the case in approximately 75% to 80% of such patients. The data also suggest that even in stage 1 breast cancer, smaller tumors do better.

I should like to now consider those patients with involved lymph nodes. It is of interest that the number of nodes involved with such small breast cancers is limited. In a recent review of patients involved in the EORTC trial of the role of a booster dose in breast-conserving therapy, 19% of patients had lymph node involvement (A. Ptaszynski, personal communication, March 1994). In 47% of such patients, only one node was involved,

22% had two nodes involved, 9% had three nodes involved, and only 22% had four or more lymph nodes involved; thus, in the entire group, only 4% had four or more nodes involved. In the Memorial series,[24] patients with one to three lymph nodes involved appeared to be cured by locoregional treatment 68% of the time. The curve became parallel with the age-adjusted peer population at approximately 13 to 15 years. The Chicago data emphasize the importance of small primary tumor size when there are only a limited number of positive nodes. In this series, size is important even when there is lymph node involvement. Small tumors that have only one positive node still have an excellent prognosis. This is also true when two or three nodes are involved. This does not appear to be true when four or more nodes are involved. Analysis of these 20-year data (Table 3.3) indicates that having only one node involved did not reduce survival for T1 breast cancer patients. Seventy-three percent of patients with two to three nodes involved survived 20 years without relapse. Only when there were four or more nodes involved was there a significant reduction in survival. These long-term data before adjuvant systemic therapy indicate that, in small breast cancers, lymph node involvement is not a marker of distant disease unless a large number of nodes are involved. When there are only a small number of nodes involved, there does not appear to be any higher

Table 3.3. Percentage Disease-Free Survival at 20 Years as a Function of Tumor Size

No. of Positive Nodes	Tumor Size (mm)		
	1–10	11–20	≥ 20
0	79	79	64
1	95	78	59
2–3	73	73	53

Data from Quiet CA, Ferguson DJ, Hellman S. The Natural History of Node-Negative Breast Cancer: A Study of 826 Patients with Long Follow-up. J Clin Oncol 13:5(May), 1144–1151, 1995. Quiet CA, Ferguson DJ, Hellman S. The Natural History of Node-Positive Breast Cancer: The Curability of Small Cancers with a Limited Number of Postive Nodes. J Clin Oncol, Vol.14, No. 12 (December), 1996, pp 3105–3111.

probability of metastastic disease. Tubiana et al.[12] show excellent results for these small tumors with limited nodal involvement and also show an independent effect of grade.

The curability, using locoregional treatment, of patients with small breast cancers and a limited number of positive lymph nodes speaks for the orderliness of disease progression in these patients. Such lymph node involvement is the first, or only, site of disease in the large number of patients cured by locoregional treatment. This suggests that the systemic hypothesis is not appropriate for patients with such small lesions. It also emphasizes the need for prompt and proper treatment, not only of the primary lesion, but of regional lymph nodes as well. While the systemic hypothesis may be correct in that tumor cells circulate very early in the natural history of the tumor, operationally it has quite different implications. Small tumors are usually amenable to local or regional treatment alone. This is true even when there is some axillary node involvement. Perhaps there is early distant dissemination of tumor cells, but, if so, presumably the host can deal with the small number of cells or these cells are insufficiently malignant to produce metastases. When tumors are larger, the likelihood for metastasis increases, perhaps both as a function of a larger number of cells seeding and possibly as the result of tumor progression.

Both the Halsted and the systemic hypotheses are too restricting. The hypothesis most consistent with the data is that breast cancer is best thought of as a spectrum of disease with increasing proclivity for metastasis as a function of tumor size, but for any tumor size there is a proportion of patients with distant metastasis. Similarly, there is a proportion with local disease alone. While lymph node involvement can be a marker of increased risk of distant disease, it may be the only site of metastasis in many patients, especially those with small tumors. We have also learned that 5-year data can be misleading and should be used with caution.

What then are the therapeutic messages of this analysis of small tumors? The proportion of the patients who present with such tumors is large and will increase with more widespread screening. The absolute curability of T1N0 breast cancer is quite high with effective locoregional treatment, and this should not be compromized. To maximize uncomplicated cure, we must develop a strategy for adjuvant systemic therapy that recognizes the excellent prognosis of these patients. The increasingly recognized importance of chemotherapy dose intensity requires a method of selecting those patients who require such treatment from the large majority cured by locoregional treatment alone. Different adjuvant therapies may affect virulence and metastagenicity differently, so that we need markers for both and should analyze mature adjuvant trials to determine which aspect of malignancy is most affected by the treatment.

This end of the century reflection on the natural history of small breast cancers then brings a synthesis to the contiguous–systemic dialectic. Both have some truth, but adherence to either alone is inadequate. The satisfactory synthesis recognizes both, within a spectrum in which for small tumors the disease is usually restricted to the primary tumor site with the possible involvement of a limited number of regional lymph nodes. Larger tumors are more likely associated with systemic disease when first observed. The lesson from all this is the value of clinical investigation to study the natural history of disease. As the philosopher of science Karl Popper[26] has emphasized, the nature of scientific truth is conditional; progress is an increasingly satisfactory approximation of truth. I believe that this synthesis is a more satisfactory approximation of truth, but it is only that—an approximation—and it is conditional on more information. This brings me to the final lesson of this *fin de siècle* discussion: that of the inappropriateness of dogma in medicine and science.[27] Halsted became dogma and, more recently, the notion of breast cancer always being systemic has become dogma. Like all dogma in science, both are too restricting. They tend to limit our inquiries and deny the conditional and approximate nature of scientific knowledge.

Acknowledgment

I have relied greatly on colleagues for much of what I have presented: my long-time colleague at the Joint Center for Radiation Therapy in Boston,

Jay Harris; my collaborators at Memorial Sloan-Kettering Cancer Center in New York, Peter Rosen, Susan Groshen, David Kinne, and Zvi Fuks; at The University of Chicago, Ralph Weichselbaum, Ruth Heimann, Coral Quiet, Donald Ferguson, and Robert Schmidt; at the Netherlands Cancer Institute, Harry Bartelink, Jacques Borger, Joop vanDongen, and Emil Rutgers; and at the EORTC, Mieke Ptaszynski, Richard Sylvester, and Pieter Clahsen. I hope I have been faithful to their data, without which this presentation would have been impossible; however, the interpretations are my responsibility. Finally, I am indebted to The University of Chicago for a leave and to the Netherlands Cancer Institute for its hospitality and intellectual stimulation.

REFERENCES

1. Halsted WS: The results of operations for the cure of cancer of the breast performed at the Johns Hopkins Hospital from June, 1889 to January, 1894. *Johns Hopkins Bull* 4:297, 1984–1985.
2. Meyer W: An improved method of the radical operation for carcinoma of the breast. *Med Rec* 46:746, 1894.
3. Halsted WS: The results of radical operations for the cure of carcinoma of the breast. *Ann Surg* 46:1, 1907.
4. Keynes G: Carcinoma of the breast, the unorthodox view. *Proc Cardiff M Soc* 40, 1954.
5. Crile G Jr: *A Biological Consideration of the Treatment of Breast Cancer*. Springfield IL, Thomas, 1967.
6. Fisher B: Laboratory and clinical research in breast cancer—A personal adventure: The David A. Karnofsky Memorial Lecture. *Cancer Res* 40:3863–3874, 1980.
7. Peer PGM, Holland R, Hendriks JHCL, et al.: Age specific effectiveness of the Nijmegen population-based breast cancer-screening program: Assessment of early indicators of screening effectiveness. *J Natl Cancer Inst* 86:436–440, 1994.
8. Tabar L, Fagerberg G, Duffy SW, et al.: Update of the Swedish two-county program of mammographic screening for breast cancer. *Radiol Clin North Am* 30:187–210, 1992.
9. Tabar L, Fagerberg G, Day NE, et al.: Breast cancer treatment and natural history: New insights from results of screening. *Lancet* 339:412–414, 1992.
10. Koscielny S, Tubiana M, Le MG, et al.: Breast cancer: Relationship between the size of the primary tumour and the probability of metastatic dissemination. *Br J Cancer* 49:709–715, 1984.
11. Tubiana M, Koscielny S: Natural history of human breast cancer: Recent data and clinical implications. *Breast Cancer Res Treat* 18:125–140, 1991.

12. Tubiana M, Koscielny S: The natural history of breast cancer: Implications for a screening strategy. *Int J Radiat Oncol Biol Phys* 19:1117–1120, 1990.
13. Rutqvist LE, Pettersson D, Johansson H: Adjuvant radiation therapy versus surgery alone in operable breast cancer: Long-term follow-up of a randomized clinical trial. *Radiother Oncol* 26:104–110, 1993.
14. Cuzick J, Stewart H, Rutqvist L, et al.: Coarse-specific mortality in long-term survivors of breast cancer who participated in trials of radiotherapy. *J Clin Oncol* 12:447–453, 1994.
15. Fisher B, Bauer M, Margolese R, et al.: Five-year results of a randomized clinical trial comparing total mastectomy and segmental mastectomy with of without radiation in the treatment of breast cancer. *N Engl J Med* 312:665–673, 1985.
16. Fisher B, Redmond C, Poisson R, et al.: Eight-year results of a randomized clinical trial comparing total mastectomy and lumpectomy with or without irradiation if the treatment of breast cancer. *N Engl J Med* 320:822–828, 1989.
17. Fisher B, Anderson S, Fisher ER, et al.: Significance of ipsilateral breast tumour recurrence after lumpectomy. *Lancet* 338:327–331, 1991.
18. Hayward JL: The Guy's Hospital trials of breast conservation, in Harris JR, Hellman S, Silen W (eds.): *Conservative Management of Breast Cancer*. Philadelphia, PA, Lippincott, 1983, pp. 77–90.
19. Harris JR, Hellman S: Observations on survival curve analysis with particular reference to breast cancer treatment. *Cancer* 57:1415–1420, 1986.
20. Harris JR, Hellman S: Natural history of breast cancer, in Harris JR, Hellman S, Henderson IC, et al. (eds.): Breast Diseases (ed 2). Philadelphia, PA, Lippincott, 1991, pp. 165–181.
21. Hellman S, Harris J: The appropriate breast cancer paradigm. *Cancer Res* 47:339–342, 1987.
22. Hellman S, Harris J: Breast cancer: Considerations in local and regional treatment. *Radiology* 164:593–598, 1987.
23. Stierer M, Rosen HR, Weber R, et al.: Long term analysis of factors influencing the outcome in carcinoma of the breast smaller than one centimeter. *Surg Gynecol Obstet* 175:151–160, 1992.
24. Rosen PP, Groshen S, Saigo PE, et al.: A long-term follow-up study of survival in stage 1 (T1M0) and stage II (T1N1) breast carcinoma. *J Clin Oncol* 7:355–366, 1989.
25. Brinkley D, Haybittle JL: Long term survival of women with breast cancer. *Lancet* 1:1118, 1984.
26. Popper K: The problem of induction, in Miller D (ed.): *Popper Selections*. Princeton, NJ, Princeton University, 1985, pp. 101–117.
27. Hellman S: Dogma and inqusition in medicine. *Cancer* 71:2430–2433, 1993.

DOGMA AND INQUISITION IN MEDICINE: BREAST CANCER AS A CASE STUDY

Republished with permission of Wiley, from "Dogma and Inquisition in Medicine," Samuel Hellman, *Cancer* volume 71, edition 7, 1993; permission conveyed through Copyright Clearance Center, Inc.

Abstract

This case study demonstrates the similarity between the development of dogma and the persecution of deviants during the Spanish Inquisition and that in medicine, using breast cancer as an example. Regarding breast cancer, the dogma of therapy became separate from the underlying hypothesis and, like the religious dogma enforced by the Inquisition, it required inflexible adherence. Apostates were publicly chastened. This serves to inhibit debate and the exploration of alternative hypotheses, both of which are essential for the advancement of scientific knowledge. Adherance to dogma is antithetical to the conditional and approximate nature of truth in science. *Cancer* 1993;71:2430–2433.

Two important centenary events to be noted during this last decade of the twentieth century bear an unexpected similarity. It was during this decade of the last century that Meyer[1] and Halsted[2] independently reported the use of the radical mastectomy first described by Moore[3] for the treatment of carcinoma of the breast. During this period, we also note the 500th anniversary of the Age of Discovery, beginning with Columbus's voyage to the New World. Less remembered in Spain at that time was the success of the united forces of Castile and Aragon in driving the Moors from the Iberian peninsula. Associated with this Spanish unification was the emergence of the Spanish Inquisition with its adherence to preserving dogma.

The Inquisition existed before 1492, but this modern Inquisition founded by Ferdinand and Isabella was promulgated and enforced by secular authorities to help unify Spain. It became an instrument of conservatism, enforcing conformity to centrally held beliefs. Most importantly, these beliefs were considered dogma, i.e., uniformly held truths not subject to question or modification.

The leaders of the Spanish Inquisition in the fifteenth century and the leaders of breast cancer treatment in the twentieth century might seem totally unrelated, yet both share an unquestioning acceptance of authoritarian dogma, which they have sought to impose over their respective domains. The acceptance of radical mastectomy was the result, not only of its effectiveness as a treatment, but also and perhaps more important, of its association with an attractive hypothesis that reinforced other values of the time. The hypothesis suggested that breast cancer was an orderly disease progressing in a contiguous fashion from a primary site by direct extension through the lymphatic vessels to the regional lymph nodes and then to distant sites. This hypothesis became fixed in medicine, and its acceptance was similar to that of the acceptance of religious dogma—that is to say, it was stated categorically, with fervor and authority. It was no longer a hypothesis; it became Truth. Deviation from these principles, especially by those assumed to be disciples, was punished. The rigidity of thinking and the zealousness of adherents to this hypothesis was remarkable. Halsted,[4] perhaps in the most doctrinaire presentation, suggested that disease even at distant sites might be the result of contiguous extension. This was a logical hypothesis of disease spread, and the surgical procedure, radical mastectomy, suited it. The early results of the operation successfully reinforced the validity of the proposed underlying mechanism of disease spread. This doctrine also was accepted because surgery had reached a stage in its development that allowed such extensive operations as en bloc dissections.

Thus, radical mastectomy became the central dogma of disease spread, giving license for the expansion of surgery, that used principles of cancer pathogenesis to develop similarly conceived operations as the appropriate treatment for cancers in many sites. Radical extirpative en bloc surgery became the apex of curative cancer treatment. Examples include contiguous dissections of primary tumors in the head and neck and corresponding draining lymph nodes, radical pneumonectomy for lung cancer, radical hysterectomy leading to pelvic exenterations, and a series of even more radical en bloc dissections, resulting in extensive tissue removal with significant functional and cosmetic loss. These operations demanded much of the surgical team, and their successful completion attested to the prowess of the practitioners. As a result, oncologic therapy became the primary province of surgeons.

Lesser but, I believe, still important supporting reasons for the emergence of the dogma of disease spread have to do with the implied characteristics of the surgeon and surgery under these circumstances. The operation became a battle with disease in which victory or defeat often could be determined as the result primarily of the operator's skill, perhaps combined with some risk taking (although the operator was not at risk). This way of looking at outcomes suggests that doctors can influence the course of malignant disease. The importance of the doctor clearly was established, and the notion that the clinical outcome was determined before therapy began was rejected soundly. Surgical technique was thought to be quite important, and many articles were written about how small technical differences could affect outcomes. Examples of this were the thinness of the flaps,[5] the size of the skin graft,[5] and the development of superradical operations that extended the en bloc dissection to the supraclavicular[6] and internal mammary regions.[7]

Medical Inquisition

In our parallel between the Spanish Inquisition, with its preservation of dogma, and the development of the dogma of cancer pathogenesis leading to a specific therapy, we might consider what happened to some practitioners during the height of acceptance of the radical mastectomy. McWhirter,[8] a Scottish radiation oncologist, suggested that, if postoperative radiation therapy were to be applied, radical mastectomy might be replaced by a lesser operation. The hypothesis of cancer spread underlying the combination of simple mastectomy with postoperative radiation was similar to that of radical mastectomy, and therefore, it was consistent with the original hypothesis. Both were regional treatments directed toward the tumor and grossly unaffected adjacent normal tissues. However, the McWhirter technique did threaten the notion of en bloc dissection that had become dogma, independent of its rationale, and his proposal aroused intense feelings because it recommended a therapeutic revision, decreasing the scope and importance of the operation. This controversy resulted in L. V. Ackerman,[9] an eminent American pathologist, reviewing the material removed from patients who had undergone McWhirter procedure because he supposed that, if the results were as good as those of radical mastectomy, it must be the result of an inaccurate diagnosis of cancer in long-term survivors. Ackerman concluded that, although he disagreed with the diagnosis of malignancy in 13 of the 719 patients, this difference did not appreciably alter the results reported by McWhirter. The main points of his review then dealt with the results he believed demonstrated greater morbidity and a poorer cure rate than the best selected surgical results. "McWhirter has not put in jeopardy the well planned radical mastectomy (p. 887)," he wrote. In this sense, the public review, implied judgment, and reaffirmation of dogma parallel the trials of the Inquisition.

The public denunciation of those thought to be apostates might, to carry the analogy further, be likened to the auto-da-fé of the Inquisition. Such "acts of the faith" were public announcements of the sentences passed by the Inquisition on those accused of heresy. They became associated with public execution of such sentences, especially the burning of heretics at the stake.

The real subjects of the doctrinaire inquisitors were surgeons who questioned the dogma of cancer surgery (first, Geoffrey Keynes[10] in Britain and then George Crile, Jr.,[11] and Bernard Fisher[12] in the United States). Although there was much orthodoxy in Britain, there were also voices from the profession presenting opposing views. Fitzwilliams[13] cautioned, "Those who have been brought up in the atmosphere of the radical operation with no experience of anything less extensive must remember that they are repeating dogma and not speaking from formed judgment. Medicine is never advanced by such action (p. 4160)." Despite this, Keynes suffered the deprecation of his colleagues. "None of us has been burnt at the stake but feelings have run pretty high (p. 40)," describes Keynes.[14] Both Crile and Fisher, in the United States, were subject to similar attacks.

The Appeal of Dogma

There appear to be powerful reasons for the persistence of dogma in medicine. Although much of medicine is empiric, basing treatment on a single paradigm becomes an extremely powerful force. It simplifies individual treatment decisions without requiring a reconsideration of the pathogenesis in each patient. If it elevates the importance and control of the physician, it is all the more powerful. Practitioners are extremely reluctant to change until they find a suitable alternative, especially one that is equally attractive. In this instance, the paradigm of cancer spread extended to all of oncology; a threat to the radical mastectomy procedure threatened accepted treatments for all local and regional cancers. A further inhibitor of change, suggested in the previous comments of Fitzwilliam,[13] is that medical and postgraduate education inculcates positions that are difficult to change during subsequent practice.

The alternate hypothesis of cancer spread was developed from the work of these surgeons. Its full expression, based on laboratory studies,[15] suggested an entirely different paradigm. In this model, breast cancer was thought to be either of the type that remains local and rarely spreads, or of the type that develops metastasis before the primary tumor is detected clinically. With either type, is there reason to use radical en bloc surgery? In the former, local treatment suffices and, if it fails, can be reapplied without risk of metastasis. In the latter, radical treatment regionally applied is inadequate because occult micrometastases already have occurred. This new hypothesis emphasized the impotence of local therapy and, therefore, that radical extirpative treatment was excessive. The disease can be affected only by a treatment that destroys the occult micrometastases.

At first considered heretical, this hypothesis of disease pathogenesis currently has become the new dogma, with a required orthodoxy of therapeutic approach. The reasons for its acceptance have much in common with the reasons for accepting radical mastectomy. The importance of adjuvant systemic therapies, both hormonal and chemotherapeutic, which are designed to affect occult micrometastases, is supported by this hypothesis of disease pathogenesis. It is interesting to note how quickly and universally this new paradigm has become accepted. Before the development of adjuvant chemotherapy, this alternative hypothesis made little headway.

We might wonder why this rapid change has occurred after such a successful defense of the older doctrine. I believe this is primarily because of the attractiveness of the therapeutic alternative, adjuvant systemic therapy. There are a number of parallels between the acceptance of adjuvant therapy based on an alternative hypothesis of cancer development to that of the Halstedian view and radical mastectomy. The new hypothesis suggests that it is medicines that are essential in the treatment of cancer because cancer is, in fact, a systemic rather than a local or regional disease, except for those few patients whose disease would never metastasize. Treatment requires a skillful use of toxic drugs at a time when medicine has developed such skills. Adherents argue, as they did in defense of the radical mastectomy, that failure may be the result of poor technique. In the current treatment, good technique requires the aggressive use of drugs at the highest dose possible.[16] Although this is consistent with the dose-response hypothesis underlying modern multidrug chemotherapy, it also has many other features supportive of the oncologist. Cancer therapy and its success require skill, courage, and risk taking (again the risks are the patient's). Most importantly, medicine is potent and, if skillfully applied, can "defeat" cancer. The medical oncologist now supplants the surgeon as the central figure in cancer management.

As we might expect, the change in dogma has not been without vigorous debate. A few adherents still zealously guard the older views,[17,18] and there are still advocates of the radical mastectomy. Despite this, acceptance of the new dogma by its adherents is as complete and uncompromising as that of the previous one. So important, it seems, are the results of new studies confirming or expanding the use of adjuvant therapies that the normal mechanisms of peer review have been abrogated to apply these results immediately. For the first time, a "Clinical Alert" was released by the National Cancer Institute.[19] It reached physicians before the peer-reviewed publications and without the full presentation of data to be published in the journals. What was presented was a governmental recommendation based on evaluation by the National Cancer Institute, which was outside the established processes by which medical information is evaluated and presented. This truly is dogma, rather than hypothesis generation and testing. Forgotten is the notion that, although the scientific method is powerful in rejecting untrue hypotheses, it cannot prove something to be true. The most that can be hoped for are successively better approximations of the truth. Current practices seem more consistent with religious excesses than with the conditional nature of scientific hypotheses and learning.

A Retreat from Dogma

A less impassioned consideration of the data would suggest that neither the old nor the new hypothesis of the pathogenesis of disease is completely true for breast cancer. Breast cancer is most likely a heterogeneous mix of conditions in which, for some patients, the disease remains only local, and for others, it has become systemic before it is clinically detectable. For a significant number of patients, the disease is local in its early manifestations and metastasizes during its clinical evolution. Evidence for this latter view is the 30% decrease in breast cancer deaths as a result of screening mammography.[20,21] The only explanation that seems appropriate for this finding is that metastasis must occur in some patients between the time of mammographic detectability and clinical detectability. Furthermore, data reveal that the likelihood for metastasis increases as a function of tumor volume, suggesting that as tumors get larger they have more opportunity to metastasize.[22] The evidence pertinent to these hypotheses is discussed in greater detail elsewhere.[23,24] It is not the purpose of this article to argue for either hypothesis or for an intermediary position (although this is clearly my view), but rather to emphasize the amount of emotion and dogmatism associated with what should be purely scientific considerations.

We should learn from this that dogma begins to develop a life of its own. It serves to enforce conservatism and inhibit new ideas or alternative views. Although a treatment begins as an extension of a hypothesis, it may become a symbol for a view of medicine and its practitioners, rather than the subject of scientific inquiry. Keynes[14] admonishes, "Orthodoxy in surgery [I would suggest all of medicine] is like orthodoxy in other departments of the mind—it starts as a tentative belief in some particular course of action but later begins almost to challenge comparison with a religion. It comes to be held as a passionate belief in the absolute rightness of that particular view (p. 40)." Despite the Inquisition, Galileo was correct. The Inquisition served primarily to restrict intellectual and scientific advance. Its parallel in medicine can have a similar deleterious effect against which we must guard.

REFERENCES

1. Meyer W. An improved method of the radical operation for carcinoma of the breast. *Med Record* 1894; 46:746.
2. Halsted WS. The results of operations for the cure of cancer of the breast performed at the Johns Hopkins Hospital from June 1889 to January 1994. *Johns Hopkins Hospital Bull* 1894–5; 4:297.
3. Moore CH. On the influence of inadequate operations on the theory of cancer. *R Med Chir Soc* 1867; 1:245.
4. Halsted WS. The results of radical operations for cure of carcinoma of the breast. *Ann Surg* 1907; 46:1–19.
5. Haagensen CD. *Diseases of the breast.* 2nd ed. Philadelphia: WB Saunders, 1971:709.
6. Dahl-Iverson E. Recherches sur les metasteses microscopiques des cancers du sein dans les ganglions lymphatiques parasternaux et susclaviculaires. *Mem Head Chin* 1952; 78:651.
7. Urban JA, Baker HW. Radical mastectomy in continuity with en bloc resection of the internal mammary lymph node chain. *Cancer* 1952; 5:992.
8. McWhirter R. Simple mastectomy and radiotherapy in treatment of breast cancer. *Br J Radiol* 1955; 28:128–139.
9. Ackerman LV. Evaluation of treatment of cancer of the breast at the University of Edinburgh (Scotland) under the direction of Dr. Robert McWhirter. *Cancer* 1955; 8:883–887.
10. Keynes GL. Conservative treatment of cancer of the breast. *BMJ* 1937; 2:643.

11. Crile G, Jr. Results of simplified treatment of breast cancer. *Surg Gynecol Obstet* 1964; 118:517–523.
12. Fisher B. Laboratory and clinical research in breast cancer: a personal adventure. *Cancer Res* 1980; 40:3863–3874.
13. Fitzwilliams DCL. A plea for a more local operation in really early breast carcinoma. *BMJ* 1940; 2:405–408.
14. Keynes G. Carcinoma of the breast, the unorthodox view. *Proc Cardiff Med Soc* 1954; 40.
15. Fisher B, Fisher ER. The interrelationship of hematogenous and lymphatic tumor cell dissemination. *Surg Gynecol Obstet* 1976; 122:791–798.
16. Hryniuk WM. The importance of dose intensity in the outcome of chemotherapy. In: DeVita VT, Hellman S, Rosenberg SA, editors. *Important advances in oncology*. Philadelphia: JB Lippincott, 1988:121–141.
17. Haagenson CD. The recent disparagement of the radical mastectomy. In: *Diseases of the breast*. 3rd ed. Philadelphia: WB Saunders, 1986:933–938.
18. Ferguson DJ. The actual extent of mastectomy: a key to survival. *Perspect Biol Med* 1987; 30:311–323.
19. National Cancer Institute. *Clinical alert*. Bethesda (MD): The Institute; 1988 May 19.
20. Shapiro S, Venet W, Strax P, Venet L. *Periodic screening for breast cancer. The Health Insurance Plan Project and its sequelae, 1963–1986*. Baltimore: Johns Hopkins University Press, 1988:90–95.
21. Tabar L, Fagerberg CJG, Gad A, Baldetorp L, Holmberg LH, Gröntoft O, et al. Reduction in mortality from breast cancer after mass screening with mammography. *Lancet* 1985; 1:829.
22. Koscielny S, Tubiana MG, Lê MG, Valleron AJ, Mouriesse H, Contesso G, et al. Breast cancer: relationship between the size of the primary tumor and the probability of metastatic dissemination. *Br J Cancer* 1984; 49:709–715.
23. Hellman S, Harris JR. The appropriate breast cancer paradigm. *Cancer Res* 1987; 47:339–342.
24. Hellman S, Harris JR. Breast cancer: considerations in local and regional treatment. *Radiology* 1987; 164:593–598.

DARWIN'S CLINICAL RELEVANCE

Republished with permission of Wiley, from "Darwin's Clinical Relevance," Samuel Hellman, *Cancer*, volume 79, edition 12, 1997; permission conveyed through Copyright Clearance Center, Inc.

Abstract

Evolutionary principles apply to malignant disease; cancers progress during their clinical phase, becoming increasingly malignant. Early diagnosis and ablation of the primary tumors are essential to a successful therapeutic strategy.

"Evolution is the dominant fact of biology," stated Nobel laureate and codiscoverer of the structure of DNA, James D. Watson[1] at a recent meeting at The University of Chicago. Although there has been a great deal of interest in the evolution of cancer, it has been focused primarily on preclinical events; however, these concepts apply as well to the clinical manifestations of cancer. To design a strategy for cancer management, one must have a model of the disease. For such a model to be useful it must be consistent with what we already know, especially with what Watson describes as "the dominant fact of biology." We must understand what evolutionary theory both states and implies before we can apply it in the clinic. What follows is a discussion of the clinical relevance of evolutionary concepts as they bear on the development of a cancer, its natural history and prognosis, and determining appropriate therapeutic strategies.

Darwin's Theory

The mechanism by which species evolve as explained by Darwin's theory of evolution is, as Ernst Mayr[2] suggests, really five related theories. First, organisms are transformed with time; they are not fixed but continue to change. The parallel in oncogenesis is the notion of cancer progression, an acquisition of the characteristics of increasing malignancy that continues throughout the natural history of the cancer. Second, all groups of organisms can be traced to a common ancestor; this, the theory of common descent, is reflected in the clonal origins of cancer. Third, species multiply, diagrammed usually as a branching tree, the result of geographically isolated founder populations and differing selection pressures. In contrast, cancer appears more like a ladder then a tree. The appropriate evolutionary analogy is called "convergent evolution." Convergent evolution means that similar selection pressures lead to similar phenotypes, but not identical genotypes. There may be similar mutations, the specific order of mutation may be different, or there may be entirely different mutations resulting in similar phenotypic expression. For oncogenesis, this is consistent with phenotypically similar tumors arising in the same tissue while allowing for the variation observed in the genotypes and in the temporal order of mutations. As Dennett suggests,[3] "convergent evolution is . . . overwhelmingly good evidence of the power of natural selection." Image-forming eyes have been found to have evolved independently numerous times in nature, perhaps 40 to 60 times in invertebrates.[4] Man and octopus have quite similar eyes, but have evolved independently. Other examples of the power of a good solution is the use of echolocation in both bats and whales as a method of sensing the environment. Arthropod respiration has evolved quite separately in different species but the phenotypic results are quite similar because, as deDuve suggests,[5] "inherited was a body plan that admitted only one solution . . . or perhaps, favored this solution over all others." A remarkable example of the power of convergent evolution is the independent evolution of three different species of periodic cicada[6] in which each has a 13- and 17-year variety. Because both 13 and 17 are prime numbers, it is suggested that these evolved in preference to, for example, a 15-year species because a parasite would be much less likely to be able to synchronize its life cycle to these prime numbers, whereas for a 15-year species, life cycles of 3 or 5 years would allow successful parasitizing of such cicada. These examples all demonstrate the power of natural selection to seek successful solutions and use them repeatedly. Similarly, the cancer phenotype has four cardinal characteristics: growth, angiogenesis, invasion, and metastasis. There are a number of mutational paths that will allow the expression of these capacities.

The fourth of the related theories comprising the theory of evolution suggests that evolution is gradual rather than saltational. This has important connotations for the nature of tumor progression. Species evolve with time to more fit organisms, more adapted to the environment. For tumors this suggests that tumor evolution is not determined by a single event but rather by a number of successive evolutionary changes, each of which must be at least neutral, but preferably contributes a competitive advantage. There is some disagreement as to how important saltational events are in evolution. Proponents argue that there are long periods of quiescence with infrequent large changes. Gould and Eldredge called this "punctuated equilibria,"[7] whereas critics have called this "evolution by jerks." Without entering this dispute, there are some oncogenic correlates of both gradual and abrupt progression. Some leukemias and sarcomas appear to be the result of one or at most a few events. This does not appear to be the case for the common carcinomas, which require a large series of genetic changes.[8-11]

The fifth related theory, according to Mayr,[2] is the theory of natural selection. Abundant production of variation and natural selection are the important engines of evolution. Darwin in his *The Origin of Species*[12] states, "as many more individuals of each species are born than can possibly survive, and as consequently there is a frequently recurring struggle for existence, it follows that any being, if it vary in any manner profitable to itself, under the complex and sometimes varying conditions of life, will have a better chance of survival and thus be naturally selected. From the strong principle of inheritance, any selected variety will tend to propagate its new and modified form." Cancer results from the abundant production of genotypic changes and selection that allows the evolving malignant clone to increase its malignant capacities.

Contributions of the New Biology

There has been an explosion of biologic information regarding carcinogenesis that should be understood and placed in a consistent framework. These discoveries offer insights into how tumors form, progress (evolve), and might best be managed. They begin with the important chromosomal abnormalities[13] and associated genetic instability[14] that are now recognized as characterizing cancer. In addition to these morphologic changes in chromosomes, specific genetic abnormalities have been identified. These include the dominant-acting oncogenes and suppressor- or recessive-acting oncogenes that are consistent with Mendelian genetics. It is presumed that a dominant lesion results from the acquisition of a new capacity, whereas a recessive lesion is the loss of some tumor-inhibiting protein. The latter requires that both genes are mutated to lose the capacity to produce the suppressor. This notion was first applied to inherited cancer in the two-hit hypothesis of Knudson.[15] He suggested that tumor predisposition requires the loss of both alleles and that hereditary cancer predisposition occurred when one of these losses was inherited. Examples of this are familial retinoblastoma observed in children and the inherited mutation in the p53 gene responsible for the various tumors observed in the Li-Fraumeni syndrome. RB, the gene associated with retinoblastoma, and p53 genes are prototypic suppressor oncogenes.

Cancer has been shown to require a cascade of mutations in which it appears that there may be significant variation in the mutations present and in their order of production. Some mutations are more important than others because not only do they result in the required phenotypes, they facilitate other phenotypic changes as well. A common type of facilitating mutation that contributes to oncogenesis is one that results in alteration in DNA repair. DNA repair deficiency has been shown to increase the likelihood of tumors in certain heredity diseases (Table 3.4). The cell cycle contains a number of "check points" at which the DNA is scrutinized for damage and either repaired or cell death initiated (apoptosis). Failure of these repair mechanisms has assumed an increasingly important role in the understanding of cancer evolution as demonstrated in the different diseases of DNA repair. The genomic surveillance allows repair but appears to favor apoptosis when the DNA damage is great or too important a cell (such as certain lymphocytes and germ cells[16]) is affected to chance incomplete repair.

Table 3.4. Oncologic Examples of the Three Required Evolutionary Activities: Mutation, Selection, and Amplification

Mutation	Selection	Amplification
Mismatch repair defect	Growth	Continued proliferation
Helicase mutation	Invasion	LOH of recessive growth
Werner's syndrome	Angiogenesis	inhibitors
Bloom syndrome	Metastatic colonization	RB
Repair defects		p53
Ataxia telangiectasia		Loss of senescence
Xeroderma pigmentosum		Telomerase
Failure of checkpoint pause		Loss of terminal
p53 Li-Fraumeni syndrome		differentiation
Loss of apoptosis		
bcl-2		
p53		

The mechanism of normal cell senescence has been related to progressive shortening of the telomere.[17] Tumor cells express the enzyme telomerase, allowing them to continue effective chromosomal replication and thus avoid senescence.[18] The appearance of telomerase is a relatively late event in tumorigenesis. Because telomerase production is a characteristic of many tumors, but few normal cells,[19] affecting telomerase function offers obvious therapeutic opportunities.

Defects in DNA repair, loss of check-point surveillance, even the loss of senescence may provide an opportunity for "hyperevolution," but increased mutations, even with the preservation of the mutations in clones not undergoing senescence, does not cause evolution to cancer without selection pressure favoring the evolving cancer. In the evolution of species there must not only be mutations, but these must be selected for and amplified. Oncogenesis has similar requirements. Cancer is characterized by growth, invasion, and metastasis. For any malignant transformation, cellular proliferation is necessary, for without such proliferation, one of the necessary conditions—growth—cannot be achieved. Increases in cell proliferation also facilitate tumor progression because they allow more opportunities for mutation. Increased proliferation can result in both increased metastagencity[20] (Table 3.4) because tumors further in their progression are more able to metastasize, and in increased tumor virulence because the more rapid proliferation will cause tumors to exhibit their malignancy over a shorter period of time. There also must be loss of senescence and a decrease in terminal differentiation, for if all cells die or mature the altered clone will die out. Terminal differentiation can be assessed clinically by histologic examination of the tumor, with grade being the accepted method of describing the state of tumor differentiation. Tumors must also invade to exhibit their malignancy and must be able to colonize at a distance. Continued growth, invasion, and metastases are the characteristics that provide cancer with a selective advantage. They all appear to require the ability to induce a blood supply (angiogenesis) (Box 3.1).

Loss of apoptosis will facilitate oncogenesis, but it is not required for it. Apoptosis serves to preserve the undamaged genotype; its loss will allow greater mutational variability to persist. Genetic instability favoring carcinogenesis can also be the result of DNA repair deficiencies. A decrease in repair allows more mutations to persist, but the likelihood and extent of mutations depend on both the presence and the fidelity of the repair process. An effective but imprecise repair process, although allowing survival, may actually favor oncogenesis because it will allow the persistence of inaccurately copied genes. Genetic alteration can be produced by a variety of both environmental and iatrogenic mutagens. It is believed

---

Box 3.1

MALIGNANCY

Virulence—pace or rate of disease growth, dissemination, and clinical manifestation

Metastagenicity—ultimate likelihood and extent of distant metastases

that the former is of major etiologic importance to the development of human cancer. The latter is demonstrated in the emergence of therapy-induced tumors in long-term survivors previously treated with radiation or chemotherapy.

Clinical Implications

TUMOR SIZE

There are important clinical implications to be appreciated when considering tumor progression in Darwinian terms. Recognition of tumors early in their evolution becomes profoundly important. The extent of tumor progression should be correlated with tumor size because the smaller tumor is likely to have had fewer of the genetic alterations in the malignant cascade. More correctly, the correlation should be with the point in the evolutionary process at which the tumor resides. Size and stage within any specific tumor type should be roughly correlated with the extent of this process. There is evidence of progression in the studies of chromosomal abnormalities and specific genetic changes in both dominant and suppressor oncogenes as a function of tumor stage that is consistent with this concept.[8-11] On average, small tumors should be more curable by radiation, chemotherapy, or hormonal treatment because there should be fewer clonogens present, they should be proliferating slowly having experienced fewer facilitating mutations, or, if they are proliferating rapidly, they should have a high cell loss due to more terminal differentiation. Because these small tumors then will be more likely well differentiated with a high cell loss and/or less proliferation, they should have less clonal expansion between therapeutic treatments, an important consideration for fractionated radiation and for chemotherapy administration. Clinical evidence is consistent with these differing characteristics of tumors as a function of size. Koscielny et al.[22] reported that as tumor size increased, the proportion of Grade 3 breast carcinomas increased and that of Grade 1 carcinomas decreased. Similar findings have been reported by Tabar et al.[23] in the two-county Swedish mammography trial. McNeal et al.[24]

demonstrated an increase in Gleason grade with increasing prostate carcinoma volume.

Small tumors are more likely to have the apoptotic mechanism preserved. p53 mutations (the most common mutation observed in cancer) are present in > 50% of human cancers. The likelihood of p53 mutations increases with tumor grade and stage.[16] Although the kinetics differ in different tumor types, the general rule of p53 mutations increasing as tumors progress is present in all types studied. *bcl*-2 and related genetic abnormalities also appear to correlate with tumor progression (Olopade, unpublished data). According to this application of Darwinism to oncogenesis, small tumors should be less likely to have metastasized because there is less progression and therefore less likely acquisition of the capabilities required for seeding and growth at a distant site. Tabar et al.[23] and Koscielny et al.[22] have shown that the likelihood of metastasis is a direct function of tumor size.

As Folkman has shown, angiogensis is central to the processes of growth and metastasis.[21] The presence of areas of angiogenesis appears to be heterogeneous within tumors and prognosis is correlated with the blood vessel density present in the most dense region.[25,26] Heimann et al. have shown that the density of these most dense regions varies directly as a function of tumor size.[27]

Such considerations of tumor progression further suggest that if metastases of small tumors have occurred they are more likely to be limited in number and location. Such oligometastases[28] are still amenable to radical treatment. The clinical implications of finding metastases with small tumors will be different than with large cancers. They are more likely to be oligometastases when the tumor is small, rather than the visible tip of the iceberg of polymetastases found with more advanced tumors. This is evidenced by the greater success of resection of metastases to the liver when the primary colon carcinoma is of an earlier stage.[29] Presumably this is because the metastases from an early stage primary tumor are more likely to be oligometastases. Similarly, lymph node metastases are more likely oligometastases when they are found associated with small primary tumors rather than, as suggested by Fisher, always being an indicator of distant disease.[30] This is the case for breast carcinoma.[20,31] The presence of 1–3 axillary lymph node metastases does not confer an ominous prognosis when the tumor is < 2 cm. This is not true when the same number of metastases is present with larger tumors. The larger tumors presumably have had more tumor progression, are therefore more malignant, and have a greater facility for distant colonization. Although small breast carcinomas can be the source of multiple distant metastases, the presence of limited lymph node disease does not predict for their presence, but rather is more likely the fledgling attempt at metastasis by this early developing cancer.

Local Control

Failure to eradicate all tumors or an intentional strategy allowing tumor persistence will have deleterious effects. Most important, it will allow the residual tumor to continue oncogenic progression. The systemic hypothesis (the basis for current therapeutic programs allowing cancer persistence) argues that tumors, when observed clinically, are of two types: they are either incapable of metastasis, or if capable of metastasis, have already metastasized.[30] This is inconsistent with the application of what we know about species evolution to cancer because it suggests that a single event causes the full malignant state or that the multiple events required have all occurred before clinical recognition, after which the phenotype is fixed without the opportunity for further malignant progression. This systemic hypothesis assumes that the final cancer phenotype is formed before clinical detectability. The continued, progressive, and gradual nature of evolutionary progression is inconsistent with this view. It is also in contrast to the proven benefit of mammography.[32,33] A 30% reduction in breast carcinoma deaths has been observed in the screening mammography trials. This reduction in death was observed even before the widespread use of adjuvant systemic treatment. This implies that the locoregional treatment administered at the time of mammographic determination was more effective because between that time and clinical detection metastases must have occurred in 30% of the patients. Because the average size of screen detected tumors is approximately 1 cm and that of clinically detected lesions ≥ 2 cm, significant tumor progression likely occurs during this part of the natural history of breast carcinoma.

That the persistence of breast carcinoma after inadequate local treatment has a deleterious effect can be observed in the comparison of lumpectomy alone with lumpectomy plus radiation or with mastectomy in the NSABP study B06.[34] There is a higher likelihood for distant metastasis associated with the higher local failure rate observed in the group having local excision only. Fisher et al.[34] state, "Significantly or nearly significantly higher percentages of patients with node negative breast cancer treated by mastectomy or lumpectomy and breast irradiation remain free of disease and free of distant disease than patients treated with node negative breast cancer treated by lumpectomy." Similarly, the Stockholm Trial[35,36] comparing mastectomy to mastectomy plus radiation has shown that the persistent local disease observed in the unirradiated group was correlated with an increased likelihood of distant metastasis. Both NSABP B-06 and this trial are consistent with the deleterious consequences of incomplete irradication of the primary tumor, allowing continued tumor progression as well as permitting a continuing potential source of metastatic cells to remain.

MARKERS OF PROGRESSION

Chronic myelogenous leukemia has a characteristic 9:22 translocation during the chronic phase, but many other genetic abnormalities are present during the acute blast crisis. Markers of tumor progression correlate with outcome and with response to therapy. This has been shown in studies of microvessel density by Wiedner and Folkman,[25,26] Gasperini et al.,[37] and Heimann et al.[27] p53 mutations appear to be related to chemoresistance.[16] Although there are many markers of proliferation, the relationship of rapid growth to progression is complicated. Proliferation should correlate with progression because with more proliferation there will be more opportunity for mutations and thus more progression. These mutations can affect cell cycle time, terminal differentiation, or other phenomena increasing cell birth or reducing cell loss. However, differing proliferation rates in equivalently progressed tumors should be reflected in increased tumor virulence but not increased metastagenicity. This is especially important when considering early stage cancers and emphasizes the need for long follow-up. For example, studies of the prognostic importance of patient age in T1 breast carcinoma reveal a greater tumor virulence in young patients, but with continued follow-up the survival becomes equivalent to older patients.[20] Similarly, proliferating cell nuclear antigen, grade, and mitotic index predict for a difference in virulence but not for metastagenicity (R. Heimann, personal communication and[38]).

Age

Because tumors evolve gradually, one would expect cancer to be a disease of later life and very uncommon in the young. The evolutionary penalty for a mutation harming a multicellular organism decreases with age, especially after the reproductive and childrearing period. Thus, there should be strong selection pressures against cancer-causing mutations in the young that decrease with advancing age. It is not an accident that cancer incidence rises steeply after the fourth decade of life. For cancers to occur early in life there should be either a profound oncogenic event or some inherited facilitating mutation such as the loss of one allele of a suppressor gene. This latter, the Knudson hypothesis,[15] appears to be correct for the hereditary cancers retinoblastoma, Wilms' tumor, and a rapidly enlarging list including early onset breast carcinoma.

Altruism

Finding an evolutionary role for the altruism observed in many species has been an interesting question for evolutionary biologists. Wilson[39] has suggested that altruism can be considered as consistent with species preservation and natural selection if it is the genome rather than the particular organism that is the object of evolution. If the sacrifice of an individual results in increasing the survival probability of a colony of organisms all sharing the same genotype, an evolutionary purpose has been served. The warrior ants in protecting the queen preserve their genes. Multicellular organisms can be considered to be the evolutionary result of altruistic behavior in which genetically identical cells stay together and develop specialized functions rather than proliferating as independent clones. This is a form of self-sacrifice by cells that become somatic and do not contribute to the next generation. Similarly, one may consider apoptosis a form of cellular altruism. In this case, a cell or even a developing embryo will be sacrificed to preserve the object of evolution: the fidelity of the genome. Although some mutational activity favors evolutionary change, most mutations are either neutral or harmful. For example, p53 has been shown to be associated with surveillance of the DNA. When at least one normal p53 allele is present, the fidelity of the DNA is monitored. If there is too much damage, apoptosis occurs. In this fashion, it acts as a guardian of the genome. Not only is loss of p53 function related to tumor progression; knockout mice in which both p53 genes are deleted have fewer abortions and a greater number of malformed offspring after X-ray exposure.[40] Thus, p53-related apoptosis suppresses not only cellular mutations but teratogenesis as well. bcl-xL, a potent inhibitor of apoptosis, is correlated with markers of tumor progression such as grade and the extent of lymph node involvement (Olopade et al., unpublished data).

The likelihood for apoptosis after exposure to radiation or chemotherapy may be the most important determinant of successful treatment. Apoptosis results in a 10–15% incremental cell kill with the usual 1.8–2.0-gray fractions.[41] This effect persists with daily administration. A 10%–15% change in fractional cell kill will have a 1000-fold difference in survival over a normally protracted radiation treatment regimen (Table 3.5).

Table 3.5. Differences in Cumulative Survival Fraction as a Function of Differences in Individual Fractional Survival

Cumulative Survival Fraction N32	Daily Survival Fraction
10–11	0.45
10–10	0.49
10–9	0.52
10–8	0.56
10–7	0.60
10–6	0.65
10–5	0.70

Similar considerations are obtained with chemotherapy and so it is not remarkable that one of the factors most correlated with successful treatment is the presence of normal p53 function.[12] Growth factor deprivation also increases apoptosis, even when the p53 gene is not functional. The importance of apoptosis provides intriguing therapeutic opportunities. It may also be relevant to the enhancement of radiation effects observed when androgen deprivation is combined with radiation therapy in the treatment of prostate carcinoma,[41] as shown in the Radiation Therapy Oncology Group trial demonstrating an improvement in both local control and progression-free survival. Androgen deprivation and other hormonal actions can cause apoptosis directly and may increase the likelihood of an apoptotic response to radiation. The theory of tumor progression and the resulting importance of early diagnosis and local tumor control are relevant to the broader current debates concerning prostate carcinoma management.

Conclusions

The important lesson of the application of Darwinism as applied to cancer is that evolutionary principles apply. As species evolve, so cancer cells progress. Mutations and selection are crucial to both speciation and cancer progression. The compelling clinical implication is that cancer is a genetic disease that changes, becoming increasingly more malignant during the clinical phase. Molecular pathology of the tumor offers the promise of prognostic information and determination of appropriate therapy. Consistent with the implications of Darwin's theory, early diagnosis is a vital tool for successful therapy. It allows treatment of a tumor with fewer clonogens and one that is less malignant because it has had less opportunity to evolve. Because clinical cancer continues to progress (evolve), maximal ablation of the primary tumor must be an essential component of any therapeutic strategy.

REFERENCES

1. Watson JD. Introduction to the Jean Mitchell Watson Lecture. Chicago [IL]: Univ. of Chicago; April 23, 1996.
2. Mayr E. *One long argument: Charles Darwin and the genesis of modern evolutionary thought*. Cambridge, MA: Harvard University Press, 1991.
3. Dennett DC. *Darwin's dangerous idea: evolution and the meanings of life*. New York: Simon and Schuster, 1995.
4. Salvini-Plawen LV, Mayr E. On the evolution of photoreceptors and eyes. *Evol Biol* 1977; 10: 207–263.
5. deDuve C. *Vital dust: life as a cosmic imperative*. New York: Basic Books, 1995.
6. Dawkins R. *The blind watchmaker*. New York: W. W. Norton, 1985.
7. Gould SJ. The episodic nature of evolutionary change. In: *The panda's thumb*. New York: W. W. Norton, 1980: 179–185.
8. Vogelstein B, Kinzler KW. The multistep nature of cancer. *Trends Genet* 1993; 8: 138–141.
9. Rinker-Schaeffer CW, Partin AW, Isaacs WB, Coffey DS, Isaacs JT. Molecular and cellular changes associated with the acquisitions of metastatic ability by prostatic cancer cells. *Prostate* 1994; 25: 249–265.
10. Schweckheimer K, Cavanee WK. Genetics of cancer predisposition and progression. *Clin Invest* 1993; 7: 488–502.
11. Reifenberger G, Reifenberger J, Ichimura K, Meltzer PS, Collins VP. Amplification of multiple genes from chromosomal region 12q13-14 in malignant gliomas. *Cancer Res* 1994; 54: 4299–4303.
12. Darwin C. *The origin of species* (1859) [reprinted]. New York: Books.
13. Mitelman F. Catalog of chromosomal aberrations in cancer. 4th edition. New York: Wiley-Liss, 1991.
14. Nowell PC. The clonal evolution of tumor cell population. *Science* 1976: 194: 23–28.
15. Knudson AG. Mutation and cancer: statistical study of retinoblastoma. *Proc Natl Acad Sci USA* 1971; 68: 820–823.
16. Ruley HE. p53 and response to chemotherapy and radiotherapy. In: DeVitaVT, HellmanS, RosenbergSA, editors. *Important advances in oncology 1996*. Philadelphia: Lippincott-Raven, 1996: 37–56.
17. Allsopp RC, Vaziri H, Patterson C, Goldstein S, Younglai EV, Futcher AB, et al. Telomere length predicts replicative capacity of human fibroblasts. *Proc Natl Acad Sci USA* 1992; 89: 10–114.
18. Harley CB, Kim NW. Telomerase and nancer. In: DeVita VT, HellmanS, RosenbergSA, editors. *Important advances in oncology 1996*. Philadelphia: Lippincott-Raven, 1996: 57–67.
19. Vaziri H, Dragowska W, Allsopp RC, Thomas TE, Harley CB, Lansdorp PM. Evidence for a mitotic clock in human hematapoietic stem cells: loss of telomeric DNA with age. *Proc Natl Acad Sci USA* 1994; 91 (21): 9857–9860.

20. Hellman S. National history of small breast cancers: The David A. Karnovsky Memorial Lecture. *J Clin Oncol* 1994; 12: 2229–2234.
21. Folkman J. Clinical applications of research on angiogenesis. *N Engl J Med* 1995; 333: 1757–1763.
22. Koscielny S, Tubiana M, Le MG, Valleron AJ, Mouriesse H, Contesso G, et al. Breast cancer: relationship between the size of the primary tumor and the probability of distant metastatic dissemination. *Br J Cancer* 1984; 49: 709–715.
23. Tabar L, Fagerberg G, Duffy SW, Day NE, Gad A, Grontoff O. Update of the Swedish two-county program of mammographic screening for breast cancer. *Radiol Clin North Am* 1992; 30 (1): 187–210.
24. McNeal JE, Bostwick DG, Kindrachuk RA, Redwine EA, Freiha FS, Stamey TA. Patterns of progression in prostate cancer. *Lancet* 1986: 1: 60–63.
25. Wiedner N, Semple JP, Welch WR, Folkman J. Tumor angiogenesis and metastasis-correlation with invasive breast cancer. *N Engl J Med* 1991; 324: 1–8.
26. Wiedner N, Folkman J. Tumor vascularity as a prognostic factor in cancer. In: DeVita VT, Hellman S, Rosenberg SA, editors. *Important advances in oncology 1996*. Philadelphia: Lippincott-Raven, 1996: 167–190.
27. Heimann R, Ferguson D, Powers C, Recant W, Weichselbaum R, Hellman S. Angiogenesis as predictor of long-term survival for patients with small node-negative breast cancer. *J Natl Cancer Inst* 1996; 88: 1764–1769.
28. Hellman S, Weichselbaum R. Oligometastases. *J Clin Oncol* 1995; 13: 8–10.
29. Hughes KS, Sugarbaker PH. Resection of the liver for metastatic solid tumors. In: Rosenberg SA, editor. *Surgical treatment for metastatic cancer*. Philadelphia: J. B. Lippincott, 1987: 101–125.
30. Fisher B. Laboratory and clinical research in breast cancer: a personal adventure: The David A. Karnovsky Memorial Lecture. *Cancer Res* 1980; 40: 3863–3874.
31. Quiet CA, Ferguson DJ, Weichselbaum RR, Hellman S. The natural history of node-positive breast cancer: the curability of small cancers with a limited number of positive nodes. *J Clin Oncol* 1996; 14: 3105–3111.
32. Tabar L, Fagerberg G, Day NE, Duffy SW, Kitchin RM. Breast cancer treatment and natural history: new insights from results of screening. *Lancet* 1992; 339: 412–414.
33. Shapiro S. Determining the efficacy of breast cancer screening. *Cancer* 1989; 63 (10): 1873–1880.
34. Fisher B, Anderson S, Redmond CK, Wolmask N, Wickerham DL, Cronin WM. Reanalysis and results after 12 years follow-up in a randomized clinical trial comparing total mastectomy with lumpectomy with or without irradiation in the treatment of breast cancer. *N Engl J Med* 1995; 333: 1456–1461.
35. Rutquist LE, Pettersson D, Johansson H. Adjuvant radiation therapy versus surgery alone in operable cancer: long term follow-up of a randomized clinical trial. *Radiother Oncol* 1993; 26: 104–110.
36. Arriagada R, Rutquist LE, Mattson A, Kramer A, Rotstein S. Adequate locoregional treatment for early breast cancer may prevent secondary dissemination. *J Clin Oncol* 1995; 13: 2869–2878.
37. Gasparini G, Weidner N, Bevilacque P, Maluta S, Della Palma P, Caffo O, et al. Tumor microvessel density, p53 expression, tumor size, and perperitumoral lymphatic

vessel invasion are relevant prognostic markers in node-negative breast carcinoma. *J Clin Oncol* 1994; 12: 454–466.
38. Stierer M, Rosen HR, Weber R, Marczell A, Kornek CV, Czerwenka E, et al. Long term analysis of factors influencing the outcome in carcinoma of the breast smaller than one centimeter. *Surg Gynecol Obstet* 1992; 175: 151–160.
39. Wilson EO. *Sociobiology: the new synthesis*. Cambridge, MA: Harvard University Press: 1975; 106–129.
40. Norimura T, Nomoto S, Katsuki M, Gondo Y, Kondo S. p53 dependent apoptosis surpresses radiation-induced teratogenesis. *Nat Medicine* 1996; 2: 577–580.
41. Pilepich MU, Sauce WT, Shipley WO, Kroll JM, Lawton CA, Grignon D, et al. Androgen deprivation with radiation therapy compared with radiation therapy alone for locally advanced prostatic carcinoma: a randomized comparative trial of the radiation therapy oncology group. *Urology* 1995; 45: 616–623.

OLIGOMETASTASES

Reprinted with permission. © 1995 American Society of Clinical Oncology. All rights reserved.

Hellman S, Weichselbaum RR. *Journal of Clinical Oncology* 1995;13(1):8–10.

Cancer treatment is based on an often unstated paradigm of disease pathogenesis. Since 1894, when W. S. Halsted[1,2] clearly elucidated a mechanism of breast cancer spread and used it to design and support the radical mastectomy, surgical and radiotherapeutic approaches to most cancers have been based on this theory. The Halsted theory proposed that cancer spread is orderly, extending in a contiguous fashion from the primary tumor through the lymphatics to the lymph nodes and then to distant sites. Radical en bloc surgery, such as radical neck dissection in continuity with removal of the primary tumor, radical hysterectomy, and primary and regional irradiation for a variety of tumor sites are all based on this notion of cancer spread. More recently, another hypothesis has gained prominence, also first suggested with regard to breast cancer.[3-5] This systemic hypothesis proposes that clinically apparent cancer is a systemic disease. Small tumors are just an early manifestation of such systemic disease, which, if it is to metastasize, has already metastasized. Lymph node involvement is not orderly contiguous extension, but rather a marker of distant disease. Systemic metastases are multiple and widespread, and when subclinical are referred to as micrometastases. Under these circumstances, treatment of local or regional disease should not affect survival.

Both the contiguous and systemic theories of cancer pathogenesis are too restricting and do not consider what is now known about tumor progression during clinical evolution. A third paradigm, one that synthesizes the contiguous-systemic dialectic, has been suggested by one of us[6] to explain the natural history of breast cancer. This thesis argues that cancer comprises a biologic spectrum extending from a disease that remains localized to one that is systemic when first detectable but with many intermediate states. Metastases are a function of both tumor size and tumor progression.

While much tumor evolution occurs during the preclinical period, we suggest that there is a progression of malignancy during the clinical evolution of a cancer. There is some evidence to support this progression of clinical cancer because pathologic grade usually correlates with tumor size, with smaller tumors being of lower grade than large ones.[7-10] Although this may be owing in part to the more rapid growth of high-grade tumors, it is also consistent with tumor progression during the clinical evolution of the tumor. Such possible tumor progression with increasing metastatic capacity during the clinically apparent period is receiving increasing support as we learn more about the multistep nature of the development of malignancy.[11-13] Once tumors become invasive, they may gradually acquire the properties necessary for efficient and widespread metastatic spread.[14] Therefore the likelihood, number, and even sites of metastases may reflect the state of tumor development. This suggests that there are tumor states intermediate between purely localized lesions and those widely metastatic. Such clinical circumstances are not accounted for by either the contiguous or the systemic hypotheses. The systemic hypothesis is binary: metastases either do or do not exist. If present, even if microscopic, they are extensive and widespread. The contiguous hypothesis considers systemic metastases to occur only after nodal disease; but when they occur, they are also blood borne, extensive, and widespread.

From considerations of these theories of cancer dissemination, in the light of the emerging information on the multistep nature of cancer progression, we propose the existence of a clinical significant state of *oligometastases*. For certain tumors, the anatomy and physiology may limit or concentrate these metastases to a single or a limited number of organs. The likelihood of the oligometastatic state should correlate with the biology of tumor progression, rough clinical surrogates of which, for many tumors, might be primary tumor size and grade. Metastasizing cells may seed specific organs as a function of the seeding tumor cell number and characteristics, as well as the receptivity of the host organ. The importance of "seed and soil" have been considered elsewhere[14,15] and will not be discussed further. Tumors early in the chain of progression may have metastases limited in number and location because the facility for metastatic growth has not been fully developed and the site for such growth is restricted (this is in contrast to micrometastases, which, although small in size, are extensive in number). With further progression, the tumor seeding efficiency increases and becomes less fastidious with regard to the location of metastatic growth. In addition to this progression of malignancy, the increasing primary tumor size and therefore cell number should also be correlated with the increasing number of cells seeding. Tumor size is the principal basis of tumor staging and, with histologic grade, correlates with the likelihood of metastases.[6-10,16] This, we suggest, is due to the number of tumor cells, the tumor vascularity, and malignant progression as tumors grow.

An attractive consequence of the presence of a clinically significant oligometastatic state is that some patients so affected should be amenable to a curative therapeutic strategy. The occasional success of surgical excision or radiation ablation of one or a small number of pulmonary, hepatic, or even brain metastases is evidence of a limited form of the oligometastatic state. The complete resection of pulmonary metastases from soft tissue sarcomas, osteosarcomas, and renal cell cancers can be curative even when they are multiple.[17] The likelihood of this for soft tissue sarcoma is correlated with tumor size and tumor grade.[18] Of 859 hepatic resections for metastatic colorectal cancer, there was a 25% 5-year disease-free survival.[19] Long-term survival decreases with the number of metastases, probably both as a function of the adequacy of the resection and the increased likelihood of occult disease. However, recurrences following hepatic resection are often restricted to the liver and, if amenable to surgical re-resection, have a likelihood for cure similar to that seen with the first resection.[20,21] Radiosurgery is being applied to solitary brain metastases with some initial success.[22] The limited effectiveness of these treatments of oligometastases has been primarily the result of an inability to recognize all metastases and the fact that these seemingly limited lesions were too often a manifestation of undetected widespread cancer. The importance of oligometastases depends on how commonly they are present. Only further study will determine this, but the frequency of their presence in the liver with colorectal cancer and in the lung with certain sarcomas offers some evidence of their clinical importance. It is estimated that of the 30% of cancer patients who develop pulmonary metastases, one-third have the primary tumor controlled and the metastases limited to the lung.[23] Similarly, one-third of all patients with colorectal cancer develop liver metastases, often as the only site of metastatic disease.[20] Effective treatment of oligometastases will require identification of all of the lesions and, most importantly, of the state of intermediate tumor progression likely to be consistent with the oligometastatic state. This must be distinguished from the circumstance in which the identified metastases are the most evident of a much larger number of widespread deposits. A special form of oligometastases recognized today as amenable to curative regional therapy is limited lymph node involvement, which is often effectively treated by surgical excision or radiation therapy.

As effective chemotherapy becomes more widely applicable, there should be another group of patients with oligometastases. These are patients who had widespread metastases that were mostly eradicated by systemic agents, the chemotherapy having failed to destroy those remaining because of the number of tumor cells, the presence of drug-resistant cells, or the tumor foci being located in some pharmacologically privileged site. Thus, effective chemotherapy may fail to be curative because of only a few metastases.

The number of metastases should reflect the biologic progression of the tumor. It will also determine the opportunities and the nature of potentially therapeutic interventions. Not only is there a spectrum of malignancy, but there is an accompanying spectrum of potentially curative treatments. Tumors early in their progression should be amenable to localized therapy. Patients with oligometastases, either de novo or following systemic treatment, should be cured by ablation of these lesions. More advanced disease will require more aggressive and effective systemic treatment.

Acceptance of this new paradigm for neoplastic pathogenesis and the resulting clinical relevance of the oligometastatic state requires the use of the most sophisticated diagnostic and therapeutic techniques. This paradigm emphasizes the importance of markers specifically related to where in the spectrum of malignancy an individual cancer is located. Truly localized, oligometastatic, and widely metastatic tumors are likely to require different strategies. New methods of surgery or radiation therapy may allow curative treatment of such oligometastases either alone or combined with systemic therapy. Their effectiveness will be critically dependent on the specificity, sensitivity, precision, and accuracy of tumor imaging. The treatment of these metastases must be equally precise and limit normal tissue toxicity. New operations for oligometastases should be devised. Such procedures—relying on the identification of appropriate patients—must excise or ablate the metastases completely while at the same time preserving normal function and structure. The likelihood of complete resection of pulmonary metastases from soft tissue sarcomas is dependent on histologic subtype, which suggests that there are differing patterns of metastatic growth for different primary tumors.[18] Knowledge of such patterns of local extension for different metastastic tumors in different sites will be necessary to any locally applied therapy of metastases. Conformal radiotherapy now being investigated for the treatment of primary tumors may find the treatment of oligometastases its most important application.[24-26] This technique allows both an increase in the tumor dose and a reduction in normal tissue toxicity by restricting, as much as possible, the radiation to the accurately imaged tumor while avoiding critical normal tissues. It requires extensive use of computers to integrate the digital information of the imaging modality to radiation treatment planning and then to deliver precise reproducible computer-controlled radiation delivery. Most critically, the integrated use of local and systemic treatment modalities requires determining where an individual tumor is located within the continuum of malignancy. This will be the challenge for the newly emerging field of molecular diagnostics.

The importance of the oligometastatic state will be dependent on the size of the group of patients for whom it offers curative prospects. Although the notion of there being some patients with limited metastases is recognized, it is thought to be quite uncommon. What is important in oligometastases is the recognition that it is not just a stochastic oddity, but rather that it is based on a state of limited metastatic capacity and is a characteristic of many tumors during their clinical evolution. The exploration of the size and nature of the oligometastatic state will profit from a careful review of past experience. Analysis of the site, number, and anatomic characteristics of metastases as a function of primary tumor size, location, and differentiation, as well as the use of newer molecular markers on paraffin-imbedded materials, should provide a great deal of information. Some of this should be available in surgical, pathologic, and medical imaging archival materials. Most importantly, while efforts are made to determine its size, recognition of the existence and implications of a state of oligometastases is necessary to invite active clinical investigation of new and potentially curative therapeutic strategies.

REFERENCES

1. Halsted WS: The results of operations for the cure of cancer of the breast performed at the Johns Hopkins Hospital from June, 1889 to January, 1894. *Johns Hopkins Bull* 4:297, 1894.
2. Halsted WS: The results of radical operations for the cure of carcinoma of the breast. *Ann Surg* 46:1, 1907.
3. Keynes G: Carcinoma of the breast, the unorthodox view. *Proc Cardiff M Soc* 40, 1954.
4. Crile G Jr: *A Biological Consideration of the Treatment of Breast Cancer*. Springfield, IL, Charles C. Thomas, 1967.
5. Fisher B: Laboratory and clinical research in breast cancer—A personal adventure: The David A Karnofsky Memorial Lecture. *Cancer Res* 40:3863–3874, 1980.
6. Hellman S: The natural history of small breast cancers. The David A. Karnofsky Memorial Lecture. *J Clin Oncol* 12:2229–2234, 1994.
7. Peer PGM, Holland R, Hendriks JHCL, et al.: Age-specific effectiveness of the Nijmegen population-based breast cancerscreening program: Assessment of early indicators of screening effectiveness. *J Natl Cancer Inst* 86:436–440, 1994.
8. Tabar L, Fagerberg G, Duffy SW, et al.: Update of the Swedish two-county program of mammographic screening for breast cancer. *Radiat Clin North Am* 30:187–210, 1992.
9. Tubiana M, Koscielny S: Natural history of human breast cancer: Recent data and clinical implications. *Breast Cancer Res Treat* 18:125–140, 1991.

10. Gleason DF, Melinger GT, Veterans Administration Cooperative Urological Research Group: Prediction of prognosis for prostatic adenocarcinoma by combined histological grading and clinical staging. *J Urol* 111:58–64, 1974.
11. Vogelstein B, Kinzler KW: The multistep nature of cancer. *Trends Genet* 9:138–141, 1993.
12. Rinker-Schaeffer CW, Partin AW, Isaacs WB, et al.: Molecular and cellular changes associated with the acquisition of metastatic ability by prostatic cancer cells. *The Prostate* 1994 Nov;25(5):249–265.
13. Schwechheimer K, Cavenee WK: Genetics of cancer predisposition and progression. *Clin Invest* 7:488–502, 1993.
14. Price JE, Aukerman SL, Fidler IJ: Evidence that the process of murine melanoma metastasis is sequential and selective and contains stochastic elements. *Cancer Res* 46:5172–5178, 1986.
15. Paget S: The distribution of secondary growths in cancer of the breast. *Lancet* 1:571–573, 1889.
16. Koscielny S, Tubiana M, Le MG, et al: Breast cancer: Relationship between the size of the primary tumour and the probability of metastatic dissemination. *Br J Cancer* 49:709–715, 1984.
17. Kern KA, Pass HI, Roth JA: Surgical treatment of pulmonary metastases, in Rosenberg SA (ed.): *Surgical Treatment of Metastatic Cancer.* Philadelphia, PA, Lippincott, 1987, pp. 69–100.
18. Gadd MA, Casper EF, Woodruff JM, et al.: Development and treatment of pulmonary metastases in adult patients with extremity soft tissue sarcoma. *Ann Surg* 218:705–712, 1993.
19. Hughes KS, Simon R, Songhorabodi S, et al.: Resection of the liver for colorectal carcinoma metastases: A multi-institutional study of the indications for resection. *Surgery* 100:278–284, 1986.
20. Hughes KS, Sugarbaker PH: Resection of the liver for metastatic solid tumors, in Rosenberg SA (ed.): *Surgical Treatment of Metastatic Cancer.* Philadelphia, PA, Lippincott, 1987, pp. 101–125.
21. Nordlinger B, Vaillant J-C, Guiguet M, et al.: Survival benefit of repeat liver resections for recurrent colorectal metastases: 143 cases. *J Clin Oncol* 12:1491–1496, 1994.
22. Flickinger JC, Kondziola D, Lunsford LD, et al.: A multi-institutional experience with stereostatic radiosurgery for solitary brain metastases. *Int J Radiat Oncol Biol Phys* 28:797–802, 1994.
23. van Dongen JA, van Sloten EA: The surgical treatment of pulmonary metastases. *Cancer Treat Rev* 5:29–48, 1978.
24. Lichtor AS: Three-dimensional conformal radiation therapy: A testable hypothesis. *Int J Radiat Oncol Biol Phys* 21:853, 1991.
25. Leibel SA, Heimann R, Kutcher GJ, et al.: Three-dimensional conformal radiation therapy in locally advanced carcinoma of the prostate: Preliminary results of a phase 1 dose escalation study. *Int J Radiat Oncol Biol Phys* 28:55–65, 1994.
26. Vijayakumar S, Myrianthopoulos LC, Rosenberg I, et al.: Optimization of radical radiotherapy with Beam's eye view techniques for non-small cell lung cancer. *Int J Radiat Oncol Biol Phys* 21:779–788, 1991.

OLIGOMETASTASES REVISITED

Ralph R. Weichselbaum and Samuel Hellman

This article was first published in *Nature Reviews Clinical Oncology* 2011;8(6):378–382.

Abstract

We previously proposed a clinical state of metastasis termed "oligometastases" that refers to restricted tumor metastatic capacity. The implication of this concept is that local cancer treatments are curative in a proportion of patients with metastases. Here we review clinical and laboratory data that support the hypothesis that oligometastasis is a distinct clinical entity. Investigations of the prevalence, mechanism of occurrence, and position in the metastatic cascade, as well as the determination of molecular markers to distinguish oligometastatic from polymetastatic disease, are ongoing.

Introduction

Current methods of cancer staging and treatment frequently separate patients into groups with tumors confined to the primary site or regional spread (lymph-node metastases).[1] These patients are usually treated with curative intent in contrast to patients with distant metastasis who are not usually considered curable by current regional treatment methods. In most adult solid cancers, the treatment for metastasis is systemic cytotoxic chemotherapy and/or hormonal manipulation. In general, distant metastases are the primary cause of cancer mortality and have led to a "leukemia-like" consideration of solid tumor metastases whereby metastases are frequently, if not always, considered extensive in number and organ site. We proposed an intermediate state of metastases termed "oligometastases."[2] In this concept, the number and site of metastatic tumors are limited. We suggested that the evolution of metastatic capacity has intermediate states in which spread may be limited to specific organs and metastases might be present in limited numbers. The clinical implication of this hypothesis is that localized forms of cancer treatment may be effective in patients with oligometastases. This is clearly the case since curative surgical resection of liver metastases from colon cancer,[3-6] lung metastases from a variety of primary sites,[7] and adrenal metastases from lung cancer[8] result in cure in some patients. A major question is the prevalence of oligometastasis. Since current research indicates that tumors evolve in their malignant capacity, the improving imaging methods (for example, MRI and PET), as well as blood-based tests (such as prostate-specific antigen levels), might identify a significant population of patients with oligometastases and afford opportunities for detecting primary tumors early in their progression, as well as permitting early diagnosis of oligometastases amenable to curative local treatment. More recently, the use of stereotactic radiotherapy, radiofrequency ablation, and MRI-guided focused ultrasound offer less invasive methods of regional treatment than surgical resection, and could offer curative potential in the treatment of oligometastases.[9-14] However, longer follow-up and larger patient numbers are required to assess the curative potential of stereotactic radiotherapy and other ablative techniques for oligometastases. We review the surgical treatment of liver and lung metastases as support for the oligometastatic concept, as well as novel laboratory investigations pertinent to the selection of appropriate candidates for localized treatment of oligometastases.

Treatment of Oligometastases

Liver Metastases

Liver metastases have a role in the mortality of many patients with cancer, in particular those of the gastrointestinal (GI) tract.[3-6] This association is partially explained by the venous drainage of the GI tract traveling through the portal vein, although tumor and host genetic factors also have a role in the tropism of GI metastases to the liver. Support for the oligometastatic state of some GI-associated liver metastases comes from data regarding the outcome of patients with colorectal cancer who underwent partial liver resection for metastasis to the liver (Table 3.6).[3-6] The curative treatment of liver metastasis has been reported for many years; however, each series was relatively small. In 1986, Hughes and colleagues compiled a registry of 607 patients from 24 institutions who had undergone curative resection for liver metastasis from colorectal cancer; 25% of these patients were disease free at 5 years.[3] Poor prognostic factors included positive surgical margins and bilobar disease.[3] In 1996, Nordlinger et al.[4] published a multi-institutional European registry study of 1,568 patients who underwent liver resection for metastasis; the 5-year survival rate was 28%. Adverse prognostic factors included a positive surgical margin of the resected metastasis, serosal or lymphatic spread of the primary tumor, large size and high number of liver metastasis, high carcinoembryonic antigen (CEA) levels, and age (< 60 years). In a single institution study that highlighted patients likely to benefit from liver resection, surgeons analyzed results from 1,001 liver resections for metastatic colorectal cancer.[5] Poor prognostic factors included the presence of extrahepatic disease, a node-positive primary tumor, size and number of metastatic lesions, a short disease-free interval between the primary tumor and metastasis, and a CEA level of greater than 200 ng/ml. The overall survival rate was 37% at 5 years, and 22% at 10 years.[5] The investigators devised risk categories based on these data and the above criteria to determine patients suitable for resection based on the number of risk factors present. In 2005, Pawlik et al.[6] analyzed 557 patients from three institutes who underwent liver resection for metastasis. These investigators identified adverse prognostic factors to be a positive surgical margin, more than three metastases and a CEA level of > 200 ng/ml. The 5-year survival rate was 58% in patients without any poor prognostic factors. Strikingly, the 5-year survival was 17% in patients with positive surgical margins compared with 63% in patients with negative margins—the width of the margin did not affect the outcome.[6] Most of these studies included patients treated before transaxial body imaging (CT and MRI) or PET was frequently used for

Table 3.6. SUMMARY OF FOUR LARGE SERIES OF RESECTION OF HEPATIC METASTASIS

Study	n	5-Year Survival Rate (%)	10-Year Survival Rate (%)
Hughes et al. (1986)[3]	607	33	No 10-year follow-up
Nordlinger et al. (1996)[4]	1,568	28	No 10-year follow-up
Fong et al. (1999)[5]	1,001	37	22
Pawlik et al. (2005)[6]	557	58	No 10-year follow-up

the detection of metastases and for staging; therefore, it is likely that these advanced imaging and molecular diagnostic techniques could be used to aid the selection of patients for curative treatment of metastatic disease. Indeed, these techniques were used in some patients in the most recent of the studies[6] and likely contributed to better patient selection and improved 5-year survival in this study compared with the other trials (Table 3.6).[3-5]

LUNG METASTASES

Pulmonary metastases are a primary cause of death from cancer.[7] As for the liver, the lung is also a primary or secondary drainage region for many frequently occurring cancers. Specific genes have been identified that are associated with lung metastases from breast cancer suggesting a genetic basis for metastatic tropism.[15,16] In addition, bone marrow-derived cells might establish a favorable microenvironment in the lung for development of metastasis.[17,18] Successful results of curative resection of lung metastases have been described for almost all types of cancer and these data were summarized in a report from the International Registry of Lung Metastases.[7] This report detailed results from pulmonary resection of 5,206 patients with pulmonary metastases with controlled primary tumors and with metastases confined to the lung from a wide variety of histological tumor types. A total of 4,572 patients underwent complete resection, 1,984 had epithelial tumors, and 1,917 had sarcomas.[7] In this study, patients who underwent complete resection of metastatic tumors had a 5-year survival rate of 36% and a 10-year survival rate of

26%. Patients with fewer metastases and a longer disease-free interval between the primary tumor and the appearance of lung metastases had 10-year survival rates as high as 40%. Similar to the liver metastases data, patients with incomplete resection had poor survival rates of 13% and 7% at 5 years and 10 years, respectively. Multiple surgeries were required in some patients and histology had a role in outcome; patients with germ-cell tumors had the best outcome, and patients with melanoma had the worst outcome. Curative resection of pulmonary metastases from sarcomas and germ-cell tumors had been reported before the report from the International Registry of Lung Metastases. A subset of patients with tumors considered to be widely metastatic in all instances, such as breast cancer and melanoma, were reported to be cured with surgical resection of lung metastases if certain clinical criteria were used for patient selection (usually the length of the disease-free interval and number of metastases).[7]

Common clinical prognostic factors emerge from these large investigations of resection and outcome in lung and liver metastasis. These include the number and size of metastasis, the interval from the treatment of the primary tumor to the appearance of metastasis, adequacy of resection of the metastatic tumors, and the presence of multiple metastatic sites. The histology of the primary tumor also seems to influence outcome. These data form the basis of clinical markers for patient selection for the treatment of oligometastatic disease.

Response to Chemotherapy

In our original article on oligometastasis,[2] we speculated that a state of oligometastasis might be created following cytoreduction as a consequence of excellent responses to systemic treatments and when local treatments might add to cure. One interesting example of this concept is the neoadjuvant chemotherapy treatment of patients with liver metastasis who then undergo resection. For example, Giacchetti et al.[19] reported that of 151 patients with liver metastasis who were unresectable (owing to the size or multi-nodularity of the metastasis) who received chemotherapy (oxaliplatin, 5-fluorouracil, and leucovorin), 77 became resectable and complete resection was achieved in 58 patients.[19] Almost all patients who were not operated on died within 5 years, but 50% of patients who achieved a response to chemotherapy and were resected were alive at 5 years. Negative predictors for survival in patients undergoing chemotherapy before liver resection included tumor progression during chemotherapy and the presence of celiac or para-aortic lymph-node metastasis even if the liver and nodal tumors were stabilized by chemotherapy.[19] Administration of cetuximab with or without chemotherapy in patients with liver metastasis who failed first-line chemotherapy resulted in a small percentage of patients sufficiently down-staged to undergo curative surgery; eight out of 11 patients who had complete surgical resection were alive at 36 months.[20]

The Biology of Metastasis

Paget first hypothesized the "seed and soil" hypothesis, which suggested that metastases were not random and were not solely dependent on circulatory patterns, but rather were an interaction between the tumor cell and the targeted organ.[21] In this concept, certain tumors have a predilection for metastasis to particular organs that support the secondary growth of cells from the primary tumor. The selective process is driven by a tumor microenvironment that is hypoxic and acidic with immune-derived cells and other host-derived cells that promote tumor growth and suppress host immunity. Tumor diversity is driven by the genetic instability of the tumor cells due to telomere erosion, mutations in tumor-suppressor and DNA-repair genes, and intrinsic tumor metabolism (aerobic glycolyis) that is toxic to surrounding normal cells.[18,22,23] The evolutionary value to the primary tumor of harboring clones that metastasize may not necessarily directly aid in the growth of the primary tumor. The capacity for metastatic spread is likely an epiphenomenon of the genetic instability of the primary tumor resulting in the capacity to grow and invade and give rise to cells capable of distant metastases.

Steps in Metastasis

Many investigators have hypothesized and have provided evidence to support the various steps in the metastatic cascade. These "discrete steps" in metastasis have been elegantly summarized by Gupta and Massagué.[24] These steps include loss of cellular adhesion, increased motility, invasiveness of the primary tumor, entry into and survival in the circulation, entry into new organs, and eventual colonization of these organs. Gupta and Massagué have defined a useful framework to categorize genes that have roles in the various stages of metastasis.[24] They term genes that confer a selective advantage to the primary tumor cells as metastasis "initiation" genes; metastasis "progression" genes are those that fulfill rate-limiting functions in colonization; and metastasis "virulence" genes are those that provide an advantage in metastasis colonization but not necessarily an advantage in the growth of the primary tumor. Metastasis colonization requires a selective advantage in the evolution of the primary tumor to be preserved and amplified during tumor progression.[24] The following characteristics of the metastatic phenotype are altered cell adhesion, intravasation, survival in the circulation, extravasation, seeding in a distant site, invasion, and development of the appropriate microenvironment in host organs. These processes have been reviewed by others in this focus issue and elsewhere. These data indicate that there are primary tumor cells that have limited capability in one or more of the necessary biological requirements for metastasis, thus the origin of oligometastases. Tumor dormancy may be a particular example of limited metastatic capacity.

Dormancy

Cells that escape from the primary tumor may be present at distant organs as cellular aggregates without forming established tumors.[25,26] Several hypotheses might explain this phenomenon:[27–29] the tumor cells fail to signal appropriate angiogenic cues or the rate of blood vessel formation equals the apoptosis in tumor endothelia and adequate neovasculature does not form; the local microenvironment does not support metastatic growth (for example, it does not have appropriate environmental growth factors or cell contact structures); and the immune system monitors tumors and eliminates incipient tumor cells (surveillance), keeps tumors at a small or microscopic size (equilibrium; perhaps analogous to dormancy), or allows escape to established tumor growth.[29] Within the context of dormancy, these processes might have an effect on the number, location, and timing of appearance of metastases; interferon signaling is a key component of these processes.[29]

Models and Molecules

Investigations of laboratory and molecular determinants of oligometastasis are limited. However, Fidler and Kripke[30] compared the metastatic ability of different tumor-cell clones derived from B16F1 melanoma. They noted a wide variation in the ability of these clones to colonize the lung (from 3.5 to 260 lung colonies per mouse) and concluded that the B16F1 cell line is heterogenous with regard to the metastasis-forming ability of preexisting tumor clones.[30] These results were confirmed and expanded upon by several investigators using KHT sarcoma cells, which varied widely in metastatic potential (lung colonization).[31,32] Cillo et al.[33] noted that clones that had a high metastatic potential were more resistant to chemotherapy than cells derived from clones of low metastatic potential. In addition, Khodarev et al.[34] used the B16F1 mouse melanoma model to show that repeated passage through the lungs evolved a more "aggressive" phenotype defined by an increase of efficiency in lung colonization and conferred resistance to radiotherapy and chemotherapy on the more highly metastatic clones; this finding is consistent with earlier reports.[34] Of interest is the finding that clones that give rise to widely metastatic tumors overexpressed genes known to be induced by interferon, which had previously been associated with resistance to radiotherapy and chemotherapy in murine models and in human databases and tumor samples.[35,36]

Considered together, these reports suggest that there are large differences between metastatic capability in tumor cells in experimental models, consistent with the concept of oligometastases. Genes that govern the metastatic process are of great interest; however, genes that govern the number of metastases have not been studied in detail. Recently, Wuttig et al.[37] used samples from 18 patients with renal cell carcinoma to identify genes that characterized "few" (less than eight) or "many" (> 16) pulmonary metastases. DNA-array analysis on fresh samples obtained from pulmonary resection of metastasis revealed 135 genes that were differentially expressed between the "few" and "many" metastasis groups. Using gene ontology enrichment analysis, the researchers demonstrated that polymetastatic tumors were enriched by genes that positively regulate the cell cycle, indicating an increase in growth potential in polymetastasis versus oligometastasis.[37] Based on a meta-analysis of these data[37] and previously published data,[38] an 11-gene classifier was established to predict the number of metastases in patients with renal cell carcinoma. Ideally, prospective trials will collect fresh-frozen tumor specimens for molecular analysis to validate this signature as well as identify other genes and gene families involved in oligometastasis.

Temporal Evolution

Recently, insights into the evolution of metastasis in pancreatic cancer were reported;[39,40] this is particularly interesting since oligometastases are rarely observed in pancreatic cancer. Two research groups analyzed somatic mutations in genes and constructed clonal evolutionary maps derived from primary and metastatic tumors.[39,40] They reported that pancreatic tumors contain geographically separate subclones within the primary tumor that are present many years before metastases become evident. As an example, it was demonstrated that long time periods existed between the appearance of the tumor and the initial metastasis. Also, different metastatic clones may appear at different time periods. It is suggested that there may be a hierarchy of metastatic sites for pancreatic cancer with peritoneal metastases occurring first, then hepatic, and finally pulmonary metastases.[40] The nature of this hierarchy is likely to vary with primary tumor histology and location; the latter because of different vascular drainage, local hypoxia, and possible local stromal interactions. For example, adrenal metastases may occur early in the process in non-small-cell lung cancer, while for colon cancer the site of early metastases is the liver, perhaps owing to the portal drainage pattern. Other examples include the lungs as an initial site for soft-tissue and bone sarcomas, perhaps because of the venous return from the tumor going first through the pulmonary circulation or from local stromal considerations. Such considerations of the sites and mechanisms of metastases early in the metastatic progression should produce opportunities for site-specific analyses of metastases from different primary tumors as well as analysis of differential gene expression as a function of the site of the primary tumor and of oligometastases. These observations put a special emphasis on the early detection of the oligometastatic state and local control of the primary tumor because if metastasis is hierarchal in time and number, ablation of "early" metastasis might be curative. Since the metastatic tumor clone arises from the primary tumor, control of the primary tumor takes on special importance in the cure of oligometastasis and perhaps also polymetastatic disease. We are conducting investigations that are ongoing to study differences between oligometastases and polymetastases in both clinical material and experimental tumor models.

Conclusions

The metastases that we define as oligometastases have long been recognized as potentially curable but were considered to be rare exceptions to the cancer metastasis paradigm. However, the oligometastatic state is becoming more frequently identified with more sensitive methods of detecting such oligometastases. As newer methods of analyzing patients with metastatic disease develop (for example, the analysis of circulating tumor cells), the oligometastatic state should be identified even earlier. As indicated earlier, new molecular analysis of pancreatic cancer suggests that there are temporal differences in the appearance of metastases based on tumor genetics. These data suggest a potential stepwise progression with intermediate stages of limited metastatic capacity. It seems quite possible that metastases from tumors with such limited capacities might be separated from those much further along in malignant progression. If this seems possible, then clinicians will be able to limit ablative local treatment to only those patients with true oligometastases. Finally, there seems to be another type of oligometastasis evolving: those limited remaining tumor deposits following successful eradication of all other apparent and occult cancer cells by systemic means. It is important to study both types of limited metastases but to recognize that the true oligometastases are present because of limited metastatic competence, while induced oligometastases following otherwise successful systemic treatment have more extensive malignant capacities and were spared from eradication by pharmacological means, local immunological conditions, or from the development of resistant clones. The strategy and tactics of treatment of these two types might be different, as well as the likelihood of therapy success.

Acknowledgments

The authors are supported by grants from the Ludwig Foundation for Cancer Research, the Lung Cancer Research Foundation, and a generous gift from the Foglia Foundation.

Author Contributions

Both authors contributed to researching data for the article, discussion of the content, and writing and editing the manuscript.

REFERENCES

1. Edge, S. B. et al. (Eds.) *AJCC Cancer Staging Manual* 7th edn (Springer, New York, 2010).
2. Hellman, S., & Weichselbaum, R. R. Oligometastases. *J. Clin. Oncol.* **13**, 8–10 (1995).
3. Hughes, K. S., et al. Resection of the liver for colorectal carcinoma metastases: a multi-institutional study of patterns of recurrence. *Surgery* **100**, 278–284 (1986).
4. Nordlinger, B., et al. Surgical resection of colorectal carcinoma metastases to the liver: a prognostic scoring system to improve case selection, based on 1568 patients. Association Française de Chirurgie. *Cancer* **77**, 1254–1262 (1996).
5. Fong, Y., Fortner, J., Sun, R. L., Brennan, M. F., & Blumgart, L. H. Clinical score for predicting recurrence after hepatic resection for metastatic colorectal cancer: analysis of 1001 consecutive cases. *Ann. Surg.* **230**, 309–318 (1999).
6. Pawlik, T. M., et al. Effect of surgical margin status on survival and site of recurrence after hepatic resection for colorectal metastases. *Ann. Surg.* **241**, 715–722 (2005).
7. Pastorino, U., et al. Long-term results of lung metastasectomy: prognostic analyses based on 5206 cases. The International Registry of Lung Metastases. *J. Thorac. Cardiovasc. Surg.* **113**, 37–49 (1997).
8. Strong, V. E., et al. Laparoscopic adrenalectomy for isolated adrenal metastasis. *Ann. Surg. Oncol.* **14**, 3392–3400 (2007).
9. Ben-Josef, E., & Lawrence, T. S. Using a bigger hammer: the role of stereotactic body radiotherapy in the management of oligometastases. *J. Clin. Oncol.* **27**, 1537–1539 (2009).
10. Salama, J. K., et al. An initial report of a radiation dose-escalation trial in patients with one to five sites of metastatic disease. *Clin. Cancer Res.* **14**, 5255–5259 (2008).
11. Rusthoven, K. E., et al. Multi-institutional phase I/II trial of stereotactic body radiation therapy for lung metastases. *J. Clin. Oncol.* **27**, 1579–1584 (2009).
12. Lee, M. T., et al. Phase I study of individualized stereotactic body radiotherapy of liver metastases. *J. Clin. Oncol.* **27**, 1585–1591 (2009).
13. Macdermed, D. M., Weichselbaum, R. R., & Salama, J. K. A rationale for the targeted treatment of oligometastases with radiotherapy. *J. Surg. Oncol.* **98**, 202–206 (2008).
14. Fakiris, A. J., et al. Stereotactic body radiation therapy for early-stage non-small-cell lung carcinoma: four-year results of a prospectice phase II study. *Int. J. Radiat. Oncol. Biol. Phys.* **75**, 677–682 (2009).
15. Minn, A. J., et al. Genes that mediate breast cancer metastasis to lung. *Nature* **436**, 518–524 (2005).
16. Minn, A. J., et al. Lung metastasis genes couple breast tumor size and metastatic spread. Proc. *Natl Acad. Sci. USA* **104**, 6740–6745 (2007).
17. Kaplan, R. N., Psaila, B., & Lyden, D. Bone marrow cells in the "pre-metastatic niche": within bone and beyond. *Cancer Metastasis Rev.* **25**, 521–529 (2006).
18. Erler, J. T., et al. Lysyl oxidase is essential for hypoxia-induced metastasis. *Nature* **440**, 1222–1226 (2006).

19. Giacchetti, S., et al. Long-term survival of patients with unresectable colorectal cancer liver metastases following infusional chemotherapy with 5-fluorouracil, leucovorin, oxaliplatin and surgery. *Ann. Oncol.* **10**, 663–669 (1999).
20. Lévi, F., et al. Cetuximab and circadian chronomodulated chemotherapy as salvage treatment for metastatic colorectal cancer (mCRC): safety, efficacy and improved secondary surgical resectability. *Cancer Chemother. Pharmacol.* **67**, 339–348 (2011).
21. Paget, S. The distribution of secondary growths in cancer of the breast. 1889. *Cancer Metastasis Rev.* **8**, 98–101 (1989).
22. Deng, C. X. BRCA1: cell cycle checkpoint, genetic instability, DNA damage response and cancer evolution. *Nucleic Acids Res.* **34**, 1416–1426 (2006).
23. Rajagopalan, H., & Lengauer, C. Aneuploidy and cancer. *Nature* **432**, 338–341 (2004).
24. Gupta, G. P., & Massagué, J. Cancer metastasis: building a framework. *Cell* **127**, 679–695 (2006).
25. Aguirre-Ghiso, J. A. Models, mechanisms and clinical evidence for cancer dormancy. *Nat. Rev. Cancer* **7**, 834–846 (2007).
26. Fokas, E., Engenhart-Cabillic, R., Daniilidis, K., Rose, F., & An, H. X. Metastasis: the seed and soil theory gains identity. *Cancer Metastasis Rev.* **26**, 705–715 (2007).
27. Uhr, J. W., Scheuermann, R. H, Street, N. E., & Vitetta, E. S. Cancer dormancy: opportunities for new therapeutic approaches. *Nat. Med.* **3**, 505–509 (1997).
28. Goss, P. E., & Chambers, A. F. Does tumour dormancy offer a therapeutic target? *Nat. Rev. Cancer* **10**, 871–877 (2010).
29. Dunn, G. P., Koebel, C. M., & Schreiber, R. D. Interferons, immunity and cancer immunoediting. *Nat. Rev. Immunol.* **6**, 836–848 (2006).
30. Fidler, I. J., & Kripke, M. L. Metastasis results from preexisting variant cells within a malignant tumor. *Science* **197**, 893–895 (1977).
31. Chambers, A. F., Hill, R. P., & Ling, V. Tumor heterogeneity and stability of the metastatic phenotype of mouse KHT sarcoma cells. *Cancer Res.* **41**, 1368–1372 (1981).
32. Harris, J. F., Chambers, A. F., Hill, R. P., & Ling, V. Metastatic variants are generated spontaneously at a high rate in mouse KHT tumor. *Proc. Natl Acad. Sci. USA* **79**, 5547–5551 (1982).
33. Cillo, C., Dick, J. E., Ling, V., & Hill, R. P. Generation of drug-resistant variants in metastatic B16 mouse melanoma cell lines. *Cancer Res.* **47**, 2604–2608 (1987).
34. Khodarev, N. N., et al. STAT1 pathway mediates amplification of metastatic potential and resistance to therapy. *PLoS ONE* **4**, e5821 (2009).
35. Khodarev, N. N., et al. STAT1 is overexpressed in tumors selected for radioresistance and confers protection from radiation in transduced sensitive cells. *Proc. Natl Acad. Sci. USA* **101**, 1714–1719 (2004).
36. Weichselbaum, R. R., et al. An interferon-related gene signature for DNA damage resistance is a predictive marker for chemotherapy and radiation for breast cancer. *Proc. Natl Acad. Sci. USA* **105**, 18490–18495 (2008).

37. Wuttig, D., et al. Gene signatures of pulmonary metastases of renal cell carcinoma reflect the disease-free interval and the number of metastases per patient. *Int. J. Cancer* **125**, 474–482 (2009).
38. Jones, J., et al. Gene signatures of progression and metastasis in renal cell cancer. *Clin. Cancer Res.* **11**, 5730–5739 (2005).
39. Campbell, P. J., et al. The patterns and dynamics of genomic instability in metastatic pancreatic cancer. *Nature* **467**, 1109–1113 (2010).
40. Yachida, S., et al. Distant metastasis occurs late during the genetic evolution of pancreatic cancer. *Nature* **467**, 1114–1117 (2010).

4

Perceptions of Cancer

COMMENTARY

Susan Sontag in her essay "Illness as a Metaphor" decries the imagery of disease as distorting reality and thereby affecting the perception of the disease. The two diseases she considers are tuberculosis and cancer. Tuberculosis is rife with romantic allusions and sensitive heroes, such as Keats and Chopin, who often engage in a rush of productivity before succumbing to the disease; cancer, on the other hand, connotes evil and even retribution for bad behavior. I was taken with this discussion of cancer and feel the differing perceptions of cancer are not limited to the culture in general but extend to the medical profession as well. In both cultures, this imagery cannot and often does not serve the best interests of the patient or of those laypeople and professionals associated with cancer prevention and care. I first presented a talk entitled "Cancer and the Elephant" to the Library Society of The University of Chicago over 10 years ago and then, more recently, in a somewhat revised form, to the Friday Club of Chicago. This talk was meant for a general audience, giving examples in the arts, politics, and media of imagery that uses cancer metaphorically to great effect but in so doing often results in distorting the perception of the disease itself. More recently, the book *The Emperor of All Maladies* by Siddhartha Mukherjee was published and then later was adapted as a PBS documentary by Ken Burns. Despite being sensitive and moving, in my judgment both works emphasize leukemia and widespread metastatic disease rather than the common tumors of the various organs, some of which are cured by local surgery or radiation, sometimes with adjuvant systemic therapy, with only limited unwanted effects. Most of the more than one-half of all cancers that are cured are treated in this manner. This is but another example of cancer presented with a point of view, and thus distorting somewhat the view of the entirety of cancer. One of the documentary episodes even uses the "Cancer and the Elephant" analogy I used in this talk more than a decade earlier. The first paper in this chapter, "Evolving Paradigms and Perceptions of Cancer," is based on that talk.

The other essay in this section is concerned with how oncologists and their patients perceive and communicate about the individual patient's disease and prognosis when cancer is so clouded by these unfortunate metaphors. This is especially an issue with medical, radiation, or surgical oncologists in training. It is further aggravated when these new physicians, so concerned with avoiding unwanted paternalism, offer only alternatives, rather than also engaging the patient in discussions as to how these alternative treatment plans apply in his or her specific circumstances. They should also indicate what plan they recommend, while making it clear that the decision is to be made by the patient. The patient must be confident in the truthfulness, faithfulness, support, and candor of the doctor if the doctor–patient relationship is to succeed. Patients have perceptions of cancer as well, and it is quite important for the caring physician to be fully cognizant of them. While they should be sought individually, great insight can come from the writings of cancer patients.

The popular war metaphor generally accepted with the passing of the National Cancer Act in 1971 is still accepted, and recent books and articles have similar bellicose tones. Currently a new but related metaphor has been used, likening expanded and directed cancer research to a "Moonshot" by President Obama to be overseen by Vice President Biden. The National Cancer Act was supposed to result in a cure for cancer by 1976, the bicentennial of the Declaration of Independence. The analogy of a "Moonshot" promises similar unrealistic goals, regardless of the resources and personnel devoted to it. Such imagery invites failure and resultant disillusionment. Cancer research and treatment should be well supported and progress will be made, but the unrealistic expectations stimulated by these analogies can distort expectations and may make the achievement of reasonable goals seem unsatisfactory. The War on Cancer begun in 1971 was not concluded with "victory" in 1976. I suspect the same to occur with the "Moonshot," with similar resulting disillusionment and pessimism. Increasing funding for the promising immunological, genetic, and technological advances should be sought, but without over-promising major improvements in cancer care. We should be modest in our claims and be pleased if we exceed them.

EVOLVING PARADIGMS AND PERCEPTIONS OF CANCER

This article was first published in *Nature Clinical Practice Oncology* 2005; 2(12):618–624.

Summary

The word "cancer" produces widely differing perceptions between the general public, and the scientific and medical communities. These different ideas lead to very diverse understandings of the disease. The paradigms affect both the focus and design of research and also impact upon patient care. The cultural perception is very pessimistic: a relentless, incurable, extremely painful disease, the treatment of which is conceived as difficult, with little chance of a simple cure. Within the medical and scientific communities, however, there are a number of quite different views of the disease. Both the orderly extension of disease described by Halsted and the systemic nature of cancer even when it appears to be localized are perceptions within the professional community. The promise of a "magic bullet" is in sharp contrast to the incremental advances seen in clinical oncology. What is needed is a clear recognition of how these varying perceptions of cancer affect and limit communication among the cancer-related disciplines as well as between these disciplines and the public. Both professionals and the general public should consider cancer as a group of diseases for which cure is related to tumor type, stage, and available treatment.

Introduction

"Cancer" is a term laden with cultural and emotional baggage, which influences how we perceive and communicate about the disease. This is true for the public and the patient, as well as for the doctor and the researcher. The public's view is the result of the metaphoric meaning of cancer, how it is reflected in the arts and media, temporized by personal experience. For the patient, cancer is immediate and ominous but, perhaps unexpectedly, for some it offers opportunities for personal growth and empowerment. Doctors have differing views about the underlying paradigm of cancer development, which produces varying conceptions of the disease and its clinical behavior, resulting in differing management strategies. For the researcher, the underlying paradigm determines the questions to be asked as well as the method of asking. For example, if a blind man were asked to describe an elephant, because he cannot see the animal in its entirety, he might feel its stout foreleg and liken the creature to a tree. Another blind man feeling its supple trunk might consider the elephant to be more like a reptile, while a third person feeling its smooth hard tusk might judge it to be similar to the exoskeleton of a sea creature, perhaps an odd mollusk or crustacean. I use this analogy because it pertains both to differing public appreciations of cancer as well as shaping the attitudes and behavior of health professionals and cancer researchers.

Cultural, Emotional, and Perceptional Views of Cancer

In her essay *Illness as Metaphor*,[1] Susan Sontag argues that the diseases that are most often culturally laden are tuberculosis and cancer: "Yet it is hardly possible to take up one's residence in the kingdom of the ill unprejudiced by the lurid metaphors with which it has been landscaped."

Cancer is associated with pessimistic connotations. If cancer develops it is seen as the ultimate health tragedy; the disease is viewed as the epitome of iniquity. "We have a cancer within, close to the presidency, that is growing," said President Nixon's advisor John Dean, during the early phase of the Watergate investigations. A growth, which could destroy the presidency, turned out to be an apt metaphor. Cancer is also commonly associated with the concept of evil. The term malignant, as in "malignant tumor," is defined as "disposed to do evil." This villainous designation of cancer influences our perception of the illness. Alexander Solzhenitsyn in *The Cancer Ward* considers the evils of the Soviet Union metaphorically as a cancer.[2] This book is also interesting for the contrasting, quite literal way in which the protagonist confronts his cancer and his would-be therapists.

Cancer, viewed as a silent, insidious, unrelenting, and inexorable entity that is not to be discussed, and for which the treatment is brutal, is the common perception in our culture. In *Miss Gee*, W. H. Auden[3] attributes the disease to repressed emotions or psychic energy. Even the word "cancer" might have magical qualities. Karl Menninger, the distinguished psychiatrist, felt that "the very word cancer is said to kill some patients who would not have succumbed (so quickly) to the malignancy from which they suffer." More recently, in November 2003, the television personality Rosie O'Donnell was quoted in *The New York Times* as stating, "Do you know what happens to people who lie? They get sick and they get cancer and they die." These images so laden the term "cancer" that it is difficult to discuss the disease in a public, social, personal, or professional encounter without dealing with the collateral images brought to the conversation by these emotionally charged perceptions. Almost every practicing physician, and probably most families, know of patients who have ignored obvious ominous clinical circumstances for as long as possible because of the fear that their symptoms and signs were those of this dreaded, incurable, and relentless disease, for which treatment would be extremely arduous and most likely ineffective.

Evolving Cancer Paradigms

Similarly, medical appreciation of cancer depends upon how the disease is thought to behave. The prevailing paradigm—first stated clearly at the end of the nineteenth century by William Stuart Halsted, then Professor of Surgery at Johns Hopkins Hospital and the leader of American surgery—was that cancer was a contiguous disease that spreads in an orderly manner from the primary site to the regional lymph nodes and only then to distant metastatic sites.[4] The corollary to this was that aggressive regional surgery was required for cancer cure. This led to the development of radical mastectomy for the treatment of breast cancer and, subsequently, to similarly conceived surgery for tumors in most accessible locations. This paradigm became completely accepted, in part because it was successful for some patients with breast cancer as reported by Halsted. The concept of aggressive radical surgery, however, was also attractive because it was promulgated in the first half of the twentieth century, a time when there were great advances in anesthesia, blood transfusion, and surgical technique that allowed the operations to be performed safely. Surgeons also championed the notion, because it made cancer management primarily their province and it emphasized the corollary that successful treatment depended on the skill of the surgical practitioner. This was highlighted by advocates of radical mastectomy as necessary for success and, when improperly applied, as an explanation for instances of failure.[5]

One interprets the world in the context of prevailing paradigms. The notion of a heliocentric solar system, rather than one that revolved around the earth, was so threatening to the established order that Galileo was considered a heretic. Similarly, despite widespread acceptance of the Halsted paradigm, after almost 50 years some began to question this thesis. Yet it had become no longer just a theory; rather, it was considered to be an accepted fact elevated to the status of dogma. Moreover, like the Ptolemaic system, it was not to be subject to question or modification. Those who disagreed were thought of as heretics to be publicly condemned. Such individuals include Robert McWhirter, the Scottish radiation oncologist, who had the temerity to suggest that, while he accepted the Halsted paradigm of contiguous extent of breast cancer, it might be possible to avoid the deformity and functional loss associated with removal of the muscles that are important for shoulder function and chest wall appearance, and to reduce the arm swelling associated with extensive dissection of the axilla. He recommended applying radiation to destroy regional disease outside the breast itself, while limiting surgery to removal of the breast (simple mastectomy) without compromising the underlying musculature or lymph drainage of the arm.[6] His reported results appeared comparable to those obtained with radical mastectomy, but with less deformity or functional loss in the arm or shoulder. This questioning of radical mastectomy—even while accepting the underlying paradigm—elicited such ire that America's leading cancer pathologist of the day, Lauren Ackerman from Washington University, was dispatched to Edinburgh to review McWhirter's cases in order to determine whether those cured were, in fact, patients who really had breast cancer. Yet even McWhirter could be forgiven to some extent, because he was not a surgeon but rather a radiation oncologist. This was not the case for the true surgical heretics, such as the British surgeon Geoffrey Keynes, who said, "none of us have been burned at the stake but feelings have run pretty high." George Crile Jr., Douglas Fitzwilliams, and, most recently, Bernard Fisher were also distinguished surgeons who evoked the ire of the surgical community for questioning the Halsted paradigm. Geoffrey Keynes (the brother of the distinguished economist) is particularly eloquent. He suggests that "orthodoxy in surgery *(I would suggest in all of medicine)* is like orthodoxy in other departments of the mind—it starts as tentative belief in some particular course of action but later begins almost to challenge comparison with a religion. It comes to be held as a passionate belief in the absolute rightness of that particular view."[7] Fitzwilliams stated, "those who have been brought up in the atmosphere of the radical operation with no experience of anything less extensive must remember that they are repeating dogma and not speaking from formed judgment."[8]

The Cancer Dialectic

Gradually the efforts of these pioneers who highlighted the inconsistencies between clinical experience and the Halsted model led to an alternative paradigm of breast cancer. Bernard Fisher formally articulated the new view that the fate of breast cancer is predetermined even before clinical detection of the disease. The tumor was thought to have one of two proclivities: if it is destined to remain local, aggressive regional treatment is unnecessary, whereas if it is destined to become pervasive, spread has occurred before clinical detection. In either case, extensive highly skilled treatment of the cancer at its site of origin does not influence ultimate outcome, but rather systemic treatment is required in order to cure the disease. This became the prevailing dogma during the last quarter of the twentieth century. The reasons for this new view becoming dominant were that systemic treatment worked, radical mastectomy was not required, and cancer care extended from the primary province of the surgeon to include that of medical and radiation oncologists. Owing to new biological information, however, and the fact that clinical experience sometimes supported the Halsted model but at other times supported the systemic model, a third paradigm has evolved—the spectrum model. This suggests that cancer is comprised of tumors with many different malignant proclivities. Some of these tumors will behave as predicted by the Halsted model, while others will be systemic from the outset. Most cancers, however, have malignant potentials in between these two extremes. The spectrum model proposes that malignant progression occurs throughout the life of a tumor, not only before, but also during, clinical detection and treatment of the cancer. Acceptance of the spectrum model requires clinicians to consider two things simultaneously: first, how to maximize local tumor control using conservative surgery and radiation for localized cancers before they develop the capacity to metastasize; and second, the importance of adjuvant systemic treatments necessary to destroy clinically undetected systemic micrometastases from those tumors that have already acquired that capacity.[9, 10]

Differing Medical Roles and How They Affect Cancer Paradigm Perception

For those not involved in this controversy, it is important to appreciate how different perceptions of cancer and the roles of medical specialties affect medical practice. Surgeons usually see patients early in the course of their disease when the cancer appears to be localized. As a consequence of inadequate local control, surgeons often observe local recurrence with subsequent metastases and, therefore, this portion of their clinical experience supports the Halsted model. They also realize, of course, that some patients, despite excellent local control of the cancer, have distant metastases, so that while the Halsted model is useful, it does not completely explain their clinical experience. Conversely, medical oncologists observe patients after clinical metastases are recognized, or they offer systemic treatment for clinically occult micrometastases. These situations assume metastases to be present, and so the medical oncologist's view of the disease is one where metastases are almost always present, supporting the systemic hypothesis. The radiation oncologist tends to see patients both early and late in the course of disease, and for this specialist the spectrum hypothesis offers the most encompassing view; this is also becoming adopted by surgeons and medical oncologists who now also see patients at varying times during this evolving clinical process.

By contrast, the pathologist all too often sees treatment failures. Unfortunately, the layman is much like the pathologist—for both, most of their attention is directed toward failed cancer treatment and widespread fatal disease. The patients treated successfully for cancer usually blend into the general population and their cancers are either unknown to others or, if known, do not offer any noticeable reminders of their former presence. Family and friends see the patient with recurrence as more typical of cancer, and so this substantiates the malign inexorability of the disease.

The great difficulties in causing a major saltation in cancer cure rates have caused some oncologists to reconsider the curative paradigm completely. They suggest that patients would be better served if cancer were considered a chronic disease for which cure is rarely the goal of treatment. They believe that physicians should concern themselves more with preventing or ameliorating tumor-induced and treatment-induced morbidity, and favor treatments that have as their goal holding cancer in check but not necessarily eliminating the tumor. Doctors, they would suggest, should observe patients carefully and deal with tumor spread promptly before it becomes a clinical problem. This prospect of the patient living with cancer as a chronic disease—which, while not cured, can have its progression and symptomatology modified—is in sharp contrast to the fact that cancer is the most curable of the serious chronic diseases. Coronary artery disease, diabetes, stroke, and multiple sclerosis are not curable at present, regardless of disease stage. Considering cancer as a disease amenable to cure is the foundation for the practices of screening, early diagnosis, prompt curative regional treatment, and adjuvant systemic therapy. These two different perceptions of the disease result in two very different cancer management strategies: one emphasizes early diagnosis and treatment to effect a cure, while the other recommends careful follow-up with therapy directed at limiting tumor growth and preventing or reducing symptoms of the disease.

Another perspective of cancer is that of basic scientists who believe that a fundamental understanding of the disease is required for successful prevention and treatment, with a corollary to this emphasizing that funding basic research should be expanded in order to acquire the fundamental knowledge required for designing effective nontoxic therapy. Within this perspective is the notion of there being a common mechanism for the development of cancer that could be the target of a potent therapy—a "magic bullet," if you will—that would be effective for all types of cancer.

To use the war analogy (which will be considered later), however, there are casualties—victims of "friendly fire" from these advocates of concentrating our efforts on finding such a panacea. The search for this universally effective therapy can subvert the more modest goals of cancer research by limiting support primarily to fundamental research on cancer, rather than to finance the more pragmatic and immediately applicable investigations.

The notion of a "magic bullet" has great appeal, and has been effective in catching the interest of legislators and policymakers. One can find much of this philosophy in the National Cancer Act enacted by the US Congress in 1971. Unfortunately, the risk of over-promise implied in the "magic bullet" concept is great, and the resulting cost for creating such illusions is subsequent public disillusionment with cancer research and treatment. The search for a "magic bullet" should continue, but not at the expense of diminished efforts to build on what is succeeding today. Perhaps a panacea will be discovered, but until that occurs, if ever, we need continued incremental improvement, building on what works.

Dealing with cancer is usually considered in the language of warfare; tumors invade and the body defenses are inadequate. Even the instruments used in cancer treatment are considered in war-like terms; the scalpel is seen as analogous to the sharp instruments used in warfare. Some of the drugs for cancer treatment were first derived from poisons designed to be used as weapons. Furthermore, radiation is seen similarly in both contexts. The National Cancer Act of 1971 was to declare war on cancer, a war that, it was optimistically hoped, would be concluded—as the result of a massive 5-year program—to coincide with the bicentennial of *The Declaration of Independence*. The war analogy permeates the National Cancer Act to the extent that the likelihood of success is assumed to be based on requirements for success in wartime: sufficient dedicated human and financial capital. The model suggests that cure will be achieved relatively quickly if a massive mobilization of resources is applied.

Private Financing of Cancer Research and Treatment

The importance of financial resources has stimulated the development of private organizations devoted to fundraising for cancer in general or for research devoted to certain types of cancer. While these groups see cancer primarily from the patient's perspective, they might also have different vantage points. Some are primarily fundraising organizations concerned with advocacy for specific groups of patients, while others provide opportunity for bonding and can serve as support groups for patients.

I had the privilege of knowing Laura Evans—the founder of Expedition Inspiration—who, as an avid mountaineer both before and after her cancer, felt that the attitude of the patient was especially important. Expedition Inspiration fosters activities for breast cancer survivors that liken mountain climbing to dealing with cancer. In both climbing a mountain and dealing with breast cancer, Laura Evans felt that patients faced their deepest fear—the reality of death. Mountaineering is an individual struggle, but it is better handled with team support. Laura Evans thought the same was true for cancer and believed that survival (literally or metaphorically) requires one small uphill step at a time. She was especially appreciative of the process, which in both cases allows a person to find out what his or her ultimate values are, and to develop a greater sense of self and self-worth.

There are also some laypeople, patients, and even physicians who believe that a patient's attitude affects his or her ultimate outcome.

Dr. Ernest Rosenbaum and his wife and professional colleague Isadora wrote: "We have often seen how two patients of similar age with the same diagnosis . . . can experience vastly different results . . . The answer seems to lie in their attitude."[11] These views, whether or not substantiated by scientific inquiry, have great appeal because they offer patients some control over their disease. Unfortunately, this empowerment can lead to feelings of guilt or personal failure when, despite the patient's best efforts, the cancer recurs.

Some, learning that genetics and environment are important in cancer causation, develop a fatalistic approach. If one has a genetic predisposition, it is believed that all is predetermined and unalterable, while if one gets a tumor without the appropriate genetic background then this is attributable to improper or irresponsible behavior. Both of these views of cancer are formidable, inevitable, and unforgiving.

Biostatisticians can offer a more aloof and pessimistic view. Requiring rigorous evidence for the reduction of cancer deaths before accepting the value of any prevention or treatment method provides a negative bias intended to limit the likelihood of accepting as useful a management method that, in reality, has no value. Unfortunately, this strategy allows, as a necessary consequence, the possibility of missing a real advance. The acceptance of the "null hypothesis" until it is formally disproved is a valid scientific method; however, when presented to the general public and often to health professionals, it can result in the perception that the unproved intervention is without value, rather than that the data provided are not sufficient to reject the null hypothesis. Such a result might be due to inadequate numbers of patients being studied, inadequate observation time, or the fact that the intervention truly is of no value in increasing survival.

Also often ignored in determinations of improvement in cancer care are those therapies that are not associated with any improvement in survival. These include improved treatments that allow the patient better functional and cosmetic results, as well as those treatments that provide better palliation. Examples of advances that do not improve survival include treatments for breast cancer that do not require removal of the breast, those that avoid amputations for tumors of the extremities, and prostate cancer therapies that offer tumor control without the loss of urinary continence or sexual potency. Appropriate cancer management goals aim not only to prevent cancer-related death but also to do so with the least possible morbidity or functional impairment.

Improving Cancer Management

In order to develop an understanding of cancer that considers this disease from as broad a perspective as possible, we should first consider what is known about cancer today. It is clear that while the disease is the result of genetic changes—both inherited and acquired during life—these changes might be required, but they are not always sufficient to produce cancer. Even for those cancers where the hereditary predisposition is great, it is just that—a proclivity that is not always expressed.

Similarly, environmental factors can influence the likelihood of cancer. In the early days of the correlation of smoking with lung cancer there was great confusion about the association. Those who doubted the etiologic importance of tobacco for lung cancer would state that since not all smokers developed the disease and not all lung cancer patients had a history of smoking, tobacco smoking could not be a cause of lung cancer. Nothing could be further from the truth. Smoking increases the likelihood of developing a lung cancer, but is neither determinative of the disease always occurring, nor is it necessarily present in all cases. Smoking is important as a causative agent because it greatly increases the incidence of the disease. This is likely to be true of most environmental agents associated with cancer. We also know that early detection of cancer profoundly affects the likelihood of cure. This is clearly demonstrated by the value of mammography for breast cancer, Pap smears for cervical cancer, and now determination of prostate-specific antigen level for prostate cancer.

While the image of cancer is as a relentless and inexorable disease, the truth is that the majority of cancer patients are cured.[12] Cancer is more properly considered as a group of diseases for which cure is related to the site of origin, the cell type, the stage of the disease and the treatment administered. Most tumors in most sites are curable in early stages. Some are curable even in advanced stages, but unfortunately some, although appearing to be in early stage, are not curable.

What about our current forms of treatment? Surgery is still responsible for most cancer cures, and the Halsted method best illustrates this. While a phase of bigger operations based on the contiguous spread thesis was observed, we are now applying more function-preserving surgery and using these limited procedures combined with other treatment modalities. Similarly, radiation therapy has become far more precise, with great efforts directed at limiting the high-dose volume to the involved areas and the use of technical innovations to reduce the radiation received by normal tissues. Cancer medicines have become more effective and their side effects are often preventable or, if not, at least they are treatable. While any of these three therapeutic modalities can be used alone as curative treatment, effective cancer management often combines treatment modalities.

The "magic bullet" is something worth striving for, but the lesson of these recent years is that the reduction in cancer deaths is the result of incremental improvement in treatment delivery and better diagnostic techniques. The improvement in diagnosing and determining tumor extent has been remarkable. We can image tumors with MRI and determine their physiology with positron emission tomography. Blood tests are being developed to screen for particular tumors using biochemical markers, such as elevated prostate-specific antigen levels to identify men who have an increased likelihood of having prostate cancer. It is possible to reduce the toxicity of treatments by using methods such as minimally invasive surgery, intensity-modulated radiation therapy, and by using agents that counteract the nausea and vomiting associated with some procedures. In addition, new classes of treatment are becoming more available; these include antibodies such as those now used in the management of lymphomas, better hormonal treatments such as those currently available for the treatment of breast cancer and prostate cancer, and improved ways of delivering externally applied focused energy within the body.[13]

Susan Sontag states, "As long as a particular disease is treated as an evil, invincible predator, not just a disease, most people with cancer will indeed be demoralized by learning what disease they have. The solution is hardly to stop telling cancer patients the truth but to rectify the conception of the disease, to de-mythicize it."[1] We must also recognize the importance of context for the health professional considering the disease. Medical dogma and paradigm are just that, but they are not necessarily true. For meaningful dialogue to exist, both within and between the various constituencies, our cultural understanding should be consistent with our medical understanding. Dogma, magical thinking, and myth must be recognized for what they are, and for what mischief can result from their acceptance. We must see cancer in its entirety rather than be like the blind men reacting to portions of the elephant, resulting in distorted impressions of the whole animal.

REFERENCES

1. Sontag S (1990) *Illness as Metaphor and AIDS and Its Metaphors.* New York: Picador, Farrar Straus and Giroux.
2. Solzhenitsyn A (1969) *The Cancer Ward.* New York: Farrar Straus and Giroux
3. Auden WH (1940) *Collected Poems by WH Auden* (Ed. Mendelson E). New York: Random House.
4. Halsted WS (1907) The results of radical operations for cure of carcinoma of the breast. *Ann Surg* 46: 1–19.
5. Haagensen CD (1986) *Diseases of the Breast*, edn 3. Philadelphia: WB Saunders.
6. McWhirter R (1955) Simple mastectomy and radiotherapy in treatment of breast cancer. *Br J Radiol* 28: 128–139.
7. Keynes G (1954) Carcinoma of the breast, the unorthodox view. *Proc Cardiff Med Soc* 40.
8. Fitzwilliams DCL (1940) A plea for a more local operation in really early breast cancer. *BMJ* 2: 405–408.
9. Hellman S (1993) Dogma and inquisition in medicine. *Cancer* 71: 2430–2433.
10. Hellman S (1994) Karnofsky Memorial Lecture. Natural history of small breast cancers. *J Clin Oncol* 12: 2229–2234.

11. Rosenbaum EH and Rosenbaum I (1998). *Cancer Supportive Care*. Toronto: Somerville House.
12. Jemal A et al. (2005) Cancer statistics 2005. *CA Cancer J Clin* 55: 10-30.
13. Jolesz FA and Hynynen KH (2005) Focused ultrasound in cancer. In *Principles and Practice of Oncology*, edn 7, 2883-2890 (Eds. DeVita VT et al.) Philadelphia: Lippincott Williams and Wilkins.

ONCOLOGISTS AND THEIR PATIENTS

(2016 unpublished)

> *The good physician knows his patients through and through, and his knowledge is bought dearly. Time, sympathy, and understanding must be lavishly dispensed, but the reward is to be found in that personal bond which forms the greatest satisfaction of the practice of medicine. One of the essential qualities of the clinician is interest in humanity, for the secret of the care of the patient is in caring for the patient.*

This quotation from Francis Weld Peabody speaking to Harvard Medical School students in 1925 is often quoted primarily for the last phrase, "for the secret of the care of the patient is in caring for the patient." Despite the many changes in medicine, this is as true today as it was then. Dr. Peabody was the founding director of the Thorndike Laboratory at the Boston City Hospital, a laboratory devoted to research, teaching, and intensive study of patients at that hospital. This was the beginning of the Harvard Medical School Department of Medicine at that hospital, which served from 1921 until 1974, when the unit closed and Harvard left that hospital.

I begin this essay with these words because I find them to be aspirational for proper behavior of all physicians and surely those caring for cancer patients. During my tenure as part of the team of health care providers caring for cancer patients, I found a number of different patterns used by good doctors trying to follow Dr. Peabody while dealing with this serious illness, which can cause an emotional rollercoaster in the health provider as well as the patient. Often the initial doctor, whether a surgeon, radiation oncologist, or medical oncologist, tries to emphasize the positive outcome that is possible while also describing the less satisfactory alternatives. This not only helps alleviate patient anxiety, but also helps the doctor deal with his or her own emotional response. How much to do this is part of the art of medicine. For me a glass is half full rather than half empty—optimistic while not being unrealistic. Sometimes this is overdone, as much for the doctor as for the patient. My son-in-law

Derek frequently comments that "the Nile [denial] is not just a river in Egypt." Alternatively, some doctors, rather than confront their emotional response, withdraw from engaging with the patient, to the detriment of the doctor–patient relationship. In 1965 when I was a regular visitor at the ward rounds at the Royal Marsden Hospital in the United Kingdom, I noted that rarely was the patient fully apprised of the nature of the illness, nor honestly of the prognosis. I was chided for having the American view of telling a cancer patient his or her diagnosis because of the emotional toll on the patient. I believe that the patients often knew they had cancer, but perceived the prognosis to be more ominous than it was. They participated in the charade in order to not upset the doctor. Earlier, as a young intern in the United States, I remember well being instructed by family members not to tell their mother of her diagnosis, only later to be told by the patient that she knew she had cancer but that I should not tell her family since it would be too difficult for them to deal with. Denial can be useful in many situations, but this kind of subterfuge is rarely helpful. Jay Katz in *The Silent World of Doctor and Patient* describes Tolstoy's Ivan Ilych as complaining that the refusal for the doctor to admit to the patient that he is dying denies Ilych the compassion, sympathy, and comforting that he much desires. The skill is to be honest but to emphasize what can be done and to assure continuity and concern for the patient by the team. We will be with her! Unfortunately, sometimes in the fractionated health care system in the United States this cannot be assured. Dealing with the end of life is a test, but a necessary part of oncologists' and most physicians' responsibility as "caring doctors." Concern with pain and other palliative care, as well as with the many fears of the patient, can be of great benefit.

All too often, the patient, when apprised of the diagnosis, considers it a death sentence. Sometimes it is, but it is well for both patient and doctor to be reminded that cancer is the most curable of the serious chronic diseases. More than half of cancer patients are cured. That is not true for coronary artery disease, diabetes, stroke, multiple sclerosis, Lou Gehrig's disease, rheumatoid arthritis, and most other serious chronic diseases. If the patient is likely to be cured, this needs to be emphasized. Cancer comprises a great variety of illnesses with different prognoses depending on the type, stage, and other circumstances. Slowly progressive disease, even when not curable, frequently can be controlled or modified, and this part of prognosis is very important to be understood.

New oncologists, be they in medical, radiation, or surgical disciplines, usually begin their training—not the best word, but what is usually used rather than "education" to emphasize the learning of the craft and art of medicine—seeing all types of patients, not just those with malignant disease. They can be helped in this transition to have some more explicit guidance as to their new role and responsibilities. While these exhortations can be expressed to many types of physicians, for me they have particular resonance in oncology.

What does the doctor offer to the cancer patient? First, he or she offers expertise in oncology in general and in the specific subtype in particular. This will be acquired during this training period so that there is a hierarchy of knowledge increasing with clinical experience. But the art of medicine is in what Peabody refers to as caring for the patient. This separation of knowledge and its application to an individual patient is essential to doctoring, especially in dealing with serious illness. I have discussed this dichotomy earlier in this book in the essay from which the volume gets its title. Knowledge may be gained in general, but to be applied to the particular patient it must be modified by considering the individual circumstances, preferences, and values.

The new oncologist should be reminded of the nature of the doctor–patient relationship. The doctor must be loyal to the obligations as a physician, and must be loyal to the patient, assuring the patient that the primary responsibility is to him or her unless explicitly limited by law. Truthfulness is essential, or the relationship founders.

The doctor must be comforting in manner, assuring his or her interest in the patient. One must be concerned with attempting to cure the patient, but also and sometimes only with ameliorating the symptoms caused by the disease. Sometimes the attempt to cure is associated with significant morbidity, even so great as to make the patient question whether the attempt to treat is worth the effort. This individual discussion requires much of the doctor in guiding and advising, but never making this decision instead of the patient. The patient needs the doctor's best judgment of the prognosis, as well as the urgency or lack thereof of a treatment decision, but must allow sufficient time for the patient to fully understand the disease and the treatment options. Too often today, young doctors present facts and alternative treatment options without a recommendation as to which they recommend. This is not enough. In trying to avoid undesired paternalism, this denies what the patient most desires. The patient wants and should receive the doctor's guidance. When this is not offered, the patient often asks something like, "what would you do if you were me." These discussions need to be realistic, while emphasizing the positives that can be achieved; for example, when cure is not possible, then the emphasis can be on the plan for palliation and the continuing involvement of the health care team extending when appropriate to terminal care. Clear delineation of the responsibilities of each of the team members is very important. The role of the doctor, as well as that of other doctors and other health care professionals, needs to be explicated and often reiterated. Cancer care is very much a team endeavor. The patient should always understand who is in charge and whom to call at each stage.

We oncologists learn much from our patients. Their views of the disease comes from a different vantage point with a different knowledge base and with much greater emotional intensity. The doctor would do well to read some of what the more articulate patients have written. Here are a few titles of books so revealing of breast cancer patients' feelings: *Why Me?*; *The Climb of My Life*; *First You Cry*. I have been fortunate—while never being involved with their care—to have known and considered both Rose Kushner (*Why Me?*) and Laura Evans (*The Climb of My Life*) to be my friends. Rose was very much a part of the feminist movement in her efforts to change the way breast cancer was treated, and to take the decision-making about this treatment from paternalistic, primarily male physicians—usually surgeons—and give it to the patient. In the book's revised edition she tells of her own diagnosis of breast cancer in June 1974. The first edition was published in September 1975, titled *Breast Cancer*, but she was told that this put people off from buying it or even carrying it with the title exposed—another example of the power of the term "cancer" evincing such a negative image, as discussed in the previous essay. The new title, *Why Me?*, appears on the 1977 revision. I much prefer it because it states the initial emotional reaction of most cancer patients. The book was meant as a guide to other women facing the diagnosis of breast cancer, as well as a cautionary tale of what she calls the male chauvinism of surgeons dominating the decision-making and treatment of newly diagnosed breast cancer patients. Later she and I were on a National Cancer Institute panel discussing the management of breast cancer, specifically, whether removal of the tumor in the breast—lumpectomy—followed by radiation therapy was a satisfactory alternative to mastectomy. She was quite outspoken and articulate as to the demeaning attitude of the surgeons to their female patients. As an aside, when one of the surgeons on the panel was interviewed on a national network news program, he said something like this: "women are like children who if you offer them milk or candy they will always take the candy even though milk is much better for them." That surely is a demeaning paternalistic description, reflecting a view of many leading cancer surgeons of that time. An unfortunate footnote to this discussion is my perception of a current return to mastectomy in some women with early stage breast cancer. In part, this must be due to the unrealistic fear associated with cancer at any stage and of any kind. In the case of small, usually mammographically discovered breast cancer, the cure likelihood is 90% with either mastectomy or breast-preserving lumpectomy and radiation. Sometimes even bilateral mastectomies are done when there is no known tumor in the opposite breast. When this is done in patients without clear evidence of a genetic predisposition or very strong family history of ovarian cancer, premenopausal breast cancer, or other uncommon indicators of excessive risk of bilateral breast cancer, this is unnecessary surgery. The cancer metaphor discussed in the preceding essay does a disservice to these patients.

Laura Evans published *The Climb of My Life* in 1996. At that time she was a skiwear designer and an avid outdoors person with a particular penchant for mountaineering. She describes finding her cancer in August 1989 and the stages of dealing with the disease diagnosis, treatment, and recovery by comparing it to climbing a mountain. Later she formed Expedition

Inspiration, which created a series of expeditions attempting to climb some of the highest mountains in many continents. She, sometimes with other breast cancer survivors on Expedition Inspiration, organized climbs to the summits that were to be reached only by these breast cancer survivors. These remarkable expeditions included climbs to Mount Rainier summit, the 16,500-foot base camp to Mount Kangchenjunga in Nepal, the summit of Mount Kilimanjaro in Kenya, Mount Elbrus in Russia, and Mount Aconcagua, the highest mountain in the Southern and Western Hemispheres. In both climbing a mountain and dealing with breast cancer, Laura Evans felt that patients faced their deepest fears. Analogously, mountaineering is an individual struggle, but it is better handled with team support. She believed that, like climbing, the experiences required of a cancer patient offered the patient a greater sense of self and self-worth.

The book has some significant literary analogies, as the chapters intersperse her breast cancer experiences with those of climbing, beginning most chapters with a quotation. A few examples: the chapter concerning the diagnosis begins, "Yesterday is already a dream, and tomorrow is only a vision" from the Sanskrit; for the chapter on side effects, from Emerson, "What lies behind us and what lies before us are tiny matters compared to what lies within in us"; the chapter on achieving the summit of Aconcagua begins with Thoreau, "If you have built castles in air, your work need not be lost: that is where they should be. Now put foundations under them." Both Kushner and Evans were extremely strong, articulate people, but I believe they convey the sentiments of many cancer patients. From these eloquent women, there is much for doctors to learn.

Frequently patients look to not completely rational techniques in dealing with the cancer doctor. A patient of mine regularly delivered a bottle of Scotch whisky to my door on the anniversary of his cancer treatment until he completed 5 years. He believed that 5 years without recurrence was tantamount to cure, so no more Scotch was needed. A distinguished college professor wrote me recently on her holiday greetings that she was referred to me by a distinguished biostatistician who stated, "Go to Hellman—his patients don't die." Would that this were so. I mention both of these as examples of looking for non-rational methods of increasing survival chances. Even the rational can and do act irrationally. Doctors need to appreciate this and watch, speak and listen to patients very carefully to be sure to understand what is really on the patient's mind.

In preparing this essay, I found an especially meaningful association. Apparently Hermann Blumgart was an early resident physician appointed by Peabody at the Thorndike. As I have mentioned in the Preface, Dr. Blumgart was the chairman of medicine at Beth Israel Hospital during my internship and a role model to many of us as to how to interact with a patient. He mixed knowledge with compassion and honesty with reassurance. So I come back full circle to Peabody, who states, "The treatment of a disease must be completely impersonal; the treatment of a patient must be completely personal."

5

Heroes

COMMENTARY

Perhaps I am too old for having heroes, but I do. By what criteria do adults decide who should be considered heroes? Conventionally, courage (especially in war) is one, as is a famous discovery, be that of new lands or new medicines. Inventors are also good hero material. In many fields these heroes are recognized with medals and prizes. Mine are quite different: one a male doctor whose name is familiar but otherwise is little known, and the other probably the most famous woman scientist ever. Marie Curie meets these conventional requirements for her identifying and purifying radium and polonium as the first known radioactive elements; but equally important in my estimation were her World War I contributions in mobilizing portable battlefield X-ray stations, her efforts to provide radium as the first nonsurgical successful cancer treatment, and finally her position as a feminist. Thomas Hodgkin was quite different. He was a considerable medical personage, but he was much more than that because of his strength of character and his demonstration of the best of what a physician engaged in issues of his time should espouse and perform. Both were important figures more than a century ago. Thomas Hodgkin was born in 1798 and died in 1866. I was first introduced to Dr. Hodgkin because of his eponymous disease. He was one of "the great men of Guy's": four physicians associated with Guy's Hospital in London, all of whom have something in medicine named after them: Thomas

Addison, Richard Bright, and Hodgkin had diseases named after them, and Sir Astley Cooper's name is associated with two ligaments. It seems to me that at least in Hodgkin's case this recognition was the least of his accomplishments, and it is for those other actions that he is my medical hero. Some of these activities are described in the following article, first published in the *Journal of the American Medical Association*. This essay uses Hodgkin's disease as the name for the disease as was appropriate for the time of its publication, but I use Hodgkin lymphoma in my recent writings included in this book since this appears to me to be the current preferred usage.

During his year in Paris, Hodgkin met many of the important intellectual figures of his time, not only within medicine but even more interesting, considering his protean interests, those important intellectual leaders of the day. Perhaps most important to him was Alexander von Humboldt, that great naturalist and discoverer, whom Hodgkin described as the "hero of my youth." As I mentioned in the Commentary to Chapter 2, Humboldt knew and influenced an astounding variety of contemporaries such as Jefferson, Madison, Bolivar, Goethe, and Schiller. Hodgkin was very much a person of his time, born at the end of the Age of Enlightenment, but very much a medical and public health leader of that age in medicine. He was truly a man for all seasons, who acted on the dictates of his moral compass on medical, national, and international venues. He met and interacted with many important personages in medicine, in both Europe and the Middle East. It was in his latter trips with Moses Montefiore that he acted as a citizen of Great Britain who had a moral commitment to the people of the colonial empire. He is the epitome of a moral and committed physician at its best.

Maria Sklodowska Curie, or "Madame Curie" as she was more popularly known, was famous for her scientific accomplishments but was reviled by some of the lay press for her personal behavior. Her scientific accomplishments were of extreme importance to physics and chemistry, as exemplified by her winning Nobel Prizes in each field. She was also important in medicine and could well have a third Nobel in this field. She was an early and committed feminist, actively involved in the movement, primarily in science. She was also a victim of discrimination and prejudice as a woman and an immigrant, and of anti-Semitism although she was not Jewish. All these condemnations came to a head when her romantic affair with a former student of her deceased husband, Paul Langevin, became known in the fall of 1910. Immediately before this she had been denied a place in the French Academy primarily because she was a woman. At the time of the exposure of the affair, she was awarded her second Nobel Prize. The affair caused great criticism of Marie even more than of Paul although he, not she, had committed adultery. There was even great pressure on her to not attend or not be invited to receive the Prize. This is discussed extensively in a 1995 biography by Susan Quinn that appeared after my article, the second essay in this chapter.

Madame Curie continued to expand her laboratory and expound on the medical use of radium, primarily in the treatment of cancer of the uterine cervix. This work continues as the Institut Curie, a cancer research and treatment organization emphasizing the use of radiation in cancer treatment. These efforts, as well as her pioneering in the use of X-rays in the war zone during World War I, and her campaigning for philanthropic funds in order to obtain radium for medical use, are discussed in my essay. This essay also considers the contributions of her daughter Irene and her husband Frédéric Joliot-Curie. Also in that article is a discussion of the cultural attitudes toward radioactivity and radium as a cautionary tale for modern biology. The final essay in this chapter discusses the similarity of the discovery and enthusiastic early use of radium with the development of new forms of targeted anti-cancer agents. Too much enthusiasm and hyperbole can, if not fully realized, result in disillusionment.

Two heroes out of many potential candidates may seem arbitrary, but not to me. They stand well above their peers not only for their scientific accomplishments, but also for their strength of character and will. They worked diligently in actually participating in the care of the sick and injured and in providing for the general well-being of their fellow humans.

THOMAS HODGKIN AND HODGKIN'S DISEASE. TWO PARADIGMS APPROPRIATE TO MEDICINE TODAY

Reproduced with permission from the *Journal of the American Medical Association* 1991;265(8):1007–1010. Copyright © (1991) American Medical Association. All rights reserved.

Abstract

Thomas Hodgkin was an investigator whose contributions extended over a wide range of medicine. While he is known for Hodgkin's disease, this was not his major interest. That this is so has more to do with his successors than him. He had a highly committed social conscience and was outspoken in advocacy of his positions. This greatly limited his professional career. The history of Hodgkin's disease is one of hypothesis generation, which allowed for its effective treatment even without an understanding of its etiology, illustrating the approximate nature of scientific discovery and the importance of chance in historical attribution. Hodgkin, as a scientist, healer, and socially committed individual, embodied the many characteristics that are desirable for today's physician, while the evolution of knowledge about Hodgkin's disease and its treatment is an instructive model for future medical advances.

This is a view of a great man of medicine and of the disease that bears his name. As one considers the exemplary life of Thomas Hodgkin, one begins to reflect on the similarities to, differences from, and lessons for physicians today. There is much that is timely and pertinent, especially during these turbulent times in medicine. The definitive biography of Hodgkin has been written by Amalie and Edward Kass[1] and the story of the development of research and our understanding of Hodgkin's disease by Henry S. Kaplan.[2] The purpose of this article is to consider both Hodgkin and his eponymous disease as models for the scholarly physician engaged in the world in which he or she lives and for our understanding of how medical practice advances and the consequences of these advances. Hodgkin and Hodgkin's disease teach us about both.

Thomas Hodgkin

An abbreviated description of Hodgkin's biography begins with his birth in 1798 into a devout Quaker family. His early interests and career choices varied but seemed to be concentrated on applied science. He first began as an apothecary's apprentice, but in 1819 he began his medical training at Guy's Hospital in London, England. While he was allowed to participate in rounds at Guy's, he was not accepted as a medical student in England because he was not a member of the Church of England. He therefore went to medical school in Edinburgh, Scotland. This was followed by study in Paris, France, where he came in contact with the great René Laënnec, from whom he learned the use of the stethoscope. While there, he also met and was greatly influenced by Alexander von Humboldt, one of the prominent scientists, explorers, and early sociologists of his day. Hodgkin returned to Britain and described some of the auscultatory findings of valvular heart disease, extensively promoted the use of the stethoscope, and published a description[3] of aortic insufficiency 3 years before that of Sir Dominic Corrigan, to whom original credit is usually given. Following European travel with Moses Montefiore, with whom he had a lifelong friendship, he began his work at Guy's Hospital as the "Inspector of the Dead and Curator of the Museum."

Hodgkin stayed at Guy's Hospital from 1825 until 1837. It is in this brief 12 years that he made the contributions most associated with him, including development of the anatomical museum, development of the specialty of pathological anatomy, the description of Hodgkin's disease, and the first application to medical problems of the improved (achromatic) microscope of Joseph Jackson Lister (the father of the initiator of aseptic surgery). He wrote on medical education, temporary insanity, and public health.

His was a remarkable life, one to be admired at many levels. I believe it can serve as the paradigm for the dedicated physician-scientist. Hodgkin was a skillful physician and dedicated student; he learned the medicine of his time. He was recognized as one of the outstanding innovators at Guy's Hospital, along with Richard Bright, Sir Astley Cooper, and Thomas Addison, who were but a few of the leaders of medicine of that day with whom Hodgkin had close association. He was a scientist who made morphological observations of the dead and associated these with diseases in the living.[4] He practiced his medicine as a physician, both treating private patients and accepting responsibilities for working in a dispensary for the indigent. In developing a collection for the museum at Guy's Hospital and organizing pathological anatomy, he wrote an important book that was influential during his time.[5] Hodgkin was a great teacher. While his opportunities were limited by discrimination, he taught at both Guy's and the new medical school in St. Thomas Hospital. He wrote extensively for medical audiences and lectured on potential curricular changes, which he was influential in bringing to fruition.

Hodgkin's relationship to Guy's Hospital ended because of his nonmedical concerns about the social welfare of Eskimos and First Nations persons as affected by the fur trade of the Hudson Bay Company in Canada.[6] Hodgkin had written to Benjamin Harrison, the powerful secretary of Guy's and a member of the Hudson Bay Company, of these concerns and his advocacy of the social responsibility of the colonial powers. The rancor he incited in Harrison resulted in Harrison's disapproval of Hodgkin's application for a vacant position as assistant physician on the staff of Guy's Hospital. Following his failure to be accepted on the attending staff, he devoted his time to writing about his social and medical concerns, which included the plight of natives of all countries and how they were treated by Western civilization, slavery, discrimination, and medical reform. He was a major advocate of the development of Liberia as a place for former slaves from the new world to develop an independent nation. He made a number of journeys with Montefiore to Europe and the Middle East, the purpose of which was to identify and, if possible, correct discrimination and public health irregularities.[7,8] He died in 1866 in Jaffa, probably of cholera, while involved in efforts to improve the plight of Jews in that area.

His social concerns were also medical. His first book was written on health promotion;[9] it was concerned with disease prevention and sanitation. Health rather than illness was the emphasis, and it is this concern to which medicine is returning today. He was also concerned with the unequal distribution of medical care. He argued against medical contracts being given to the lowest bidder because he believed that business techniques were not applicable to medicine. He did not believe that the patient would obtain adequate care if the lowest price was the only criterion. He wondered whether price should be considered when determining a plan for health care. This problem is, of course, with us today as we consider methods of providing health care to ensure that it is distributed uniformly, universally, and that it is of adequate quality.

He was also concerned with the question of an individual's responsibility for his or her actions as evidenced by his involvement in the early considerations of "moral insanity" as a plea in court as a defense for one's actions. This involved his defending an attempted assassin of Queen Victoria and Prince Albert. Hodgkin's argument was that moral insanity could be possible in a person who was unable to distinguish right from wrong, even if he or she were not overtly insane.

Thus, we find Thomas Hodgkin a Renaissance physician of his time. He was a healer, teacher, scientist, innovator, great discoverer, as well as a concerned and committed human being—an exemplary role model for contemporary physicians.

Hodgkin's Disease

I should like to turn from a discussion of Thomas Hodgkin to a consideration of the history of the discovery and treatment of the disease that bears his name. Hodgkin's study,[10] published in 1832, is based on a pathological review of six of his patients and one who was described illustratively to him by a colleague, Robert Carswell. He modestly suggests that his discovery is not an entirely new finding, but that it must have been apparent to many other physicians practicing at the time. The original specimens are preserved in the museum created by Hodgkin, and recent studies indicate that three of the patients probably did have Hodgkin's disease. Considering that his observation was based purely on gross morphology, unaided by the microscope, this was a remarkable finding. He first presented these findings to the Medico-Chirugical Society of London in January 1832, but between this presentation and the formal publication, a colleague pointed out to him that Malpighi[11] had described a patient with such a condition in 1668. Hodgkin, in his typically deferential manner, not only refers to this in his article, but emphasizes that his own finding is not unique. The disease was then subsequently mentioned by Bright[12] and by Wilks,[13] who described the disease once again. Curiously, between the time of Wilks's writing what he thought to be an original insight and the final publication, he found an earlier reference by Bright indicating Hodgkin's description of the disease. In his classic article in 1865, Wilks gives the disease the eponymous name that it now bears.

The next important event has to do with the ability to further study the disease using the microscope. This was probably first described by Greenfield[14] in 1878, embellished on by Sternberg[15] in 1898, and finally most clearly described and illustrated by Reed[16] in 1902. It is for the latter two investigators that the multinucleated giant cell, considered pathognomonic for the disease, is named. Throughout its history, the disease has sometimes been thought to be infectious, sometimes malignant, and sometimes both. While it is clearly malignant, it is still unclear how important an infectious component of the disease might be. Epidemiologic studies suggest that socioeconomic conditions that limit early exposure to infectious agents may predispose persons to Hodgkin's disease later in life.[17] This suggests a pathogenesis similar to that seen with poliomyelitis, where early infection is usually asymptomatic but confers long-lasting immunity, while infection later in life may be associated with the devastating, paralytic disease. Infectious agents have been suggested, but no clear etiologic agent has been found. Hypotheses as to pathogenesis have also suggested mechanisms that explain the immune suppression of the disease as well as its malignant nature.[18-20] These hypotheses have suggested that there is an infectious agent to which there is an exuberant immune proliferative response that eventually gives rise to the emergence of the clone of malignant cells involved in the prolonged and protracted reaction. This malignancy has been thought to be of B-cell, T-cell, histiocytic, or other cell origin and only now, using monoclonal antibody techniques, is it being elucidated.

With the discovery of roentgen rays by Wilhelm Röntgen in 1895, early radiologists began to treat Hodgkin's disease with some success. The first report of disease remission was by Pusey[21] in 1902. Many observers suggested that the disease spread in a contiguous fashion, but the clearest exposition of this, as well as a technique for treatment based on this, was described by the Swiss radiologist Gilbert[22] in the 1930s. He believed that the disease spread in a contiguous fashion and therefore should be treated with large curative doses to the known disease, and treatment should be applied prophylactically to adjacent, seemingly noninvolved areas. His results were curative for many patients with localized Hodgkin's disease. These techniques were greatly expanded by Peters,[23,24] who based her treatment on this notion of pathogenesis and presented evidence for cure by reporting on patients who were followed up for 20 years. It is important to understand that the disease was the model of the chronically recurring incurable disease. Thus, the results from Toronto, Ontario, were disbelieved by many who were positive that with further follow-up, these patients would eventually succumb to the disease unless another morbid condition should intervene, a theme that many espouse concerning cancer in general. The long-term data of the Toronto group began to dispel this, as did an influential report by Easson and Russell[25] in 1963, provocatively and prophetically entitled "The Cure of Hodgkin's Disease." This was followed by the extensive and careful study of the Stanford Group, led by Kaplan and Rosenberg.[26] They presented clinical evidence of the distribution of lymph node involvement that documented the contiguous nature of the disease and developed therapeutic techniques using the modern linear accelerator, which treated all potentially involved areas with tumoricidal doses. Use of the linear accelerator was possible as a result of the new equipment that was able to deliver high doses of radiation to deep-seated structures without damaging the skin, something not available to Gilbert or Peters. It also required careful collimation of the radiation beam to limit the exposure to normal tissues. The target volumes were determined by careful tumor imaging by radiological means or by direct surgical observation.

These latter points deserve further comment. Kaplan was quick to appreciate the importance of radiological imaging in determining tumor location and greatly expanded the technique of lymphangiography to help determine tumor location in the retroperitoneal area. He recognized the difficulty in ascertaining whether the disease had involved the spleen, liver, or lymph nodes of the upper abdomen, and thus the Stanford Group embarked on systematic laparotomy, splenectomy, and celiac lymph node and liver biopsy in order to elucidate the locations of the disease. They then fashioned therapeutic prescriptions based on this information. This radical approach of targeted treatment after extensive tumor localizing procedures was new to the treatment of what was thought to be a universally fatal, disseminated malignancy. It has proved a model for the careful staging of cancer as a required prerequisite to the design of therapy, which is a hallmark of oncological practice today. Finally, a new therapeutic modality became available: multidrug chemotherapy. DeVita and his colleagues[27] at the National Cancer Institute began a protocol for patients with advanced, previously incurable Hodgkin's disease using four drugs together, which were known to be effective in treatment of the disease when used individually, in an aggressive curative approach. This approach had not been previously used in cancer chemotherapy of solid tumors because of the strongly held belief that, while drugs were useful for the symptomatic relief of this seemingly inexorably fatal disease, they should be used sequentially and only in low doses so as to maximize their effectiveness. It was accepted that they offered no hope for cure. This revolutionary curative approach transformed the treatment of the disease.

I believe there are several lessons to be learned in the history of the description, understanding, and treatment of Hodgkin's disease. First, we should learn something about the nature of scientific precedent. Who was it who first described the disease? Probably Malpighi. Hodgkin gets most of the credit, despite his mentioning Malpighi's early observation, because Wilks named the disease "Hodgkin's disease," thus emphasizing the importance of Hodgkin's contribution. Whether this was a generous or necessary assignment by Wilks is described in an interesting article by Nuland[28] that is primarily concerned with the prevalence of the notion of contiguity. In any case, it suggests that it is difficult to assign full credit for scientific discovery to any single individual. That scientific discovery is a continuum is noted in the description of the disease, its pathogenesis, as well as the acceptance of the cell thought to be pathognomonic of the disease. Greenfield[14] described the multinucleated giant cell, and Hodgkin identified the contiguity of the disease. Nevertheless, the cell is known as the Reed-Sternberg cell, and contiguity is usually attributed to Kaplan or Gilbert. This attribution of discovery suggests that the time must be right for acceptance of a new conclusion. Malpighi was first, but there was not a sufficient body of observation, so that there was no further discovery until Hodgkin, Bright, and Wilks. Historical credit may be an accident, generosity, or persistence.

A second lesson to be learned from the history of Hodgkin's disease is that truth in scientific discovery is of an approximate nature, for only three of his six patients actually had Hodgkin's disease. It is interesting to observe that effective treatment of Hodgkin's disease is available without our understanding the etiology of the disease. This is important to consider in this day of extensive fundamental research in medicine. Much can be done by careful observation and pragmatic therapeutic experimentation, even without the advantage of understanding the disease's etiology. What may be necessary is an adequate hypothesis on which to base treatment. In this case, the most important hypothesis was that the disease was curable and not inexorably fatal. That previous hypothesis was, of course, a self-fulfilling prophecy that led to low doses of radiation or, later, single-agent chemotherapeutic treatment applied sequentially. Both of these strategies were based on the notion that the patient should be treated gently and that the limited normal tissue tolerance should be saved because the disease was hopelessly incurable. The goals of such treatment were comfort rather than cure. Most important, then, was acceptance of the hypothesis that the disease was curable. Second, a new model or, more properly, the acceptance of an older paradigm of the disease was required, i.e., that the disease was localized and that it spread in a predictably contiguous fashion. The next important hypothesis was that by using multiple drugs, one could overcome resistance of cells to any single drug. If one could use drugs in adequate doses without overlapping toxic effects, then the cells resistant to any single drug should fall prey to other drugs in the mixture to which they might be sensitive. This hypothesis has been vital to the curative treatment of cancer by chemotherapeutic agents. It was first described in the treatment of childhood leukemia and quickly applied to Hodgkin's disease. Another lesson to be learned in studying this disease is the importance of technological advance. Radiation therapy was limited until linear accelerators became available, and marked improvement in curability rapidly followed the use of this technical advance. Similar technological advances resulted in improved tumor localization and most recently in the development of new cancer chemotherapeutic agents.

Despite the success in the treatment of Hodgkin's disease, this treatment is not always successful and has far more morbidity than we would like there to be. All too often this is the nature of medical treatment. The "Magic Bullet" of Ehrlich is not often at hand, but rather effective toxic therapy has a real place in medicine. We should learn from the history of treating Hodgkin's disease that when we have such a moderately effective but morbidity-producing treatment, we should be amenable to change as we better learn how to use these treatments or develop new ones. The evolution of therapy has been characterized by many modifications after the large innovation was made that further improved the treatment. Physicians must be prepared to change their techniques easily and quickly without excessive dogmatic adherence to previous approaches. Adequate treatment requires a careful understanding of current medical developments, and there are many problems determining what is the best treatment currently available. Should one's emphasis be on maximizing cure or minimizing complications? These risk versus gain discussions are complicated and have important theoretic and practical consequences in medicine. The current treatments are expensive, perhaps far more expensive than simple definitive treatments might be, yet despite this, they are clearly of value. A disease that was curable perhaps 10% or 15% of the time 30 years ago is now being cured 75% or 80% of the time.

With these cures, we begin to see the undesirable long-term consequences of such treatment: iatrogenically induced leukemia, cardiovascular disease, sterility, growth arrest, and many other consequences that may follow such toxic treatment and must now be studied and treated in these "cured" patients. Treatment techniques must be modified as much as possible to reduce these complications while preserving therapeutic efficacy.

Today's Physicians

The role of the physician today is being reconsidered within and outside the profession, and science is emerging as a dominant factor, with scientific method a requirement for medical discovery and scientific training essential for the scholarly physician. The physician is considered an applied scientist from whom great technical assistance is expected. While Hodgkin was such a scientist, he was also a great deal more; the ethical responsibilities of the profession find expression in his life and work. Not only did he hold moral convictions, he acted on them and accepted the consequences of these actions.

We live in a multifaceted world, and our concerns should be wide-ranging, including advances in science, the provision of health care, and the important societal issues of today. Hodgkin considered these all to be his concerns, and they formed a continuum of behavior that defined him as a person. Similarly, the physician today should continue in the roles of scientist, healer, and humanist. He or she must understand and interpret science for the public and apply this to the art of medicine to heal and, if possible, to prevent disease. However, this is not the end of our charge. Because of the exposure to evolving scientific discovery, as well as the essentials of the human condition as seen in clinical practice, the physician must combine intellectual strength with moral leadership. The perception that the physician is concerned primarily with the scientific and the material may explain some of the public's current disaffection with the profession. Hodgkin should serve as a paradigm to emulate if we are to restore the physician to the appropriate societal role.

REFERENCES

1. Kass A, Kass E. *Perfecting the World: The Life and Times of Thomas Hodgkin (1798–1866)*. New York, N.Y.: Harcourt Brace Jovanovich Publishers; 1988.
2. Kaplan HS. *Hodgkin's Disease*. 2nd ed. Cambridge, MA: Harvard University Press; 1980.
3. Hodgkin T. On the retroversion of the valves of the aorta. *London Med Gaz.* 1829;3:433–442.
4. Hodgkin T. On the object of post-mortem examinations. *London Med Gaz.* 1828;2:423–431.
5. Hodgkin T. *A Catalogue of the Preparations of the Anatomical Museum of Guy's Hospital*. London, England: R Watts; 1829.
6. Kass EH, Carey AB, Kass AM. Thomas Hodgkin and Benjamin Harrison: crises and promotion in academia. *Med Hist.* 1980;24:197–208.
7. Rosenblum J. An interesting friendship—Thomas Hodgkin, M.D., and Sir Moses Montefiore Bart. *Ann Med Hist.* 1921;3:381–386.
8. Sakula S. Dr. Thomas Hodgkin and Sir Moses Montefiore Bart—the friendship of two remarkable men. *J R Soc Med.* 1979;72:382–387.
9. Hodgkin T. *Promoting and Preserving Health*. London, England: Cornhill Darton & Harvey Highley Fry; 1835.
10. Hodgkin T. On some morbid experiences of the absorbent glands and spleen. *Medico-Chirurgical Trans.* 1832;17:68–97.
11. Malpighi M. De Viscerum Structura Exexcitato Anatomica Bononiae. *J Montij.* 125–156. Translated in: *Ann Med Hist.* 1925;7:245–263.
12. Bright R. Observations on abdominal tumors and intumescence, illustrated by cases of disease of the spleen. *Guy's Hosp Rep.* 1938;3:401–409.
13. Wilks S. Cases of enlargement of the lymphatic glands and spleen (or Hodgkin's disease), with remarks. *Guy's Hosp Rep.* 1865;11:56–67.
14. Greenfield WS. Specimens illustrative of the pathology of lymphodenoma and leukocythemia. *Trans Path Soc Lond.* 1878;29:272–304.
15. Sternberg C. Ueber eine eigenartige unter dem Bilde der Pseudoleukaemie verlaufende Tuberculose des lymphatischen Apparates. *Ztschr Heilk.* 1898;19:21–92.
16. Reed D. On the pathological changes in Hodgkin's disease: with especial reference to its relation to tuberculosis. *Johns Hopkins Hosp Rep.* 1902; 10:133–196.
17. Gutensohn N, Cole P. Childhood social environment and Hodgkin's disease. *N Engl J Med.* 1981;304:135–140.
18. Kaplan HS, Smithers DW. Autoimmunity in man and homologous disease in mice in relation to the malignant lymphomas. *Lancet.* 1959;2:1–4.
19. Order SE, Hellman S. Pathogenesis of Hodgkin's disease. *Lancet.* 1972;1:571–573.

20. DeVita VT. Lymphocyte reactivity in Hodgkin's disease: a lymphocyte civil war. *N Engl J Med.* 1973;289:801–802.
21. Pusey WA. Cases of sarcoma of Hodgkin's disease treated by exposure to x-rays. *JAMA.* 1902;28:166–169.
22. Gilbert R. Radiotherapy in Hodgkin's disease. *AJR Am J Roentgenol.* 1939;41:198–240.
23. Peters MV. A study of survivals in Hodgkin's disease treated radiologically. *AJR Am J Roentgenol.* 1950;63:299–311.
24. Peters MV. The place of irradiation in the control of Hodgkin's disease. In: *Proceedings of the Fourth National Cancer Conference.* Philadelphia, Pa.: JB Lippincott; 1960:571–584.
25. Easson EC, Russell MH. The cure of Hodgkin's disease. *BMJ.* 1963;1:1704–1707.
26. Kaplan HS, Rosenberg SA. The management of Hodgkin's disease. *Cancer.* 1975;36:796–803.
27. DeVita VT, Serpick A, Carbone PP. Combination chemotherapy in the treatment of Hodgkin's disease. *Ann Intern Med.* 1970;73:891–895.
28. Nuland SB. The lymphatic contiguity of Hodgkin's disease: a historical study. *Bull N Y Acad Med.* 1981;57:776–786.

CURIES, CURE, AND CULTURE

Copyright © 1992 Johns Hopkins University Press. This article was first published in *Perspectives in Biology and Medicine* 1992; 36(1):39–45. Reprinted with permission by Johns Hopkins University Press.

As we come close to the end of the first century following the discovery of radioactivity, it is interesting to reflect upon what can be learned from the story of this discovery, of the discoverers, and of its acceptance by society. It is difficult to exaggerate the profound effect of this finding of a new power and of the lionization of its discoverers. This great revelation, with its folk heroes, was accompanied by great expectations and, unfortunately, some subsequent disillusionment. Perhaps we can profit from the consideration of this experience as we enter a similar time of discovery and expectation about the results of the new biology.

My interest in the Curies and their discoveries is both professional and personal, stimulated by my medical specialty (radiation oncology) and by my admiration for a remarkable and dedicated individual, Maria Sklodowska Curie, and her family. There are three interesting and quite different biographies worth your attention: the French biography, *Une Femme Honorable,* by Françoise Giroud [1], which has been translated into English and retitled *Marie Curie—A Life* [2]; the highly personal and adulatory biography *Madame Curie* by Marie's daughter, Eve Curie [3]; and the most recent one, *Grand Obsession*, by Rosalynd Pflaum [4]. The latter is of special interest because it also includes biographical information on Irene Curie (Marie's other daughter) and her husband, Frédéric Joliot. Because Joliot was actively involved in and was the leader of the study of atomic energy and its application in France, this family story allows us to trace radioactivity from its discovery through some of its potential and realized societal applications.

One might ask whether this is appropriate for a medical journal. I believe that the answer is yes, since in almost every instance the purposes and consequences of the discovery of radioactivity, either intended or not, were primarily medical. It was the medical uses of radium that stimulated the hysteria for this "wonder drug," and the popularity of Madame Curie, in large measure, resulted from the therapeutic indications for radium use. Radioactivity brought to us the artificial radioactive isotopes so much a part of past and present medical research, clinical laboratory tests, and medical imaging, isotopes that are, for the radiation oncologist, essential weapons in the therapeutic armamentarium. The undesired consequences of radiation exposure were only realized later. Both Marie and Irene became martyrs to their discoveries, for they both died of the hematopoietic consequences of exposure to ionizing radiation. Today, of course, the untoward health consequences of exposure to radioactive substances are a feared sequel to the widespread use of atomic energy.

While most of the original benefits as well as the subsequently discovered complications of radioactivity and its uses are medical, the implications of the story are far greater. It reveals a great deal about society's response to discovery, new knowledge, and disillusionment. It also reveals a profound fear and antipathy to certain areas of scientific research thought to be tampering with essentials of nature, which, it is argued, one should better leave alone. This type of antiscience is embodied in the Frankenstein story, where the doctor, despite good intentions, is driven by ambition to experiment in forbidden areas, thus unleashing evil. A similar view is of concern today as we consider genetic engineering and other applications of the biological revolution. The story of the Curies and their discoveries is interesting history and can teach us much about other great discoveries and how they may be accepted by society.

Curies

Maria Sklodowska was born in 1867, in Warsaw, Poland, the fifth child of Vladislav and Bronislawa Sklodowski, who were impoverished members of the lesser nobility. Vladislav was a physics and mathematics professor. The death of Madame Sklodowska from tuberculosis when Marie was eleven was a great tragedy for the family, but it helped create a strong bond between the children and Professor Sklodowski as he sought to raise them. Marie's early life was characterized by strong filial devotion, as well as by close bonds to her siblings, and especially to her sister, Bronya. Because of their penurious situation it was not possible for both Bronya and Marie to be educated simultaneously. Marie convinced Bronya that she should go to Paris to study medicine while Marie worked as a governess to help support her. As soon as Bronya was able, she arranged for Marie to come to Paris and live with her while she helped support Marie. Marie studied both physics and chemistry, becoming the first woman to receive a master's and, eventually, a Ph.D. in France. She was dedicated, introverted, and humorless. Even by today's standards, her feminism was well declared and expressed.

Marie's marriage to Pierre appears to have been a grand romance. He was a dreamer with accomplishments in many fields and, perhaps, had true genius. He studied crystallography and was fascinated by symmetry in crystals and in all of nature. In this he was the physical science counterpart of his contemporary D'Arcy Thompson, whose studies of symmetry in biology were so important. Pierre Curie discovered piezoelectricity, the current produced in crystals when subject to pressure. This was the basis of the very sensitive electrometers so important to their early work. The Curies' marriage came to an abrupt end after only eleven years when Pierre was run over and killed in an accident involving a horse-drawn wagon.

During their period of scientific collaboration, the Curies discovered polonium and radium, and Marie suggested that the source of radioactivity was the atomic nucleus. They shared the Nobel Prize in 1904 with Becquerel, for their discovery of these radioactive elements and for his initial discovery of radioactivity. Marie eventually ascended to the chair previously occupied by her husband, and she continued her dedicated study of the chemistry of radium and accumulated the metal for medical use. She won her second Nobel Prize alone, this time in chemistry, for this work.

Marie was lionized at the time because it was already appreciated that radium could be used as a cancer therapy, not only for skin cancers, but by interstitial or intracavitary insertion for a variety of malignant tumors of the head and neck, breast, uterus, and uterine cervix. It was also used as a source of external radiation. In fact, Marie's appeals for funds for radium were successful for the most part because of these applications for use in women with cancer. These appeals included a tour of the United States, largely organized by American women, to raise money for the purchase of a gram of radium for medical use, primarily for the treatment of gynecologic and breast tumors.

During World War I, Marie spent much of her time organizing and actively participating in the development of diagnostic radiologic facilities for the wounded. She and her daughter Irene set up and taught physicians how to use these X-ray machines. Madame Curie, as she was known to all but her intimates, was slow to appreciate the harmful effects of radiation. Since she was a keen observer, one must assume that this was largely her reluctance to accept these unfortunate consequences, rather than failure of her observational insight. She suffered considerable damage to her hands and fingers from her contact with radioactive materials. At the age of fifty-four she required extensive surgery for cataracts, almost certainly brought on by her work, and, finally, she succumbed to the hematopoietic consequences of radiation exposure.

Irene was very much her mother's daughter. She, too, became educated in physics and chemistry and continued a career quite similar to her mother's. She married Frederick Joliot, and they worked together for a number of years, resulting in their joint discovery of artificial radioactivity, the production of new radioactive elements by the bombardment of stable isotopes with nuclear particles produced by the decay of polonium and radium. This resulted in their being awarded the Nobel Prize in 1935. Like her parents' work had, the Joliot-Curies' work separated somewhat. Irene was concerned primarily with the chemical determination and isolation of the radioactive products, while Frederick was concerned with radioactive decay, the energy released, and chain reactions. It is interesting to note that Frederick took the Curie name as his own after their marriage. While some have suggested that his motive in doing this was less than noble, at the least it indicates the strong influence and common purpose within the family.

In order to study atomic physics before the cyclotron was invented, radioactive materials were required as the source of both alpha particles and neutrons for the bombardment of other elements. When cyclotrons and Van de Graaff generators became available, Frédéric continued to work with these. However, it was radium and, perhaps more importantly, polonium, an almost pure alpha emitter, that allowed the study of radioactivity and led to the discovery of artificial radioactivity. Frédéric was not only a brilliant scientist but also an effective organizer, who appreciated early the potential use of controlled chain reactions for energy production. This was especially important in France where hydrocarbon-based fuel had to be imported. The postwar development of the peaceful use of atomic energy in France was led by Frédéric until he was relieved of this position because of his communist affiliations. Irene followed her mother in becoming a martyr to radioactivity, dying of leukemia. Frédéric died of liver failure ascribed by some to post-hepatitic cirrhosis, while others believed the cause of his hepatic failure to be the result of the chronic ingestion of polonium.

Cure

It is difficult to overemphasize the importance of the discovery of radium on the general public. The discovery of X-rays had fired the imagination of all; some people were sure that the new discovery could be used to see the naked body under clothes and, in general, to see what society had determined should be hidden. Radium followed the discovery of X-rays and was the first "wonder drug." Its cancer cures were visible and remarkable. It was thought to be a valued addition to health potions and tonics of all descriptions. It was widely accepted as an important constituent in a variety of over-the-counter medications used to invigorate the recipient. Radium baths were considered healthy and desirable. In the early 1970s, while attending an international cancer meeting, a large number of us stayed outside Florence (where the meeting was held), in the spa town of Montecatini. I remember well reading in the hotel brochure about the baths for which Montecatini was noted. The brochure emphasized that radium was present in these warm baths and was an important source of their medical benefit.

The hazards of radiation were only slowly appreciated, and the first recognition came with the cutaneous lesions seen by those original workers with the material. Pierre described skin changes in places where the radium was in close contact, but it was not until the radium dial painters' internal ingestion of radium that the dangers associated with radioactive isotopes were appreciated. The death of millionaire Eben Byers from radium toxicity prompted governmental consideration of the hazards of radium ingestion [5].

Encapsulated radium salts and radon seeds formed an essential part of cancer therapy in the 1920s through the 1940s. They were gradually replaced in the 1950s and 1960s by artificial radioactive isotopes. Teletherapy, using X-ray machines, was restricted by both the limited penetration of the radiation produced and by severe acute and late skin and soft tissue changes. As it became possible to increase the energy of the radiation, resulting in increased doses at depth and skin sparing, the therapeutic efficacy of this treatment improved. The most widely applied high-energy radiations were the gamma rays produced by ^{60}Co, an isotope produced as one of the products of the atomic age. While this has gradually been replaced by the linear accelerator, it was ^{60}Co that allowed modern radiation therapy to develop much of its therapeutic potential.

We take for granted the successful treatment of carcinomas of the oral cavity, oral pharynx, breast, and, especially, uterus and uterine cervix, but this was not the case before radium. What a medical revolution this produced! Not only were patients cured, but function and cosmesis were often preserved. Physicians from all over the world came to Paris to learn the techniques of Regaud and his disciple Coutard, both working at the Radium Institute founded by the Curies. They returned to their home countries to develop centers for radium therapy that became the foundation for many of the world's current cancer centers.

Culture

Marie Curie was a pioneer. Her feminism was expressed in achieving what previously had been done only by men. She was clear in asserting her position and rights and in assuring such opportunities to other women. She was friendly with Herta Ayrton, the well-known British physicist and activist for women's rights. Marie taught in a women's school to prepare women for careers in science.

The great enthusiasm for radium as a cure began to be reversed with the understanding of some of the hazards of radiation exposure; however, the greatest fear and repugnance came from the association of atomic energy with nuclear holocaust, both in the form of a bomb and as accidents at power plants (*The China Syndrome* and Chernobyl). This fear of radioactivity, in any form and for any purpose, is currently an almost visceral response, sometimes quite excessive for the individual use proposed or amount of material being considered. The fear of nuclear explosion, as well as the potential environmental hazards of radioactive products, has become the stuff of major political discussions. It is not the purpose of this essay to discuss atomic energy but rather to note the intensity of the feeling concerning all things radioactive and the extension of these views to the medical uses of radioactive materials.

What are we medically to learn from the initial enthusiastic acceptance and subsequent fear and rejection of the use of radioactivity? The first lesson is that great expectations can breed great disappointment, especially if the initial beneficial effects are exaggerated and occur significantly before the deleterious effects are appreciated. The price for having illusions is disillusionment. We should remain aware of this as we discuss the great promise of the current revolution in biology. If the application of new discoveries falls short of the initial promise, we run the risk of society being disillusioned and unable to appreciate the limited but important gains that are made.

This is a lesson that is being painfully relearned in the "war against cancer." Radiation therapy has made and continues to make significant progress in the treatment of cancer. While it is not the panacea originally hoped for, its uses are considerable. The advances in molecular biology offer promise of "designer drugs" specifically engineered to destroy or prevent cancer without damaging normal tissues. And the products of biological discovery have potential far beyond cancer and even beyond medical uses. While we may hope for such results, it is important to be cautious in our promises lest disillusionment mask what may be considerable gains. The cross-cultural effects of strongly felt apprehension and aversion are amazing. Physicians supposedly knowledgeable of the hazards of radioactive material may appear to have a great fear of its use, while they are much more accepting of the hazards of exposure to harmful chemicals such as anesthetic agents and of workplace exposure to pathogens. In fact, there is very little balancing of the relative risks of different kinds of hazards. Some are societally acceptable, while some clearly are not.

The most important lesson to be learned is from the Curies' dedication and perseverance to a mission. The goals of both altruism and ambition have served well as a stimulus for discovery and are seen in the life of the Curies. Scientific discovery has tremendous power to change the world. Our time, with the explosion of discoveries in molecular biology, has great similarity to those early heady days of radioactivity. Today, like the beginning of the century, new discoveries and their potential medical benefits are found on the front pages of the newspapers, and companies are being founded to exploit the potential therapeutic benefits of new discoveries. This happened with radium as well. However, the enthusiasm for radium led to overpromising and overuse and then, with the appreciation of the hazards, came disillusionment. The intended beneficial medical uses of the new biology also have accompanying societal concerns. We should learn from the Curies and the history of radioactivity how to balance these, and thus avoid both great expectations and their attendant potential for disillusionment.

REFERENCES

1. GIROUD, F. *Une Femme Honorable.* Paris: Librarie Arthene Fayard, 1981.
2. GIROUD, F. *Marie Curie—A Life,* translated by L. DAVIS. New York: Holmes and Meier, 1986.
3. CURIE, E. *Madame Curie,* translated by V. SHEEAN. Garden City: Doubleday, 1937.
4. PFLAUM, *Grand Obsession.* New York: Doubleday, 1989.
5. MACKLIS, R. M. Radithor and the Era of Mild Radium Therapy. *JAMA* 264:614–618, 1990.

THE FIRST CENTURY OF CANCER CHEMOTHERAPY

Reprinted with permission. © 1998 American Society of Clinical Oncology. All rights reserved.

Hellman, S. *Journal of Clinical Oncology* 1998;16(7):2295–2296.

Ehrlich promulgated the notion of a "magic bullet," a chemotherapy that would be effective against microorganisms while not affecting the host. In 1909, he synthesized arsphenamine for the treatment of syphilis to be such a magic bullet. Although it was hoped to be specific for the spirochete, it was neither very effective nor very specific. The American Heritage Dictionary defines chemotherapy as "(1) the treatment of cancer using specific chemical agents or drugs that are selectively destructive to malignant cells," and "(2) the treatment of disease using chemical agents or drugs that are selectively toxic to the causative agent of the disease, such as a virus, bacterium or other microorganism." The second definition applies to Ehrlich's magic bullet, whereas the first emphasizes that it is anticancer agents rather than antibiotics that the public thinks of as chemotherapy. Such has been the perceived importance of cancer chemotherapy.

The treatment of cancer using a specific chemical agent started before arsphenamine. One hundred years ago in December of 1898, Marie and Pierre Curie reported the discovery of radium. This was adapted quickly for medical treatment and was recognized as the first effective nonsurgical cancer treatment. Its properties are consistent with the primary definition of chemotherapy. Also, like current cancer chemotherapy, it relies on tumor and normal tissue biology, physiology, differential efficaciousness, and repair. Just 5 years after the discovery of radium, the Nobel Prize was awarded to Marie and Pierre Curie. Marie won a second Nobel Prize for the chemistry of radium in 1911. Two Nobel Prizes awarded so soon after the discovery of radium gives us some idea of the importance attributed to this event. In 1935, the Curies' daughter, Irene, and her husband, Frédéric Joliot, won the Nobel Prize for the discovery of artificial radioactivity. They produced radioactive isotopes by bombarding targets with radiation produced by radium and, more importantly, by the alpha particles in polonium. Five Nobel Prizes in one family (Marie [2], Pierre, Irene, and Frédéric) is highly unlikely to be exceeded.

This centenary of the discovery of radium in 1898 causes me to digress briefly to consider a few other events in that remarkable year, considered to be the beginning of the American century. It was the year of the Spanish-American War; a 10-week war that resulted in the ceding of Puerto Rico, Guam, and the Philippines to the United States, and Cuba gaining its independence. The United States also annexed Hawaii in 1898. British Imperialism continued with Britain getting a 99-year lease on Hong Kong (how times flies) and Kitchener defeating the Mahdist Revolt at Omdurman in the Sudan. These acts of imperialism—America just beginning and the United Kingdom in late maturity—bespeak a sense of manifest destiny, of cockiness and optimism. Similarly, the discovery of radium was expected to be a general panacea. Radium was considered to be the first wonder drug.

Effective radium treatment of cancer was performed by applying the radium directly to the affected area or by interstitial or intracavitary treatment. This treatment, brachy-therapy, was both the first chemotherapy as well as the beginning of modern radiotherapy. It was the first chemotherapy because chemical salts were used to selectively destroy cancer cells and allow for normal tissue reconstitution. Although there was great enthusiasm for radium in the treatment of cancer, there were other benefits attributed to radium when used in different forms. While attending the International Union Against Cancer meeting in Florence, Italy, in the 1970s, I was lodged in the spa town of Montecatini. I well remember the hotel offering warm baths and enemas using the spa waters said to be beneficial because of the presence of radium in the water.

The internal use of radium-laced mixtures was recommended as a general health tonic as well as for the treatment of a variety of diseases. The hazards of internal radium ingestion were not appreciated until osteosarcomas were noticed in radium watch-dial painters who moistened the tip of the brush in their mouths to maintain a fine point and the death of millionaire E. M. Byers from radium poisoning induced by an over-the-counter nostrum.

As we celebrate the centenary of this chemotherapy, we should reflect on the lessons of radium use. Ehrlich's wish for therapeutic selectivity is difficult to obtain for cancer. Currently, only antibiotics meet the rigorous requirements because bacterial cells are so different from the mammalian cells, offering targets not present in mammalian cells. Unfortunately, anticancer agents face a much greater challenge because of the similarity of tumor cells to normal cells and the adaptability of cancer to modify in response to treatment. Evolution in the plant world favors the production of antibacterials, but not of anticancer agents; therefore, searching plant products is more difficult, although some of our most effective chemotherapies are natural products or their derivatives.

We also should be reminded of the Manichean nature of medical therapies. Effective agents in other circumstances are agents of destruction. The deft surgical scalpel is to be contrasted with the violent use of cutting instruments. Medicines are chemicals used effectively, whereas poisons often are the same or similar chemicals used in entirely different ways. Radium showed that ionizing radiation could be an effective therapy; however, we need to look no further than the hazards of radioactivity and the use of nuclear weapons to see its misapplication. In their enthusiasm, the early users of radium minimized the risk of localized and generalized radiation exposure. Both Marie Curie and her daughter, Irene, died of the hematologic consequences of their close contact with radium.

We should learn from radium that overpromise, which produces excessive enthusiasm, may result in an aversion that overshadows the benefits of careful, appropriate use. This is an important lesson for this new era of "designer drugs." Although we are optimistic, we must recognize the similarity between normal and malignant cells and the tumor's capacity for adaptation. The experience with radium should temper the dialogue within the medical-scientific community, but even more importantly, between medical science and the public, lest false illusions breed disillusionment. The hubris of manifest destiny is mirrored in the confidence, enthusiasm, and cockiness of many of the advocates of molecular medicine's value in cancer treatment. Santayana commented that "those who cannot remember the past are condemned to repeat it." As we reflect on the enthusiasm with which radium was accepted and then the disillusionment, we should remember that in the reporting of new cancer treatments, the good news always comes first.

This has been an eventful 100 years for medicine as well as for the world. Science has become the basis of medicine, resulting in many new treatment opportunities; however, despite the great promise of new information and technology, we must neither overpromise nor underestimate the difficulty of our challenge. Wonder drugs are hard to come by.

Summing Up

I began considering this project with the notion of examining my life in order to determine what I have learned during this half century replete with tremendous changes in medical science and practice, as well as what it may offer for a future certain to have even more remarkable opportunities and conundrums. I have collected my essays and a few speeches relevant to these changing circumstances. Included are only those articles that I believe would be accessible to the general reader. Some were expressly written for such an audience; though others were addressed to a medical audience, the thrust of the essays makes them worth the attention of readers interested in how medical science is designed and evaluated, and its implications in the light of available theories. With these essays, I have tried to give the general sense of some of the research articles related to breast cancer, metastatic spectrum, and stem cells. While these may contain scientific and medical jargon, I believe the essence of the essay or scientific paper is either clear or is clarified in the accompanying Commentary.

My professional activity does not occur in a vacuum, and it is in the context of my personal, family, and everyday living that my work has been done. There is also chance. Being lucky is very important and I have been very fortunate, most importantly in my family life. While I have had two bouts with cancer, I am still here and doing well "on an age-adjusted basis," as an economist friend is fond of conditioning his response to "how are you." If you have read this far you will know that I have had the opportunity to participate in times of great changes in biological science, medical practice, and the technological and pharmaceutical modalities available. These have led to significant changes in my profession, mostly for the better, but there are far more to come, which will challenge medicine as a profession, as well as the evolving ethics associated with how to learn from our patients and how and whether to do all that the new science and technology will allow.

Philosophic thinking is an essential part of medicine. How knowledge is gained, how trustworthy it is, and how valuable it is when applied to a specific patient are dependent upon epistemological values. Theories are just that, not dogma or received truth, but rather subject to revision or even rejection by further scientific evidence. Medical ethics as a field began during my working life. It is not fixed, but rather is evolving. What was accepted earlier is being questioned today and, I believe, will be even more so in years to come. From the Tuskegee willful study of untreated syphilis to the intentional infection of children at the Meadowbrook State School for the Retarded using fecal material from other patients to the randomized clinical trial, what is considered acceptable has changed. While the Tuskegee episode was begun in the 1930s, it caused revulsion when it was exposed in the 1970s. Similarly, the Meadowbrook experiments were considered exemplars of research methods when the principal investigator was awarded the Lasker Prize in 1983. These surely would not be tolerated today. I have expressed my concerns about the ethics of randomized trials as early as 1979. While they are still considered ethically acceptable in clinical research, I note that recently Doctors Without Borders refused to cooperate in a randomized vaccine trial during the recent Ebola epidemic. We are becoming more rights-based in our attitudes toward patients, and the utilitarian views are less compelling. For the doctor caring for a patient, loyalty to that patient must be paramount.

My personal experience required ethical reflection when considering when, whether, and how randomized clinical trials could be acceptable. Health care distribution and quality require ethical considerations as well as pragmatic ones. I do not believe this can or should be done based on a competitive marketplace model as presented by the Clintons in the failed Health Security Act or by President Obama in the Affordable Care Act.

Even the change of names of the acts is discouraging. Health Security has a nice ring, but Affordable Care connotes the primacy of cost rather than universal availability or quality. These acts are far too complicated—the result of political bargaining, lobbying, and other considerations, rather than accepting that adequate health care is a fundamental right that must be delivered to all. This social good is primary; its delivery, while subject to overall practical resource availability, cannot be determined by the lowest cost or other purely utilitarian considerations. The doctor dealing with the individual patient—except when limited by formal governmental restrictions—must have that patient's best interests held paramount. The doctor's deliberations are fraught with conflicting values when the roles of physician and medical investigator are combined in a single individual. This is often the case in clinical investigation, especially in random allocation clinical trials. It is my hope that this method will be used less often and with greater skepticism as to its appropriateness in the future. When done, these dual roles of the doctor and investigator need to be placed in different individuals who are clearly demarcated.

I believe that each individual in our society has rights both *to* and *in* health care. The rights to adequate health care require equitable distribution to all persons. The rights in health care include personal care that recognizes the patient's individuality; loyalty of the physician to that patient; fidelity to the ethical precepts and codes of medicine; reassurance, compassion, and support.

The messages of my research appropriate for the nonscientific public are many. Humans are very complicated; while basic research can be very useful, its applicability to man must be contextualized within the layers of complexity of organ physiology and whole organism behavior. Basic research is necessary but far from sufficient. We learn differently from many different kinds of information. Some are from formal experiments, while some are evaluation of past experience; some are easily accepted, while others depend on discarding previously accepted knowledge. How this learning is done in medical science must respect and value all forms of knowledge acquisition. My research on blood-forming stem cells is not the most fundamental since it was studied in the whole organism—in this case, the mouse. But its direct application to man presumes much similarity despite the different species, markedly different life spans, and the nature of the experimental design. The breast cancer research is quite different since it studies the clinical experience gained from review of patients' disease extent, treatment, and eventual clinical outcome. These studies are limited by the lack of knowledge of how the patients studied were chosen, as well as by considerations of the quality of the care delivered. These qualifications on my laboratory and clinical investigations or that of others are necessary limitations of all inductive reasoning. What we learn in medical science is tentative and subject to modification or rejection in the future. It is gained from a great variety of methods, including but not limited to expert opinion, past personal experience, and that reported in the literature, by colleagues, and by formally conducted basic and clinical experiments. It is leavened implicitly as well as explicitly by the observer using previously acquired information and judgment in order to determine how to apply this knowledge to a specific circumstance. I consider my research studies to be of value but primarily as a part of the general progress in these fields. Many feel that science moves in fits and starts, with major saltations occurring uncommonly in the midst of what is referred to as "ordinary science." I am not convinced of this dichotomy. So-called ordinary science, as long as its path is forward, is necessary to develop the foundation for a significant change. Watson and Crick did not work in a vacuum when studying how DNA could provide a method for inheritance; rather, they made an important jump but just a little ahead of others; so did Darwin, so did most acclaimed scientists and doctors. We love heroes and our custom is to treat them as a breed apart. Prizes and medals are given to a few, but most often their efforts are the culmination of a great deal of "ordinary work." A personal example for me is the study of stem cells. My work and that of many others provide some of the necessary foundation for larger advances to come when the accumulated knowledge of stem cell basic biology and systems physiology will be sufficient to allow their application to clinical medicine. Then our studies of how the cells function in animals under various conditions will be again relevant. We live in a time of reductionism in medical science, but in order to know about how a cell-renewal system functions we need to study it in the context of its environment when responding to the needs of the organism. Our studies were directed to these areas.

I have seen great changes in clinical oncology. Radical surgery was accepted as the most effective cancer treatment, and the consequences of these large extirpative procedures were considered unfortunate but necessary. When I began my postgraduate medical training in radiation oncology in the early 1960s, linear accelerators were just becoming available for precise radiation therapy. Combination chemotherapy for childhood leukemia was just being reported. By the time of this writing, great improvements in radiation therapy delivery have resulted in widespread use of this technique for cancer treatment. Combination chemotherapy has now become a major therapy both alone and when combined with radiation or limited surgery in the curative treatment of many cancers. Radical surgery has had an ever-decreasing role with greater emphasis on limited surgery, often utilizing newer techniques such as laparoscopic and robotic surgery.

Research has expanded greatly during this period. A major expansion was due to the National Cancer Act of 1971. This promised tremendous success by the two hundredth anniversary of the Declaration of Independence in 1976. This hyperbole was far too optimistic, but I am excited about two revolutionary new approaches to the systemic treatment of a wide variety of cancers that are on the forefront of cancer treatment. Utilizing the discovery of genetic alterations in many cancers, drugs have been designed to target these abnormalities. Tumors have been shown to have mechanisms to inhibit normal anti-cancer immunity. When the body is allowed to have the capacity to immunologically attack cancer, these tumors are often reduced or destroyed. These two new approaches bode well for the future. But during my career, I have seen all too often initial enthusiasm lead to overpromise and subsequently disillusionment. I am cautiously optimistic that this will not be the case with genetically-targeted pharmaceuticals or with the restoration and even enhancement of host anti-cancer immunity, but we shall have to wait and see the long-term status of patients receiving these new treatments. As my friend, Ted

Phillips, a noted radiation oncologist cautions "in cancer the good news always comes first."

My clinical efforts in treating breast cancer while preserving the breast and normal shoulder and arm function was the culmination of the work of many who preceded me in developing the methods and, even more importantly, in changing the paradigm of cancer spread and thus the appropriate treatment. Often these pioneers were vilified, but their work and advocacy provided the bases for the changes that I championed to succeed. Many of these early efforts were done abroad and thus were not easily accepted in America. Part of my function was to build on them and use the "bully pulpits" of my positions at Harvard and then at Memorial Sloan-Kettering to present and advocate conservative (really, preservative) management of breast cancer. At the same time, there were important cultural changes occurring that made efforts to change breast cancer treatment much easier. Feminism was gaining steam and in its vanguard were women who rejected the paternalism of doctors, usually men, who were dismissive of the importance of a women's body image and who as doctors thought they knew best and should be in control. This paternalism in medicine has diminished greatly, and these changes in the patient's relationship with the doctor gained great strength from these controversies about breast cancer treatment while also synergizing the movement for therapeutic methods that preserved the breast.

The paradigm of centrifugal spread of cancer via the lymphatics championed by Halsted led to dogma that was first replaced by the notion of metastases, if they are to be present, to occur before clinical detectability. This alternative systemic theory has not become dogma but still has very vociferous advocates. My place in the breast cancer disagreements was at a time ready for re-evaluation of the underlying science and resulting theories. The spectrum theory that my colleagues and I espouse attempts to explain breast cancer's natural history and includes some of both the centrifugal theory, as well as the notion that cancer is either local only or systemic at the time of clinical detection. This reconsideration of how cancer spreads no longer dichotomizes cancer but rather claims that cancer comprises a continuum of disease of increasing malignancy between some cancers being present only at the site of origin to some being widespread with many intermediate malignant states. This view of the spectrum of cancer behavior seems to be becoming more widely accepted.

It is well to remember that a doctor's goal should be to cure the disease and return the patient as much as possible to the pre-diseased state. This preservative management of breast cancer is far closer to that goal than the previously accepted radical mastectomy. The spectrum theory has also led to the notion that within the evolution of cancer there is a state of limited metastatic potential that we call oligometastases. These metastatic deposits are limited in number and location and may be cured by treatments directed at these individual sites. We have shown that oligometastatic spread is associated with certain molecular markers, which should allow physicians to direct different treatment to this form of metastases.

In considering the great advances in molecular medicine, it is important to also appreciate the tremendous technological advances that occurred in medicine during my half-century of involvement. When I was in medical school little attention was given to molecular biology, but it was also a time when there were only rudimentary radiological instruments. Computed axial tomography (CAT scans), magnetic resonance imaging (MRI), and positron emission tomography (PET scanning) were in the realm of science fiction, if imagined at all. Today they are used early in the evaluation of a patient, and are much more precise in the detection of cancer and in determining its extent. There is much more to come. So both biology and technology are advancing rapidly and in step.

While a simple panacea that can cure all cancers without significant toxicity is a worthy goal, it is unlikely to be found any time soon since this disease is the result of a distortion of essential human functions. In the meantime we must not allow this desire for a simple cure detract from continued steady improvement such as that seen in my half-century as an oncologist. The perfect must not be the enemy of the good.

Medical practice has also changed markedly during my career. My view of a medical practitioner when I entered medical school was that of a single doctor in the general practice of medicine being the dominant medical caregiver. That has changed markedly with the great expansion of group practice and of the medical specialties. With Medicare, Medicaid, and now with the Affordable Care Act, there is much more government involvement and more access to health care. All of this is for the good; my only caution is to remind us that the social contract of the doctor to the patient requires that the doctor's primary responsibility is to the individual patient in her or his care.

Being in academic medicine means teaching. I performed this at many levels, from college undergraduates to graduate students, medical students, and postdoctoral fellows, but mostly for postgraduate doctors in all the oncologic specialties. These young physicians must learn to deal with cancer patients, with their symptoms and prognosis, with compassion, honesty, and reassurance. She or he should advise and guide the patient throughout the cancer experience, but must assure that the patient rather than the doctor makes the decisions consistent with the values, preferences, and circumstances of the individual patient. Teaching provided pleasure while doing and great joy in seeing the accomplishments of many of my former students. I was fortunate to have participated in the education of a dean, chairmen, good and even outstanding scientists, and most importantly, excellent oncologists, as well as many other medical practitioners. I bask in their reflected accomplishments. I remain convinced of the importance of a liberal education as the necessary predicate to medical education. I am equally convinced of the importance of modern biology in the education of all students. You can't knowledgeably participate in discussions of genetic engineering of foods or humans if you don't really understand genes and heredity.

Unfortunately the term "cancer" congers up images and exaggerations, which not only may increase anxiety, but also may deter or delay patients from seeking care. Differing perceptions of cancer also occur within medicine practitioners, resulting in quite different attitudes toward the disease by the various medical specialties. Patients, doctors, and the general society would be helped greatly by demythologizing cancer. Rather than the diagnosis of cancer always being a death knell, we should remember that there are many different types and stages of cancer with a great spectrum of outcomes, from cure easily attained to inexorable fatal disease with distressing symptoms and with many patients in between. Currently cancer best fits the glass half full, half empty analogy. I urge both doctor and patient to be in the half-full camp: positive about what can be done, but realistic as to the likely outcome. This will occur more easily if we reduce the single image of cancer as an ominous, incurable disease. Surprising as it may appear, cancer is the most curable of the serious chronic diseases, and progress continues to be made. Much can be learned from the patient. I was particularly fortunate to learn from a number of my most articulate and insightful patients, as well as from the writings and conversations with cancer survivors, to whom I am greatly indebted.

While I believe that medicine should be central to a university, often it is marginalized. Its faculties are large and its finances great and complicated, both feared by leaders and boards to distort or put the university at risk. While these characteristics need attention, they should not result in holding medicine at arm's length. Medicine was very early a part of the university. Its inclusion is even more important today since both its costs and benefits are much greater. Having the capacity to do something does not determine whether it should be done. The deliberations concerning the uses of scientific advances require the wisdom derived from many parts of the university. The consequences of these decisions may impact on our basic conceptions of human life.

While research, teaching, and patient care were primary early in my career and continued to be so, medical leadership became a major emphasis later in my career. I very much enjoyed this phase as it related to cancer care and research. I was very fortunate to have the opportunity to develop the Joint Center for Radiation Therapy and to establish the Department of Radiation Oncology at Harvard. There was great joy in doing research during that time of adequate funding for research both basic and clinical. Perhaps the pinnacle of my career was as physician-in-chief at Memorial Sloan-Kettering Cancer Center (MSKCC). Here my leadership was completely congruent with my clinical and research interests. Being a dean/vice president of the Division of Biological Sciences and of the Pritzker School of Medicine at The University of Chicago was more complicated. But being in this latter position in an integrated and collaborative university caused me to reflect on how we teach biology and medicine not only to doctors-to-be but also as a part of a general education. I also realized and responded to the importance of medicine to the university and vice versa. All this occurred while medicine was changing rapidly in how research was supported, how medical care was organized, and how it was financed. I remain convinced that the application of market principles to medicine is not in the best interests of patients, health care professionals, or society at large. Managed competition reduces collaboration, the lowest price does not result in the best care, efficiency is good but should not be the final determinant, and equitable care must be a right available to all.

I have selected two heroes, Thomas Hodgkin and Marie Curie. Both have made very important contributions, but I have selected Hodgkin for his many other salutary activities, and Curie not only for her professional activities but also for her important war efforts and pioneering feminism. They are heroes not only because of their great discoveries; rather, it is the whole of their activities for the benefit of mankind that must be considered. My review of their lives as well as their scientific contributions has made them paragons to me.

I have had an extremely fulfilling professional career. Hopefully these essays and remarks have given the reader a sense of its nature. I have also acquired some of what I consider good advice:

- A rough restating of Hippocrates' famous quotation is "to try to do good but if you are unable to help then at least do no harm." It is only the last phrase that is usually presented, but it should be seen in this larger context. This is good advice in medicine and serves well in life in general.
- Medical science is general, but patient care is given individually. The essence of the "art of medicine" is in applying that medical knowledge to each unique patient.

The doctor in general and the oncologist in particular should provide knowledge with compassion and honesty with reassurance.

Beware of mediocrity; the pressure to be average is great but must be eschewed. There is a great difference between competence and excellence.

Love and value what you do.

Have epistemological modesty; don't be too sure!

INDEX

academic health center
  dean of, 144
  hospital board of, 148
  innovation by, 102–3
academic medicine
  diversity of, 158
  Freedberg for, 157
  teaching in, 304
Ackerman, Lauren V., 201–2, 251–52
action analysis, 142
Adelberg, Edward, 167
adjuvant therapy
  "Clinical Alert" against, 164–65, 204–5
  dogma for, 204–5
Advisory Committee on Human Radiation Experiments, 90
Affordable Care Act
  healthcare by, 36–37
  by President Obama, 298–99
age of patient
  breast cancer influenced by, 191–92, 191t
  cancer influenced by, 218
Age of Discovery, 199
AIDS
  considerations for, 12–13
  ethics and, 51
"The Aims of Education" (Whitehead), 5–6
Allegheny College
  "A Doctor's Dilemmas" for, 20

Kern from, 24
Shafer from, 24
altruism
  doctor-patient relationship and, 78
  evolution of, 218–19
  by patient, 60, 63
Americans, education of, 6
American Society of Clinical Oncology, Presidency of, 170
American Society of Therapeutic Radiology and Oncology, 173
anatomy, 72–73
angiogenesis, 215
antiangiogenic treatment, 108
apoptosis
  for oncogenesis, 213–14
  for treatment, 219–20
architecture, 8
arsphenamine, 292–93
atomic energy, 284, 287–88
atomic physics, 287–88
Auden, W. H., 250
autonomy, 61–62
autopsy, 133–34

B16F1 melanoma, 238
basic right, healthcare as, 96–97, 299
Baum, Michael, 74
Beecher, Henry
  on consent, 88
  "Ethics and Clinical Research" by, 82–83

Belmont Report of 1979, 88–89
Beth Israel Hospital, 150–52, 154
biological revolution
  acceptance of, 25, 70
  at Beth Israel Hospital, 154
  commercialization of, 103–4
  early years of, 154
  "The End of Inevitability, or Frankenstein and the Biological Revolution" on, 25
  ethics of, 104, 135, 140
  of human genome, 132
  implication of, 104, 128–29
  for innovation, 106
  of oncology, 176
  physician of, 138
Biological Sciences Division (BSD) at The University of Chicago
  development of, 126
  for tumors, 166–67
biology
  of cancer, 125
  of cell cycle, 181
  in education, 9–10, 128
  knowledge of, 137–38
  medicine and, 125
  for radiation therapy, 177–78
  of tumors, 210–11
biomedical model, 26
biostatisticians, 257
Bloedorn, Fernando, 172–73
Blumgart, Hermann, 268
body preservation, 302
bone marrow transplant, 64–65
Brady, Luther, 178
breast cancer
  age influence on, 191–92, 191t
  Baum on, 74
  body preservation for, 302
  chemotherapy for, 54–55
  diagnosis of, 186–87
  dogma of, 199
  Ewing on, 171
  Fisher and, 163–64
  interest in, 163–64
  Journal of the American Medical Association on, 28–29
  locality of, 203–4
  metastases of, 187–88
  pathogenesis for, 205–6
  "preservative" treatment for, 163–64
  radiation therapy for, 113–14, 189–90
  radical mastectomy for, 199, 200–201
  randomized clinical trial for, 68–69
  Rosen on, 192–93
  screening for, 189–90
  spectrum theory for, 164–65, 195, 303
  systemic-dissemination model for, 185–86, 187–88, 224
  tumors of, 107
Bronx, 1–2
Brookings Review, 100
Brown, John Seeley, 133
Browning, Robert, 17
BSD. *See* Biological Sciences Division

cancer. *See also* breast cancer; prostate cancer; small breast cancer
  amplification of, 212t
  by Auden, 250
  biology of, 125
  biostatisticians on, 257
  chemotherapy for, 161–62
  chromosomal abnormalities of, 210–11
  as chronic disease, 254–55
  "convergent evolution" of, 208–9
  curing of, 259, 263–64
  Darwinism of, 220
  doctor-patient relationship for, 262–63
  environmental factors influence on, 258
  fundraising for, 256
  genetics and, 257
  hematopoiesis influence on, 168–69
  lung metastases from, 234–35
  malignancy of, 227–28
  medical oncologist perception of, 253–54
  Menninger on, 250
  mutations of, 211, 212t
  O'Donnell on, 250

oligometastases of, 225–26
paradigm of, 248–49
pathologist and, 254
patient age influence on, 218
perceptions of, 245–46, 248, 250
pessimistic connotations of, 249–50
Phillips on, 301–2
Principles and Practice of Radiation Oncology on, 178
public view of, 248–49, 304–5
radiation oncologist perception of, 253–54
radiation therapy for, 161–62, 290–91
research for, 161
stem cell research for, 168–69, 298–300
surgeon perception of, 253–54
surgery for, 259
"traffic" of, 182–83
understanding of, 258
career
  advice for, 306–7
  of Curie, M., 270–271
  of Curie, I., 285, 287–88, 294
  of Freedberg, 157
  of Hodgkin, 16, 273
  in leadership, 305–6
  sociology for, 129
  undergraduate education for, 17–18
caregiver role, 33–34
Casper, Gerhard, 125–26
cell cycle
  biology of, 181
  of tumors, 182
cell resistance, 279–80
cellular aggregates, 237–38
chemotherapy
  for breast cancer, 54–55
  for cancer, 161–62
  experimental treatment of, 55–56
  intensity of, 55
  for liver metastases, 235–36
  for oligometastases, 227
  for pediatrics, 172
  randomization process of, 57, 60
  randomized clinical trial for, 55–56

reasoning for intensive chemotherapy, 58
Chicago, 8–9
childhood
  in Bronx, 1–2
  of Curie, M., 285–86
chromosomal abnormalities, 210–11
chronic disease
  cancer as, 254–55
  modification of, 27–28
chronic myelogenous leukemia, 217–18
Cincinnati project, 89–90
The Climb of My Life (Evans), 265–67
"Clinical Alert," 164–65, 204–5
clinical equipoise
  ethics by, 65
  by Freedman, 71, 74
Clinical Ethics Series, 35–36
clinical investigation
  consent for, 95–96
  cost of, 70
  willful blindness in, 86–87
clinical research
  methods of, 3
  "On First Looking into Kutcher's *Contested Medicine*" about, 34–35
  utilitarianism in, 90
clinical scientist, 44–45
Clinton, Hillary, 36–37, 93, 298–99
Clinton, William Jefferson
  Advisory Committee on Human Radiation Experiments by, 90
  Health Security Act of 1993 by, 36–37, 93, 298–99
Coley, William, 170–71
colleagues
  collaboration of, 196–97
  of dean, 144
commencement, 18
"Comments on the Presentation by President Don Randel, The University of Chicago Symposium, "University of the Future," 132

commercialization
  of biological revolution, 103–4
  of medicine, 156
community. *See also* culture; society
  Casper on, 125–26
  doctor-patient relationship
    influenced by, 41
  resources allocated by, 97–99
  undergraduate education for, 18
  of The University of Chicago, 9, 125–26
consent
  Beecher on, 88
  for clinical investigation, 95–96
  as patient right, 49
conservatism, 206
Contested Medicine (Kutcher), 79
  about Cincinnati project, 89–90
  ethics by, 84
control group, 39–40
"convergent evolution," 208–9
Copernican view, 26
Crick, Francis, 2
Crile, George, Jr., 202–3
culture, 143
Curie, Eve, 284
Curie, Irene
  career of, 285, 287–88, 294
  Joliot-Curie and, 271, 284,
    287, 292–93
Curie, Marie
  biographies on, 284
  childhood of, 285–86
  Curie, P., and, 286
  feminism of, 289–90
  as hero, 269–70, 306
  lessons learned from, 291
  Nobel Prize for, 286, 292–93
  polonium identification and
    purification by, 286
  radiation effects on, 287
  radium identification and purification
    by, 286
  scientific accomplishments of, 270–71
Curie, Pierre
  Curie, M., and, 286

Nobel Prize for, 292–93
  on radium, 289
"Curies, Cure, and Culture," 284

Dana-Farber Cancer Institute, 56, 150–52
Darwinism
  of cancer, 220
  evolution by, 208–9
"Darwin's Clinical Relevance," 208
dean
  of academic health center, 144
  colleagues of, 144
  decision-making by, 145–46
  against mediocrity, 145
  prevention of, 149
  as psychiatrist, 144
  responsibilities of, 145
Dean, John, 249–50
decision-making, 145–46
Declaration of Geneva, 34–35
Department of Defense, 81–82
dermatology, 155–56
DeVita, Vincent, 162, 172, 278
diagnosis
  of breast cancer, 186–87
  evolution and, 208
  by technology, 179
diagnostic imaging, 172–73
digital revolution, 133
dignity, 45–46, 84–85
discovery
  of radiation, 284
  of Reed-Sternberg cell, 278–79
  in science, 27
  value of, 21
"discrete steps," of metastases, 237
disease-free state, 194–95, 194*t*
disease risk, 25, 26
diversity, 158–59
DNA repair, 212–13
doctor. *See* physician
doctor-patient relationship
  altruism and, 78
  basis of, 129–30
  for cancer, 262–63

INDEX 313

circumstances of, 22–23
comfort of, 264–65
community influence on, 41
economics of, 75–76, 77–78
essence of, 49
Fried on, 95
healthcare influence on, 76, 104, 303–4
importance of, 4–5
individuality of, 95, 106
loyalty of, 1, 264
managed care and, 93
randomized clinical trial and, 58–59
rationing influence on, 101
society and, 88–89
Toon on, 71
treatment from, 70–71
"A Doctor's Dilemmas," 20
dogma
    for adjuvant therapy, 204–5
    of breast cancer, 199
    conservatism and, 206
    Crile, Jr., against, 202–3
    Fisher against, 202–3
    Fitzwilliams on, 202–3, 251–52
    Keynes against, 202–3, 206, 251–52
    of medicine, 203
    of radical mastectomy, 200
    surgeon against, 202–3
    of surgery, 200–201
    systemic-dissemination model as, 302–3
"Dogma and Inquisition in Medicine: Breast Cancer as a Case Study," 199
dormancy, 237–38
drugs
    for cell resistance, 279–80
    "off label" use of, 63–64

economics
    of doctor-patient relationship, 75–76, 77–78
    of medicine, 130–31
education. *See also* lifelong learning; undergraduate education
    aims of, 11–12, 17

of Americans, 6
answers from, 23
biology in, 9–10, 128
glossary terms for, 10–11
Hutchins on, 13
interdisciplinary collaboration in, 11
knowledge and, 10–11, 15, 100
memory in, 10–11
of physician, 1, 110, 131, 143
stages of, 6–7
use of, 20
of Vesalius, 133–34
Ehrlich, Paul, 292
emotional state
    of patient, 73
    of physician, 262–63
"The End of Inevitability, or Frankenstein and the Biological Revolution," 25
Enlightenment, 134
environmental factors, 258
EORTC. *See* European Organization for Research and Treatment of Cancer
epistemology, 5
equitably, 93
ethics. *See also* "right-based ethics"
    AIDS and, 51
    Belmont Report of 1979 for, 88–89
    of biological revolution, 104, 135, 140
    by clinical equipoise, 65
    by *Contested Medicine*, 84
    "Ethics and Clinical Research" on, 82–83
    "Ethics of Randomized Clinical Trials" on, 33–34, 54
    evolution of, 91
    field of, 2–3
    by Kutcher, 79
    Nuremberg Code of 1947 for, 82
    of patient-centered care, 74
    of radiation therapy, 79–80, 84
    of randomization process, 48, 65
    of randomized clinical trial, 33, 38, 42–43, 44, 47, 298–99
    of research, 83
    Smith on, 46–47, 91
    of Tuskegee study, 83–84

"Ethics and Clinical Research"
 (Beecher), 82–83
"Ethics of Randomized Clinical Trials,"
 33–34, 54
European Organization for Research
 and Treatment of Cancer
 (EORTC), 191–92
Evans, Laura
 The Climb of My Life by, 265–67
evolution. *See also* "convergent evolution"
 of altruism, 218–19
 by Darwinism, 208–9
 diagnosis and, 208
 of ethics, 91
 gradualness of, 210
 Mayr on, 208–9
 natural selection of, 208–9
 of oligometastases, 228–29,
  240–41, 303
 "punctuated equilibria" of, 210
 of tumors, 214–15, 224–25
 Watson on, 208
"Evolving Paradigms and Perceptions of
 Cancer," 248
Ewing, James
 on breast cancer, 171
 of oncology, 170–71
 for systemic-dissemination
  model, 172
 treatment by, 171
Expedition Inspiration, 256–57
experimental treatment
 of chemotherapy, 55–56
 health insurance against, 141
 "off protocol" of, 67

faculties, 27
false positive, 115–17
Fauci, Anthony
 on clinical scientist, 44–45
 on randomized clinical trial, 46–47
fee-for-service medicine, 94
feminism, 289–90
fertility, 54
fin de siècle, 185

"Fin de siècle medicine. Avoiding the
 unintended consequences of health
 care reform," 100
"The First Century of Cancer
 Chemotherapy," 292
Fisher, Bernard
 breast cancer and, 163–64
 against dogma, 202–3
 systemic-dissemination model by, 107,
  164–65, 185–86, 252–53
Fitzwilliams, Douglas, 202–3, 251–52
Folkman, Judah, 215
fossils, 147
fractional cell kill, 219, 219t
Frankenstein (Shelley), 25, 30–31
Freedberg, Irwin
 for academic medicine, 157
 career of, 157
 dermatology by, 155–56
 friendship of, 127
 molecular science by, 154–55
 in New York, 156–57
Freedman, Benjamin, 71, 74
Fried, Charles, 95
friendship
 of Freedberg, 127
 of Fuks, 127, 158–59
 of Johanson, 127, 158–59, 167
 of Peckham, C., 127
 of Peckham, M., 127
Fuks, Zvi, 127, 158–59
funding
 for cancer, 256
 of research, 139–40, 155, 156

gastrointestinal (GI) tract, 232–33
gating techniques, 180
genetic engineering, 28–29
genetics
 by Adelberg, 167
 cancer and, 257
 by Watson and Crick, 2
German university, 134
Gilbert, René, 277–78
Giroud, Françoise, 284

INDEX

GI tract. *See* gastrointestinal (GI) tract
glossary terms, 10–11
government regulation, 99
Gowans, James, 128–29, 132–33, 182–83
Grand Obsession (Pflaum), 284
Gray, Hanna, 133–34
Great Britain, 170, 173–74
Guy's Hospital, 273–74

"halfway technology," 102
Halsted, William Stewart, 107, 165–66, 224, 250–51
Halsted model
    by Halsted, 107, 165–66, 224, 250–51
    for radical mastectomy, 185–87
harm, 66, 130, 306
Harrison, Benjamin, 16, 274
healthcare
    Affordable Care Act for, 36–37
    as basic right, 96–97, 299
    competition for, 152
    doctor-patient relationship influenced by, 76, 104, 303–4
    epistemology of, 5
    government regulation for, 99
    Hodgkin on promotion of, 275
    hospital competition by, 151
    Managed Care Consumer Protection Act for, 99
    patient rights and, 35
    by physician, 105
    for public good, 74–75
    reform of, 36–37, 100, 101, 106, 140
    restrictions for, 139–40
    revolution of, 25, 70
    Siegler on, 101
    society for, 97
health insurance, 140–41
Health Security Act of 1993, 36–37, 93, 298–99
hematopoiesis, 168–69
hepatitis transmission study, 83
hero. *See also* role model
    criteria for, 269–70
    Curie, M., as, 269–70, 306

Hodgkin, T., as, 123–24, 269–70, 306
hierarchy, 111–12
Hill, Sir Austin Bradford, 73
Hippocrates
    on harm, 66, 130, 306
    on patient-centered care, 129
Hodgkin, Thomas
    career of, 16, 273
    contributions by, 16, 272
    at Guy's Hospital, 273–74
    as hero, 123–24, 269–70, 306
    Hodgkin's disease and, 15, 272–73, 275–76
    humanity of, 16–17, 274
    life of, 15, 273–74, 281–82
    for moral insanity, 275
    New World natives and, 15–16
    promotion of healthcare by, 275
    for von Humboldt, 134, 270
Hodgkin Lymphoma
    first findings of, 275–76
    "halfway technology" for, 102
    by Hodgkin, 15, 272–73, 275–76
    lessons of, 278–80
    microscope for, 276–77
    morbidity of, 280–81
    pathogenesis of, 276–77
    side effects of, 281
    treatment for, 160–62
Hodgkin's disease. *See* Hodgkin Lymphoma
homogeneous group
    patient consolidation by, 72
    of randomized clinical trial, 113
honesty, 61
hospital. *See also* Beth Israel Hospital
    healthcare competition of, 151
hospital board, 148
host organ quantification, 72–73
Hudson Bay Company, 16, 274
human genome, 132
humanity, 16–17
Hutchins, Robert Maynard, 13

"Illness as Metaphor" (Sontag), 245–46, 249
Ilych, Ivan, 262–63
immune system, 183
individuality
   of doctor-patient relationship, 95, 106
   Montgomery on, 119–20
individual rights, 90–91
inductive learning, 37
inherited disease, 28–29
innovation
   by academic health center, 102–3
   biological revolution for, 106
   cost influence on, 103
   research and, 101
   in surgery, 27–28
"The Intellectual Quarantine of American Medicine," 135
interdisciplinary collaboration
   in education, 11
   of university, 142
   by The University of Chicago, 133
international communication, 159
The Invention of Nature (Wulf), 123–24
"Irwin Freedberg and the Changing Times of Academic Medicine," 154
"Ivar, Michael, and Zvi: Celebrating the Diversity of Our Friends and Colleagues," 158

James, William, 8–9
JCRT. *See* Joint Center for Radiation Therapy
Johanson, Ivar, 127, 158–59, 167
Joint Center for Radiation Therapy (JCRT)
   collaboration of, 150–51
   dissolution of, 127, 150–53
   by Lee, 150
Joliot-Curie, Frédéric
   atomic energy by, 284, 287–88
   Curie, I., and, 271, 284, 287, 292–93
Journal of Clinical Oncology, 33–34, 54
Journal of Investigative Dermatology, 154
Journal of the American Medical Association, 28–29
judgment, 64

Kant, Immanuel, 45–46, 84–85
Kaplan, Henry S., 278
"Karnofsky Memorial Lecture. Natural History of Small Breast Cancers," 185
Katz, Jay, 262–63
Kern, Alfred, 24
Keynes, Sir Geoffrey, 202–3, 206, 251–52
knowledge. *See also* tacit knowledge
   of biology, 137–38
   conditionality of, 109–11
   education and, 10–11, 15, 100
   medicine influenced by, 136, 299–301
   NICE for, 111–12
   by physician, 264
Kushner, Rose, 265–66
Kutcher, Gerald
   Contested Medicine by, 79, 84, 89–90
   ethics by, 79
   medical background of, 80
   radiation therapy by, 80–81

Laënnec, René, 123–24
"A Lamentation on the Death of Collaboration," 150
Lasker Prize, 83
leadership
   career in, 305–6
   Laënnec on, 123–24
"Learning While Caring: Medicine's Epistemology," 37, 109
Lee, Sydney, 150
lifelong learning, 110
liver metastases
   chemotherapy for, 235–36
   GI tract and, 232–33
   oligometastases of, 232–33
   survival rate of, 233–34, 234*t*
loyalty
   of doctor-patient relationship, 1, 264
   for patient, 89
lung metastases, 234–35
lymphangiography, 278
lymph nodes
   small breast cancers and, 195
   treatment of, 190, 193–94

Machiavelli, Niccolò, 24
Madame Curie (by Curie, E.), 284
"magic bullet"
   by Ehrlich, 292
   of treatment, 255, 259–60
magnetic resonance, 179
malignancy
   of cancer, 227–28
   of tumors, 191, 213–14
managed care
   doctor-patient relationship and, 93
   fee-for-service medicine replaced by, 94
"Managed Care and the Doctor-Patient Relationship: A Ménage à Trois," 93
Managed Care Consumer Protection Act, 99
Manichaean, 130
Mayr, Ernst, 208–9
McWhirter, Robert, 251–52
McWhirter technique
   Ackerman on, 201–2, 251–52
   for tumors, 201–2
mechanical life-sustaining assistance, 21
medical care
   equitable distribution of, 93
   cost of, 22, 135, 150
   by The University of Chicago, 126–27
medical cost
   by physician, 97–98
medical oncologist, 253–54
medical school
   incorporation of, 8, 123–25
   Rhodes on, 136–37
   specialization influence on, 20
medical science
   necessity of, 4
   society influence on, 23
Medicare, 36–37
medicine. *See also* academic medicine; fee-for-service medicine; molecular medicine
   biology and, 125
   changes in, 142–43
   commercialization of, 156
   in culture, 143

   dogma of, 203
   economics of, 130–31
   international communication for, 159
   knowledge influence on, 136, 299–301
   as Manichaean, 130
   philosophy and, 298
   progress in, 185
   reductionism of, 132–33
   science for, 295
   technology for, 117–19, 303
   university and, 123–24, 128, 136–37, 305
"Medicine: A University," 128
Memorial Sloan-Kettering Cancer Center, 12–13
memory, 10–11
Menninger, Karl, 250
meta-analysis, 113–14
metastases. *See also* oligometastases
   of breast cancer, 187–88
   "discrete steps" of, 237
   dormancy of, 237–38
   of pancreatic cancer, 239–40
   primary tumors as source of, 188–89, 188*f*, 212–13, 212*t*, 215–16, 227
   prognosis of, 235
   "seed and soil" hypothesis of, 236
   theories on, 165
   "traffic" of, 183–84
microscope, 276–77
molecular medicine
   host organ quantification by, 72–73
   treatment by, 70–71
molecular science
   by Freedberg, 154–55
   for radiation therapy, 180–81
Montgomery, Kathryn, 119–20
morbidity, 280–81
mutations
   of cancer, 211, 212*t*
   of chronic myelogenous leukemia, 217–18

National Cancer Act
   for research, 301–2
   war metaphor relating to, 246–47

National Institute for Health and Care Excellence (NICE), 111–12
natural selection, 208–9
Nature Clinical Practice Oncology, 159
   "Ivar, Michael, and Zvi: Celebrating the Diversity of Our Friends and Colleagues" in, 158
   "Premise, Promise, Paradigm, and Prophesy" in, 107
Nature Medicine, 70
neoplastic pathogenesis, 227–28
New England Journal of Medicine, 33–34, 44
New World natives, 15–16
New York, 156–57
NICE. *See* National Institute for Health and Care Excellence
Nobel Conference 2000, 177
Nobel Prize, 286, 292–93
normal tissue, 182
null hypothesis, 115–17
Nuremberg Code of 1947, 35, 82
nurse practitioner, 56–57

Obama, Barack
   Affordable Care Act by, 298–99
   on treatment, 246–47
observer bias, 51–52
"off label," 63–64
"off protocol," 67
"Of Mice but Not Men: Problems of the randomized clinical trial," 33–34, 44
oligometastases
   B16F1 melanoma and, 238
   of cancer, 225–26
   chemotherapy for, 227
   as clinical entity, 231
   evolution of, 228–29, 240–41, 303
   experimental models for, 239
   of liver metastases, 232–33
   therapy for, 226–28
   Weichselbaum on, 165–66
"Oligometastases," 224
"Oligometastases Revisited," 231
oncogenesis, 213–14

"Oncologists and their Patients," 262
oncology
   biological revolution of, 176
   Ewing on, 170–71
   procedures of, 301
   specialties of, 174, 175–76
   training for, 264
"On First Looking into Kutcher's *Contested Medicine*," 34–35
oxygen concentration, 181

paclitaxel, 67
pancreatic cancer, 239–40
paradigm
   of cancer, 248–49
   against Copernican view, 26
   of neoplastic pathogenesis, 227–28
past experience
   of physician, 112
   Santayana on, 130
pathogenesis. *See also* neoplastic pathogenesis
   for breast cancer, 205–6
   of Hodgkin's disease, 276–77
pathologist, 254
patient
   altruism by, 60, 63
   attending to, 4–5
   emotional state of, 73
   by homogeneous group, 72
   individuality of, 119–20
   loyalty for, 89
   treatment of, 14
   trial participation by, 65–66
   with tumors, 231–32
   vantage point of, 265–66
"The Patient and the Public Good"
   on caregiver role, 33–34
   in *Nature Medicine*, 70
patient-centered care
   ethics of, 74
   Hippocrates on, 129
   Peabody on, 129, 262, 268
   for public good, 77

INDEX

randomized clinical trial and, 71
treatment by, 74, 119–20
patient rights
   Clinical Ethics Series on, 35–36
   consent as, 49
   healthcare and, 35
   Physician's Oath for, 50
   waiver of, 48–49
   willful blindness of, 85–86
Peabody, Francis Weld, 129, 262, 268
Peckham, Catherine, 127
Peckham, Michael, 127
pediatrics, 172
peer review, 82, 84
Perez, Carlos, 178
personal life, 297–98
Peters, Mildred Vera, 277–78
Pflaum, Rosalynd, 284
phenotypes, 181–82
Phillips, Ted, 301–2
philosophy
   medicine and, 298
   science and, 9–10, 20–21, 23
   of utilitarianism, 84–85
Philosophy in Literature (Ross), 20
physician
   of biological revolution, 138
   for cancer, 2
   continuous education of, 110, 131, 143
   differences of, 73
   of doctor-patient relationship, 38
   education of, 1, 110, 131, 143
   emotional state of, 262–63
   healthcare by, 105
   honesty by, 61
   knowledge by, 264
   lifelong learning by, 110
   medical cost by, 97–98
   past experience of, 112
   postgraduate for, 1–2
   prognosis by, 166
   for public good, 75
   rationing by, 94
   role of, 64, 104–5, 139, 281–82
   as scientist, 45–46
   as technical expert, 100–101, 138–39
   utilitarianism of, 46
   willful indifference by, 87
physician-in-chief, 12–13
physicians, 201–2
Physician's Oath, 50
polonium, 286
Polanyi, Michael, 111–12
Popper, Karl, 196
postgraduate, 1–2
postoperative radiation therapy, 113–14
practitioner *vs.* medical scientist, 61
"Premise, Promise, Paradigm, and Prophesy"
   on inductive learning, 37
   in *Nature Clinical Practice Oncology*, 107
"preservative" treatment, 163–64
Principles and Practice of Radiation Oncology, 178
profession, 297–98
prognosis
   of metastases, 235
   by physician, 166
   randomized clinical trial influenced by, 63
prolonging life, 29–30
prostate cancer, 115
protocol. *See* "off protocol"; research protocol
proximate utility, 117–19
psychiatrist, 144
public good
   healthcare for, 74–75
   patient-centered care for, 77
   physician for, 75
public view, 248–49, 304–5
"punctuated equilibria," 210

quantum theory, 132–33

"Rabbi ben Ezra" (by Robert Browning), 17
radiation
   Clinton, W., for, 84
   Curie, M., affected by, 287

radiation (*cont.*)
  discovery of, 284
  hazards of, 289
  for treatment, 289
radiation oncologist
  of American Society of Clinical Oncology, 170
  cancer perception by, 253–54
  in Great Britain, 170, 173–74
  technology of, 177
  van der Schueren as, 80–81
radiation therapy
  biology for, 177–78
  Bloedorn on, 172–73
  for breast cancer, 113–14, 189–90
  for cancer, 161–62, 290–91
  by Dana-Farber Cancer Institute, 56, 150–52
  for diagnostic imaging, 172–73
  ethics of, 79–80, 84
  expansion of, 178
  future of, 175
  gating techniques for, 180
  giants of, 173
  justification for, 88
  by Kutcher, 80–81
  molecular science for, 180–81
  normal tissue influenced by, 182
  oxygen concentration for, 181
  by Saenger, 81–82
radical mastectomy
  for breast cancer, 199, 200–201
  dogma of, 200
  fin de siècle of, 185
  Halsted model for, 185–87
  McWhirter against, 251–52
  physicians influenced by, 201–2
radioactivity
  for atomic physics, 287–88
  fear of, 285, 290, 291
  for medicine, 284–85
  for treatment, 271
radium
  Curie, P., on, 289
  identification and purification by Curie, M., 286
  lessons of, 294–95
  for treatment, 271, 286–89, 292–93
randomization process
  argument against, 47–48
  of chemotherapy, 57, 60
  ethics of, 48, 65
  for meta-analysis, 113–14
  of randomized clinical trial, 47
randomized clinical trial
  advantages of, 41–42
  alternatives to, 52, 69
  for breast cancer, 68–69
  for chemotherapy, 55–56
  control group of, 39–40
  doctor-patient relationship and, 58–59
  ethics of, 33, 38, 42–43, 44, 47, 298–99
  Fauci on, 46–47
  Hill on, 73
  homogeneous group of, 113
  information by, 51
  justification for, 67–68
  limitations of, 113
  null hypothesis of, 115–17
  for observer bias, 51–52
  patient-centered care and, 71
  preference of, 40–41
  prognosis influence on, 63
  proof from, 62
  for prostate cancer, 115
  randomization process of, 47
  repetition of, 50
  for scientific confirmation, 40
  selection of, 51–52
  size of, 42
  treatment by, 13–14, 38–39
rationing
  doctor-patient relationship influenced by, 101
  by physician, 94
reductionism
  Gowans on, 128–29, 132–33, 182–83
  of medicine, 132–33

Reed-Sternberg cell, 278–79
"Reflections of a Radiation Oncologist as President of the American Society of Clinical Oncology," 170
research. *See also* clinical research; stem cell research
   for cancer, 161
   ethics of, 83
   funding of, 139–40, 155, 156
   on humans, 13–14
   innovation and, 101
   message of, 299–301
   National Cancer Act for, 301–2
   Rockefeller, L., for, 170
   for treatment, 161, 255
research protocol, 67
resources
   community allocation of, 97–99
   of therapy, 66
   in treatment, 13
revolution. *See* biological revolution; digital revolution
Rhodes, Frank, 136–37
"right-based ethics," 68, 109, 117, 129
Rockefeller, John D., Jr., 170
Rockefeller, Laurance, 170
role model, 268
Röntgen, Wilhelm, 100, 277–78
Rosen, Peter, 192–93
Rosenbaum, Ernest, 257
Ross, Julian, 20
Rothman, David, 82–83

Saenger, Eugene, 81–82
Santayana, George, 130
Shafer, Raymond, 24
Schrödinger, Erwin, 132–33
science. *See also* medical science; molecular science
   discovery in, 27
   for medicine, 295
   philosophy and, 9–10, 20–21, 23
scientific advancement, 30–31
scientific confirmation, 40

scientific truth, 196
scientist, 45–46. *See also* clinical scientist
screening, 189–90
"seed and soil" hypothesis, 236
selection, of cancer, 212t
self-realization, 17–18
senescence, 212–13
senior faculty, 149
setting, of interaction, 62–63
Shelley, Mary, 25, 30–31
Siegler, Mark
   Clinical Ethics Series by, 35–36
   on healthcare, 101
single-payer system, 36–37
small breast cancers, 187
   hypotheses of, 192–93
   lymph nodes and, 195
   natural history of, 189, 196
Smith, Rebecca Pringle, 46–47, 91
society
   doctor-patient relationship and, 88–89
   for healthcare, 97
   medical science influenced by, 23
   against scientific advancement, 30–31
sociology, 129
Sontag, Susan
   "Illness as Metaphor" by, 245–46, 249
   on perception, 260
Spanish Inquisition
   acts of faith for, 202
   history of, 199–200
specialization
   medical school influenced by, 20
   of oncology, 174, 175–76
   reduction of, 104–5
   for treatment, 174–75
spectrum theory
   acceptance of, 302–3
   for breast cancer, 164–65, 195, 303
   of tumors, 252–53
stem cell research
   for cancer, 168–69, 298–300
   of tumors, 168–69
   at Yale, 167

Strangers at the Bedside (Rothman), 82–83
surgeon
    cancer perceptions by, 253–54
    against dogma, 202–3
surgery
    for cancer, 259
    dogma of, 200–201
    innovations in, 27–28
survival rate
    of liver metastases, 233–34, 234t
    of lung metastases, 234–35
    of treatment, 257–58
systemic-dissemination model
    attractiveness of, 204
    for breast cancer, 185–86, 187–88, 224
    Coley for, 170–71
    as dogma, 302–3
    Ewing for, 172
    by Fisher, 107, 164–65, 185–86, 252–53
    for tumors, 216

tacit knowledge, 111–12
"Tales of the Unnatural: Return From the Dean(d)," 144
"targeted" pharmaceuticals, 107–8
TBI. *See* total body irradiation
teaching, 304
technical expert, 100–101, 138–39
technology. *See also* "halfway technology"
    diagnosis by, 179
    for medicine, 117–19, 303
    proximate utility of, 117–19
    of radiation oncologist, 177
    for tumors, 179–80
    ultimate utility of, 117–19
"Technology, Biology, and Traffic," 177
telomere, 212
The University of Chicago
    architecture of, 8
    community of, 9, 125–26
    German university for, 134
    President Gray of, 133–34
    interdisciplinary collaboration, 133
    medical care by, 126–27
    undergraduate education at, 7–8

therapy. *See also* adjuvant therapy
    Manichean nature of, 294
    for oligometastases, 226–28
    resources of, 66
    war analogy for, 255
"Thomas Hodgkin and Hodgkin's Disease. Two Paradigms Appropriate to Medicine Today," 272
Toon, Peter, 71
total body irradiation (TBI)
    Department of Defense for, 81–82
    peer review of, 82, 84
"traffic"
    of cancer, 182–83
    of immune system, 183
    of metastases, 183–84
treatment. *See also* antiangiogenic treatment; experimental treatment; "preservative" treatment
    anatomy influence on, 72–73
    apoptosis for, 219–20
    arsphenamine for, 292–93
    bone marrow transplant as, 64–65
    collaboration for, 175
    from doctor-patient relationship, 70–71
    EORTC trial for, 191–92
    by Ewing, 171
    false positive of, 115–17
    fractional cell kill from, 219, 219t
    by Gilbert, 277–78
    by "halfway technology," 102
    health insurance coverage of, 140–41
    for Hodgkin Lymphoma, 160–62
    judgment on, 64
    localization of, 216–17
    of lymph nodes, 190, 193–94
    "magic bullet" of, 255, 259–60
    medical school for, 2
    by molecular medicine, 70–71
    Obama on, 246–47
    of patient, 14
    by patient-centered care, 74, 119–20
    by Peters, 277–78
    radiation for, 289
    radioactivity for, 271

INDEX

radium for, 271, 286–89, 292–93
by randomized clinical trial,
    13–14, 38–39
research for, 161, 255
resource distribution in, 13
specialization for, 174–75
survival rate of, 257–58
theory for, 162–63
for tumors, 231–32
war analogy of, 255–56
tuberculosis, 245–46
tumors
    biology of, 210–11
    of breast cancer, 107
    cell cycle of, 182
    cellular aggregates of, 237–38
    disease-free state influenced by,
        194–95, 194t
    evolution of, 214–15, 224–25
    gradualness of, 210
    localization of, 190
    magnetic resonance for, 179
    malignancy of, 191, 213–14
    McWhirter technique for, 201–2
    metastatic, 188–89, 188f, 212–13, 212t,
        215–16, 227
    patients with, 231–32
    phenotypes of, 181–82
    size of, 190–91, 215, 225–26
    spectrum theory of, 252–53
    stem cell research of, 168–69
    systemic-dissemination model for, 216
    "targeted" pharmaceuticals for, 107–8
    technology for, 179–80
    treatment for, 231–32
Tuskegee study, 83–84

ultimate utility, 117–19
undergraduate education
    as career preparation, 17–18
    commencement of, 18
    for community, 18
    experience of, 7
    purpose of, 10

self-realization in, 17–18
at The University of Chicago, 7–8
Une Femme Honorable (Giroud), 284
university
    action analysis by, 142
    of Enlightenment, 134
    interdisciplinary collaboration by, 142
    medicine and, 123–24, 128, 136–37, 305
University of Bologna, 133–34
utilitarianism
    in clinical research, 90
    philosophy of, 84–85
    physician as, 46
    "right-based ethics" against, 68, 109,
        117, 129

van der Schueren, Emmanuel, 80–81
vantage point, 265–66
Vesalius, 133–34
von Humboldt, Alexander
    contributions by, 15–16, 123–24
    influence on Hodgkin, 134, 270
vulnerability, 61

war analogy, 255–56
Watson, James Dewey
    for antiangiogenic treatment, 108
    on evolution, 208
    genetics by, 2
Weatherall, Sir David, 61
Weichselbaum, Ralph, 165–66
Whitehead, Alfred North, 5–6
Why Me? (Kushner), 265–66
willful blindness
    in clinical investigation, 86–87
    of patient rights, 85–86
willful indifference, 87
World Medical Association, 34–35
Wulf, Andrea, 123–24

x-ray, 100, 277–78

Yale, 167
Yeats, William Butler, 153